Global Health and Pathology

Editor

DANNY A. MILNER Jr

CLINICS IN LABORATORY MEDICINE

www.labmed.theclinics.com

Editor-in-Chief
MILENKO JOVAN TANASIJEVIC

March 2018 • Volume 38 • Number 1

ELSEVIER

1600 John F. Kennedy Boulevard • Suite 1800 • Philadelphia, Pennsylvania, 19103-2899

http://www.theclinics.com

CLINICS IN LABORATORY MEDICINE Volume 38, Number 1
March 2018 ISSN 0272-2712, ISBN-13: 978-0-323-58158-5

Editor: Stacy Eastman
Developmental Editor: Laura Fisher

Reprints. For copies of 100 or more, of articles in this publication, please contact the Commercial Reprints Department, Elsevier Inc., 360 Park Avenue South, New York, New York 10010-1710. Tel. 212-633-3874, Fax: 212-633-3820, E-mail: reprints@elsevier.com.

Clinics in Laboratory Medicine (ISSN 0272-2712) is published quarterly by Elsevier Inc., 360 Park Avenue South, New York, NY 10010-1710. Months of issue are March, June, September, and December. Business and Editorial offices: 1600 John F. Kennedy Blvd., Suite 1800, Philadelphia, PA 19103-2899. Periodicals postage paid at NewYork, NY and additional mailing offices. Subscription prices are $263.00 per year (US individuals), $507.00 per year (US institutions), $100.00 per year (US students), $347.00 per year (Canadian individuals), $617.00 per year (Canadian institutions), $185.00 per year (Canadian students), $402.00 per year (international individuals), $617.00 per year (international institutions), $185.00 (international students). Foreign air speed delivery is included in all Clinics subscription prices. All prices are subject to change without notice. POSTMASTER: Send address changes to *Clinics in Laboratory Medicine*, Elsevier Health Sciences Division, Subscription Customer Service, 3251 Riverport Lane, Maryland Heights, MO 63043. **Customer Service: 1-800-654-2452 (US). From outside of the US and Canada, call 1-314-447-8871. Fax: 1-314-447-8029. E-mail: journalscustomerservice-usa@elsevier.com (for print support) or journalsonlinesupport-usa@elsevier.com (for online support).**

Clinics in Laboratory Medicine is covered in *EMBASE/Exerpta Medica, MEDLINE/PubMed (Index Medicus), Cinahl, Current Contents/Clinical Medicine, BIOSIS and ISI/BIOMED.*

Contributors

CONSULTING EDITOR

MILENKO JOVAN TANASIJEVIC, MD, MBA
Vice Chair for Clinical Pathology and Quality, Department of Pathology, Director of Clinical Laboratories, Brigham and Women's Hospital, Dana-Farber Cancer Institute, Associate Professor of Pathology, Harvard Medical School, Boston, Massachusetts, USA

EDITOR

DANNY A. MILNER Jr, MD, MSc(Epi), FASCP, FASTMH
Chief Medical Officer, Center for Global Health, American Society for Clinical Pathology, Chicago, Illinois USA; Adjunct Lecturer, Harvard T. H. Chan School of Public Health, Affiliate, Global Health and Social Medicine, Harvard Medical School, Boston, Massachusetts, USA

AUTHORS

TIMOTHY K. AMUKELE, MD, PhD
Department of Pathology, The Johns Hopkins University School of Medicine, Baltimore, Maryland, USA; Clinical Core Laboratory at Infectious Diseases Institute, MU-JHU Research Collaboration, Makerere University-Johns Hopkins University, Kampala, Uganda

LINDA R. ANDIRIC, MT(ASCP), MSc, EdD
Center for Global Health, American Society for Clinical Pathology, Chicago, Illinois, USA

FABIENNE ANGLADE, MD
Partners In Health, Boston, Massachusetts, USA; United States and Canadian Academy of Pathology, Evans, Georgia, USA; University Hospital of Mirebalais, Centre Department, Haiti

FAY BETSOU, PhD, HDR
Chief Scientific Officer, Integrated BioBank of Luxembourg, Luxembourg, Luxembourg

JANE E. BROCK, MBBS, PhD
Assistant Professor of Pathology, Brigham and Women's Hospital, Boston, Massachusetts, USA

LAWRENCE A. CHAVEZ, PhD
Center for Global Health, American Society for Clinical Pathology, Chicago, Illinois, USA

FRED CHIMZIMU, BS
UNC Project Malawi, Tidziwe Centre, Lilongwe, Malawi

OLIVER D. COHEN, MD, PhD
AGEIS EA 7407 Laboratory, Professor, Medical School of Grenoble, Joseph Fourier University, La Tronche, France

ISHAAN K. DESAI, BA
Partners In Health, Department of Global Health and Social Medicine, Harvard Medical School, Boston, Massachusetts, USA

BAL MUKUNDA DHUNGEL, MBBS, MD
Kamuzu Central Hospital, Tidziwe Centre, Lilongwe, Malawi

MOHENOU ISIDORE JEAN-MARIE DIOMANDE, MD, FWACP (Lab Med)
Professor of Pathology, Président de la Société Ivoirienne de Pathologie, Laboratoire d'Anatomie Pathologique, UFR Sciences Médicales, Abidjan, Côte d'Ivoire

QUENTIN EICHBAUM, MD, PhD, MPH, NNHC, JD
Associate Director of Transfusion Medicine, Director, Transfusion Medicine Fellowship Program, Professor, Department of Pathology, Microbiology, and Immunology, Vanderbilt University Medical Center, The Vanderbilt Clinic, Nashville, Tennessee, USA

PAUL E. FARMER, MD, PhD
Partners In Health, Department of Global Health and Social Medicine, Harvard Medical School, Boston, Massachusetts, USA

YURI FEDORIW, MD
Associate Professor, Director of Hematopathology, Department of Pathology and Laboratory Medicine, University of North Carolina at Chapel Hill School of Medicine, Lineberger Comprehensive Cancer Center, Chapel Hill, North Carolina, USA

ANDREW S. FIELD, MBBS (Hons), FRCPA, FIAC, DipCytopath (RCPA)
Associate Professor, The University of Notre Dame, School of Medicine, Deputy Director and Senior Consultant, Department of Anatomical Pathology, St Vincent's Hospital Melbourne, Sydney, New South Wales, Australia

JOHN S. FLANIGAN, MD
Senior Adviser for Non-Communicable Diseases, Center for Global Health, National Cancer Institute, National Institutes of Health, Rockville, Maryland, USA

WILLIE GITHUI, PhD
Chief Research Officer and Head, Mycobacteriology Research Laboratory, Centre for Respiratory Diseases Research, Kenya Medical Research Institute, Nairobi, Kenya

SATISH GOPAL, MD, MPH
UNC Project Malawi, Tidziwe Centre, Lilongwe, Malawi; UNC Lineberger Comprehensive Cancer Center, Chapel Hill, North Carolina, USA

LAUREN A. GREENBERG, BA
Partners In Health, Boston, Massachusetts, USA

MARTIN HALE MB ChB, FCPath, (ANAT) SA
Professor and Chair, Department of Anatomic Pathology, National Health Laboratory Service, University of the Witwatersrand, Johannesburg, Johannesburg, South Africa

MARIANNE K. HENDERSON, MS
Senior Advisor on Biobanking and Division Resources, National Cancer Institute, National Institutes of Health, Department of Health and Human Services, Bethesda, Maryland, USA

E. BLAIR HOLLADAY, PhD, MASCP, SCT (ASCP)^CM
Chief Executive Officer, American Society for Clinical Pathology, Chicago, Illinois, USA

ANDRÉ M. ILBAWI, MD
Technical Officer, Management of Noncommunicable Disease Unit, Department for Management of Noncommunicable Diseases, Disability, Violence and Injury Prevention, World Health Organization, Geneva, Switzerland

YAWALE ILIYASU, MBBS, MD, FMCPath(Nig), FICS, MIAC, IFCAP, FCPath(ECSA)
Associate Professor, Department of Pathology, Faculty of Medicine, Ahmadu Bello University, Smaru, Zaria, Kaduna State, Nigeria

MICONGWE MOSES ISYAGI, BDS, MMed, FCPath(ECSA)
Dental Surgeon and Oral Pathologist, Legacy Specialty Clinics, Kigali, Rwanda

LOUISE C. IVERS, MD, MPH
Partners In Health, Department of Global Health and Social Medicine, Harvard Medical School, Center for Global Health, Massachusetts General Hospital, Boston, Massachusetts, USA

MIRA JOHNSON, BA
Center for Global Health, American Society for Clinical Pathology, Chicago, Illinois, USA

RAPHAEL M. KALENGAYI, MD, MMedSc, SpPath, PhD
Professor of Pathology, Department of Pathological Anatomy, Faculty of Medicine, University of Kinshasa, Kinshasa, Democratic Republic of Congo

SIMEON KALYESUBULA-KIBUUKA, MD, MPH
M&E Technical Advisor, Uganda National Health Laboratory Services, Kampala, Uganda

COXCILLY KAMPANI, BS
UNC Project Malawi, Tidziwe Centre, Lilongwe, Malawi

ROBERT KRYSIAK, MS
UNC Project Malawi, Tidziwe Centre, Lilongwe, Malawi

STEVE KUSSICK, MD, PhD
Chief Medical Officer, PhenoPath Laboratories Clinical Assistant Professor, University of Washington, Department of Laboratory Medicine, Seattle, Washington, USA

KENNETH LANDGRAF, MSc
Center for Global Health, American Society for Clinical Pathology, Chicago, Illinois, USA

RITA T. LAWLOR, PhD
Research Centre Coordinator, ARC-Net Applied Research on Cancer Centre, Verona University, Verona, Italy

MARIA P. LEMOS, PhD, MPH
Staff Scientist, Fred Hutchinson Cancer Research Center, Seattle, Washington, USA

ROBERT LUKANDE, MBChB, MMed, FCPath(ECSA)
Lecturer, Department of Pathology, College of Health Science, Makerere University, Kampala, Uganda

YEHODA M. MARTEI, MD
Instructor, Department of Medicine, Division of Hematology-Oncology, University of Pennsylvania, Abramson Cancer Center, Philadelphia, Pennsylvania, USA

NEIL A. MARTINSON, MBBCh, MPH
Perinatal HIV Research Unit (PHRU), MRC Soweto Matlosana Collaborating Centre for HIV/
AIDS and TB, University of the Witwatersrand, Johannesburg, Johannesburg, South Africa;
Johns Hopkins University, Center for Tuberculosis Research, Baltimore, Maryland, USA

MARTIN MATU, PhD, MSc, MBA
Senior Laboratory Specialist, Regional Project Director, ECSA Health Community,
Arusha, Tanzania

SUZANNE M. McGOLDRICK, MD, MPH
Seattle Genetics, Seattle Children's Hospital, Fred Hutchinson Cancer Research Center,
Seattle, Washington, USA

MAIMUNA MENDY, PhD
Group Head, Laboratory Services and Biobank Group, International Agency for Research
on Cancer, Lyon, France

MANOJ MENON, MD, MPH
Assistant Member, Global Oncology, Vaccine and Infectious Disease and Clinical
Research Division, Fred Hutchinson Cancer Research Center, Assistant Professor,
Department of Medicine, University of Washington, Seattle, Washington, USA

DANNY A. MILNER Jr, MD, MSc(Epi), FASCP, FASTMH
Chief Medical Officer, Center for Global Health, American Society for Clinical Pathology,
Chicago, Illinois USA; Adjunct Lecturer, Harvard T. H. Chan School of Public Health,
Affiliate, Global Health and Social Medicine, Harvard Medical School, Boston,
Massachusetts, USA

NONHLANHLA N. MKHIZE, PhD
Centre for HIV and STIs, National Institute for Communicable Diseases (NICD),
National Health Laboratory Service (NHLS), Faculty of Health Sciences, University of
the Witwatersrand, Johannesburg, Johannesburg, South Africa

MALCOLM E. MOLYNEUX, MD, FRCP
Liverpool School of Tropical Medicine, Liverpool, United Kingdom

NATHAN D. MONTGOMERY, MD, PhD
Department of Pathology and Laboratory Medicine, University of North Carolina at Chapel
Hill School of Medicine, Chapel Hill, North Carolina, USA

ELIZABETH A. MORGAN, MD
Brigham and Women's Hospital, Boston, Massachusetts, USA

MAURICE MULENGA, MBBS, MD
Kamuzu Central Hospital, Tidziwe Centre, Lilongwe, Malawi

ANN MARIE NELSON, MD, FASCP
Professor of Pathology (Visiting), Duke University School of Medicine, Durham, North
Carolina, USA; President, InPaLa Consulting, Washington, DC, USA

JOHN NKENGASONG, PhD, MSc
Director, Africa Centers for Disease Control and Prevention, African Union Headquarters,
Addis Ababa, Ethiopia

JUAN DANIEL OROZCO, DPH
Partners In Health, Boston, Massachusetts, USA

MICHAEL K. OWINO, MPH
UNC Project Malawi, Tidziwe Centre, Lilongwe, Malawi

LYDIA E. PACE, MD, MPH
Instructor, Department of Medicine, Division of Women's Health, Brigham and Women's Hospital, Boston, Massachusetts, USA

ERIC POWERS, BA
Department of Pathology and Laboratory Medicine, University of North Carolina at Chapel Hill School of Medicine, Chapel Hill, North Carolina, USA

JULIE RANDOLPH-HABECKER, PhD
Pacific Northwest University of Health Sciences, Yakima, Washington, USA

PETER H.J. RIEGMAN, PhD
Department of Pathology, Director, The Erasmus MC Tissue Bank, Rotterdam, The Netherlands

SARAH RILEY, PhD
Department of Pathology, Saint Louis University, St Louis, Missouri, USA

JULIA ROYALL, BA, MA
(Ret.) Chief, Office of International Programs, US National Library of Medicine, National Institutes of Health, Dubois, Global Health Information Specialist, Washington, DC and Dubois, Wyoming, USA

BELSON RUGWIZANGOGA, MD, MMed (Path)
Department of Clinical Biology, School of Medicine and Pharmacy, University of Rwanda College of Medicine and Health Sciences, Kigali, Rwanda

DEOGRATIAS RUHANGAZA, MD
Ministry of Health, Butaro Hospital, Rwanda

SHAHIN SAYED, MMed(Path)
Department of Pathology, The Aga Khan University Hospitals, Nairobi, Nairobi, Kenya

MIRIAM SCHNEIDMAN, MA, MPH
World Bank, Health, World Bank, Washington, DC, USA

LAWRENCE N. SHULMAN, MD
Professor, Department of Medicine, Division of Hematology-Oncology, University of Pennsylvania, Abramson Cancer Center, Philadelphia, Pennsylvania, USA

SHANNON L. SILKENSEN, PhD
Program Director, Center for Global Health, National Cancer Institute, National Institutes of Health, Rockville, Maryland, USA

KELLY ARAUJO SILVA, MBA, MPH
Lacliv – Laboratorio de Analises Clinicas de Valenca, Valenca, Bahia, Brazil

ANDREA STRITMATTER, BA, HTL(ASCP)
Focus Histopathology LLC, Seattle, Washington, USA

TERRIE E. TAYLOR, DO
College of Osteopathic Medicine, Michigan State University, East Lansing, Michigan, USA; Blantyre Malaria Project, University of Malawi, College of Medicine, Blantyre, Malawi

MERIH T. TESFAZGHI, PhD
Department of Pathology, Washington University School of Medicine in St. Louis,
St Louis, Missouri, USA

TAMIWE TOMOKA, MD
UNC Project Malawi, Tidziwe Centre, Lilongwe, Malawi

ANNE LINDA VAN KAPPEL, MSc, PhD
Managing Director, IMV Technologies, l'Aigle, France

ADRIANA VELAZQUEZ-BERUMEN, MSc
Senior Advisor on Medical Devices, Innovation, Access and Use Unit, Essential Medicines
and Health Products Department, World Health Organization, Geneva, Switzerland

EDDA VUHAHULA, DDS, PhD, FCPath
Department of Pathology, Muhimbili University of Health and Allied Sciences (MUHAS),
Dar es Salaam, Tanzania

NICHOLAS G. WOLF, BA
CRTA Fellow, Center for Global Health, National Cancer Institute, National Institutes of
Health, Rockville, Maryland, USA

Contents

and outlines the necessary elements for training and sustaining a robust workforce in pathology and laboratory medicine. The authors provide several case studies of institutions around the continent that include expansion of existing programs, a de novo program, South-South collaborations, and skill building for the existing workforce.

The shared practice of pathology via the Internet holds great potential for pathologists in sub-Saharan Africa (SSA) and their global partners. Application of the Internet is constrained by issues of bandwidth, cost, and power. The penetration of mobile telephony and the arrival of smartphones have changed the use of Internet and social media in Africa and therefore the work of the 4 African pathologists featured in this article. As pathology in SSA struggles for visibility and usefulness, the Internet and its electronic applications provide a critical infrastructure as well as a podium for pathologists across the continent.

The process of conducting pathology research in Africa can be challenging. But the rewards in terms of knowledge gained, quality of collaborations, and impact on communities affected by infectious disease and cancer are great. This article reviews 3 different research efforts: fatal malaria in Malawi, mucosal immunity to HIV in South Africa, and cancer research in Uganda. What unifies them is the use of pathology-based approaches to answer vital questions, such as physiology, pathogenesis, predictors of clinical course, and diagnostic testing schemes.

The care of patients with lymphoma relies heavily on accurate tissue diagnosis and classification. In sub-Saharan Africa, where lymphoma burden is increasing because of population growth, aging, and continued epidemic levels of human immunodeficiency virus infection, diagnostic pathology services are limited. This article summarizes lymphoma epidemiology, current diagnostic capacity, and obstacles and opportunities for improving practice in the region.

The diagnostic laboratory is essential to patient care and to the achievement of health equity. Through the development of quality laboratories in settings burdened by poverty and weak health systems, Partners In Health has demonstrated the critical contributions of clinical laboratories to the care of patients with HIV, tuberculosis, and cancer, among other conditions. The lessons learned through the organization's experience include the importance of well-trained and well-supported staff; reliable access to supplies, reagents, and diagnostic equipment; adequate facilities to provide diagnostic services; the integration of laboratories into networks of care; and accompaniment of the public health sector.

Miriam Schneidman, Martin Matu, John Nkengasong, Willie Githui, Simeon Kalyesubula-Kibuuka, and Kelly Araujo Silva

Laboratory networks are vital to well-functioning public health systems and disease control efforts. Cross-country laboratory networks play a critical role in supporting epidemiologic surveillance, accelerating disease outbreak response, and tracking drug resistance. The East Africa Public Health Laboratory Network was established to bolster diagnostic and disease surveillance capacity. The network supports the introduction of regional quality standards; facilitates the rollout and evaluation of new diagnostic tools; and serves as a platform for training, research, and knowledge sharing. Participating facilities benefitted from state-of-the art investments, capacity building, and mentorship; conducted multicountry research studies; and contributed to disease outbreak response.

Linda R. Andiric, Lawrence A. Chavez, Mira Johnson, Kenneth Landgraf, and Danny A. Milner Jr

The Strengthening Laboratory Management Toward Accreditation (SLMTA) program and subsequent Stepwise Laboratory Quality Improvement Process Toward Accreditation (SLIPTA) checklist were a response to the need for high-quality laboratories to combat the human immunodeficiency virus (HIV) epidemic and provide patients with the highest-quality care. The two tools work together to create a culture of quality in laboratories and allow the identification of gaps. The ultimate goal for any laboratory is to achieve a standard benchmark for quality, and these programs have been highly successful in initially affecting the HIV epidemic but continuously improving laboratory quality across all diseases.

Nathan D. Montgomery, Tamiwe Tomoka, Robert Krysiak, Eric Powers, Maurice Mulenga, Coxcilly Kampani, Fred Chimzimu, Michael K. Owino, Bal Mukunda Dhungel, Satish Gopal, and Yuri Fedoriw

Across much of Africa, there is a critical shortage of pathology services necessary for clinical care. Even in settings where specialty-level clinical care, such as medical oncology, is available, access to anatomic pathology services has often lagged behind. Pathology laboratories in the region are challenging to establish and maintain. This article describes the

Maimuna Mendy, Rita T. Lawlor, Anne Linda van Kappel, Peter H.J. Riegman, Fay Betsou, Oliver D. Cohen, and Marianne K. Henderson

Biobanks provide a critical infrastructure to support research in human health. Biospecimens and their accompanying data are increasingly needed to support biomedical research and clinical care. The original text was initially published in the Handbook for Cancer Research in Africa. The value of this publication is great because it underlines the importance of biobanks in Africa as a key resource to increase quality scientific research and participate in global health research. Therefore, a revision to extend these principles to other low resource contexts, include updated material and references, and add the topic of biobank sustainability was relevant.

CLINICS IN LABORATORY MEDICINE

Preface

Pathology: Central and Essential

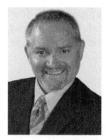

Danny A. Milner Jr, MD, MSc(Epi)
Editor

There is no other portion of a health care system that links patients to more diagnoses and treatment plans than the laboratory, and diagnostic tests determine more than 70% of all health care decisions. Communicable and noncommunicable diseases alike rely on parts, or in some diseases states like cancer, nearly all of the laboratory to provide crucial details for establishing a diagnosis and creating a feasible treatment plan. Regardless of whether a person is born in New York City, rural Oklahoma, Rio de Janeiro, Accra, Mumbai, Moscow, or Hanoi, high-quality laboratories are essential for diagnosing their symptoms accurately and rapidly. That only the privileged or the wealthy (relative or actual) who can afford laboratory testing is a "fact of life" is simply a travesty and a tragedy. As social justice advocates opine that "health care is a human right," they do not mean only medical doctors or only nurses or only surgeons. They mean health care is a system, and such a system only functions with a laboratory at its center to provide the essential bridge to appropriate care that every patient deserves.

The challenge of laboratories is not in knowledge but in access. A successful laboratory test requires trained personnel, equipment, reagents, reporting system, controls, quality control, and stable environment. These are all based in real dollar costs or functioning systems that require constant vigilance. It is not good enough to say that a laboratory is doing a perfect job 99% of the time. If we used that logic with airplanes, 1 in 100 would crash. Patients, no matter where they live, deserve 100% high-quality laboratory testing at all times. Thus, our challenge in meeting the needs of patients around the world is to insure they have access and that their laboratorians have access to all the tools that are needed to return a useful laboratory result. This starts with government recognition of the power and value of laboratory professionals and their laboratories. This includes recognition at all levels from government, through hospitals, to clinicians, and last, with patients of the laboratory and the laboratory professionals who use their expertise every day to save lives. This ends with the patient

Clin Lab Med 38 (2018) xv–xvi
https://doi.org/10.1016/j.cll.2017.11.001
0272-2712/18/© 2017 Published by Elsevier Inc.

labmed.theclinics.com

who is ultimately saved or unfortunately dies because all the pieces of the puzzle that make up a functioning health care system were or were not in place. The laboratory, its personnel, and their tools make up a vast number of pieces and, in all cases, complete the puzzle for best patient care.

In this issue, we take a detailed look at several different aspects of the laboratory and global health from personnel training through research. We have perspectives from clinicians as well as laboratorians, including voices from the field. There is a very great and positive future for the lowest resourced places on the planet if we just take the time to think outside the box and recognize that no human should suffer a disease simply because of where they were born.

Danny A. Milner Jr, MD, MSc(Epi)
American Society for Clinical Pathology
Harvard T. H. Chan School of Public Health
33 West Monroe Street, Suite 1600
Chicago, IL 60603, USA

E-mail address:
dan.milner@ascp.org

Laboratories as the Core for Health Systems Building

Danny A. Milner Jr, MD, MSc (Epi)*,
E. Blair Holladay, PhD, MASCP, SCT (ASCP)ᶜᴹ

KEYWORDS

- Laboratory • Health systems • Diagnostics • Personnel standards • Telepathology
- Cancer • HIV

KEY POINTS

- Access to medical care, including diagnostics and treatment, is a universal human right.
- Laboratories play a central role (70%) in medical care decisions.
- Building health systems through single disease programs or silos is antiquated and should be avoided.
- The diagnostic laboratory for cancer has a central role in building overall health systems because of the logistics, coordination, overlapping resources, and networks that are required to make it functional.

BACKGROUND

We live in a time of great strides in medicine and patient care in the arenas of knowledge, technology, and information. We see breakthroughs in diagnostics and treatment virtually every day. The historical challenge of our time is to deliver high-quality, impactful health care to every human being on the planet.

While the United States is in turmoil over political assignment of payer systems, much of Europe and Canada strike a balance between private care and highly functioning socialized medical systems. Similar systems, strategies, and debates are ongoing throughout the world. No country has a perfect system; in no country are all patients covered all the time, for a variety of reasons. However, 2 principal conclusions can be deduced from the authors' observations of the current debates: (1) health care is a universal right that should be provided to all people and/or (2)

Disclosure Statement: The authors of this article have no conflicts of interest associated with the material presented.
American Society for Clinical Pathology, 33 West Monroe Street, Suite 1600, Chicago, IL 60603, USA
* Corresponding author.
E-mail address: Dan.Milner@ascp.org

Clin Lab Med 38 (2018) 1–9
https://doi.org/10.1016/j.cll.2017.10.001
0272-2712/18/© 2017 Elsevier Inc. All rights reserved.

health care is a commodity available to those who can afford it. We may find that these two conclusions can be in agreement if we modify the statements to the following: Basic health care is a universal right for all people, whereas advanced personalized medicine is available to those who can afford it. However, this statement creates an ethical conundrum that only be resolved by arriving at a single conclusion, namely, high-quality, impactful health care is a universal human right. If we start with that principal mantra, we are faced with the challenge of delivering high-quality care to everyone.

Global health has many meanings, most of which have crested and troughed with the success or failure of a range of historical and current interventions across the globe. The authors would not begin to assign a definition that should be considered universal or appropriate for everyone who functions in this space domestically or internationally. For the purpose of this article, the authors define global health, in their context, as "the practice of providing health care system solutions adapted to the disease spectrum, environment, and socioeconomic demographics of the populations served." Using this definition, we see very quickly that the system of care for a 65-year-old woman in rural southern Alabama may be as different from the one serving a woman of the same demographic in New York City, as both are from the system used by the same woman in rural Madagascar.

Communicable diseases are a product of environment and human population stability, which includes the infrastructure and economy. There is no need for cattle ranchers in Texas to be concerned about *Trypanosoma brucei* infection of their stocks or themselves, whereas vast stretches of land in multiple African countries are unusable because of the tsetse fly. However, Texans and Africans may similarly have hypertension, diabetes, cancer, glomerulonephritis, or acral-lentiginous melanoma. Shockingly for those outside of global health, the rates of these 5 diseases are similar among these groups, although the incidence and prevalence vary highly with economic status. So we are left to ask, what constitutes a basic or essential package of health care? There is a need to cover all noncommunicable diseases affecting populations while at the same time accounting for systems that also must combat communicable diseases, such as African sleeping sickness, human immunodeficiency virus (HIV), tuberculosis, malaria, schistosomiasis, filariasis, and rickettsiosis. Is the logical solution to create one health care system in African countries based solely on communicable diseases and a second system in Texas based largely on noncommunicable diseases? Obviously, it is not. Both places need a system of health care that addresses patients' comprehensive needs.

An example the authors have used many times in discussion and recount here is the malaria backpack proposition. If one would like to lower mortality from malaria in a rural village in Africa, one need only put a backpack on one person filled with rapid diagnostic assays for malaria along with a second backpack on a second person filled with artemisinin combination therapy (ACT). With basic training, those two people can enter a village, respond to any fever that is present with a rapid diagnostic therapy, and treat those who are positive with an ACT. In short, mortality from malaria will end.

There are 2 problems with this scenario. The first is that mortality from other fever-causing diseases will not end. The authors have used a silo approach focused on malaria, although the village certainly has fevers due to virus, bacteria, parasites, noncommunicable disease, and so on for which malaria drugs are of no value. Still, if we only measure malaria mortality, we look very successful. In truth, we must enter this village with a range of tools to deal with fever and a range of drugs to treat those fevers. In short, we will have to add a few more backpacks—and perhaps a large truck.

The second problem with this scenario is that if we solve the fever problem, our population is now healthier, grows older, and the incidence and prevalence of noncommunicable diseases will increase. We now need a backpack of diagnostics for cancer as well as a backpack of treatments for the same. Cancer represents hundreds and hundreds of unique heterogeneous diseases affecting different organs, requiring dozens and dozens of different drugs arranged in complex protocols, not to mention surgery and radiation therapy. To take a biopsy of tissue from a suspected tumor and turn it into a diagnostic histology slide (currently essential to treating almost all cancers), we require at least one large truck full of equipment along with electricity, reagents, and supplies. Thus, to tackle the cancer epidemic in a remote village, we need a few trucks and several dozen people to begin to have an impact on patients' lives. Regardless of cancer, there are other noncommunicable diseases, such as hypertension, diabetes, cardiovascular disease, and strokes, just to name a few, that also must be diagnosed and treated.

When we consider the myriad approaches that have been taken to health care in low- and middle-income countries (LMICs), we see either syndrome-based approaches (such as with fever) or single-entity interventions (such as for HIV and tuberculosis). That way of thinking about disease has come and gone; now we must face the reality that populations have spectrums of diseases and only a comprehensive health system can meet the needs of these individuals. Tackling a single disease can no longer work. But where do we start?

As stated in the preface of this issue, more than 70% of all medical decisions are based on results from the medical laboratory. Thus, if we desire to move a health system far along in its development, a core principle should be that a high-functioning, high-quality medical laboratory must be accessible. A laboratory, however, can only perform a test if a health care worker is knowledgeable enough to request one. The good news is that worldwide initiatives like the US President's Emergency Plan for AIDS Relief (PEPFAR) recognized early on the value of the medical laboratory in the care and treatment of HIV-infected individuals and embarked on a plan to strengthen laboratories in heavily affected countries. Today, the results of this highly successful initiative are, for some countries, highly trained laboratory professionals, standardized laboratory practices, process improvement strategies, specimen transportation networks, and established laboratory spaces, including large central reference medical laboratories. More importantly, this process of strengthening is published, established, and can be implemented by any country. The second part of the good news is that there are now innumerable community health care workers (CHWs), products of PEPFAR as well as tuberculosis and malaria programs, among others, who are at the interface of patients with the system, usually in the most remote villages. Although originally built for communicable diseases, this existing infrastructure of laboratories and workers can be adapted to deal with diseases, such as diabetes and hypertension (with the CHW as the local driver) as well as cancer (with the central reference laboratory and services as the driver). The connectivity of the CHW and the central laboratory (along with all the health care staff and smaller laboratories in between) can be the movement of trucks or motorcycles on a regular schedule. In addition, there is now the real opportunity to use unmanned drones as needed. Consider for a moment that almost every village in Africa has access to Coca-Cola, which is purchased by the end user. Many of these end users have mobile phones. Why then is it so difficult for that end user to access appropriate health care? Transportation and communication systems do not seem to be the issue. The missing piece is highly trained personnel at both locations who understand the system and respond to patients' needs.

In this issue, the collected articles attempt to present a broad picture of pathology and laboratory services in the context of global health. Because of the current pressing disease burdens, many of the articles focus on Africa and/or malignancy; however, these should be considered living examples and much of the strategy presented throughout can address myriad complex human diseases. There are discussions of how to meet personnel needs (including volunteers, training, social media, and telepathology) and to provide context-specific care (including the diagnoses of lymphoma, breast cancer, and the use of cytopathology). Several articles will delve into the need for research in pathology specific to populations, how such research can be funded, and the increasing value of extremely high-quality, population-specific biorepositories for all diseases. Finally, the concept of health systems and networks is discussed with 2 specific example stories along with guiding documents on general laboratory improvement and a recently published essential equipment list for cancer. The remainder of this article focuses on cancer in Africa as an example of complex human diseases, only to be tackled with a systems-based approach, including an example of an initiative to do just that.

SOLVING THE PROBLEMS OF CANCER IN AFRICA

In Africa, it is estimated that about 650,000 people develop cancer every year. Because of limited treatment, almost 510,000 die of cancer each year (approximately 80%). By 2030, because of aging and growth of the population,[1] these figures will more than double to 1.28 million new cancer cases and 970,000 deaths every year. Currently, more than a third of cancer deaths in Africa are from cancers that, if detected early, can be easily treated. Although these statistics are appalling, the actual epidemiologic data will likely reveal, when systems are in place to properly collect and properly estimate, that the incidence of cancer is likely much higher. It is well known that currently noncommunicable diseases are highly underreported, cancer among them. Most importantly, regarding Africa as a single entity is fallacy. It is made up of more than 50 countries with very diverse geography, population structure, economic resources, and disease epidemiologic case mix. Some countries are equipped to combat cancer much more quickly than others. However, all countries have patients with cancer and all patients require access to diagnosis and treatment.

In many sub-Saharan African countries and in the region overall, cervical cancer is the number one cause of cancer death for women, with most patients diagnosed only when the malignancy is far advanced. The number of cases per 100,000 for the 20 countries with the highest rates (75% of which are in Africa) ranges from 38 to 76.[2] Contrast those statistics with a high-income country (HIC) like the United States, where human papillomavirus (HPV) vaccination, HPV testing, and cytologic analysis of cervical samples are available systematically, and note that the mortality rate for cancer overall in the United States is 36% and 33% for cervical cancer; but the number of cases per 100,000 is 4.[3] Even in the United States, 1 in 3 patients with invasive cervical cancer will die. Prevention (HPV vaccination) and/or early detection (removal of precancerous lesions before cancer develops), not treatment, are the keys to success with the disease. A huge gap clearly exists between LMICs and HICs for cervical cancer; however, unrestricted use of HPV vaccination, along with referral systems and early detection and treatment, can essentially eliminate cervical cancer death from populations. But what about the remaining cancers, which are waiting to take the lead?

Pathology is vital for diagnosing and treating cancer; but LMICs in sub-Saharan Africa lack pathologists and trained laboratory personnel, infrastructure, and opportunities for professional training. Without adequate numbers of pathologists and medical laboratory professionals, these countries cannot keep up with routine diagnostics, and patients wait longer and longer before ever receiving a diagnosis. A key component of any laboratory test for any disease is simple: turnaround time. There is a window during which any test is very valuable for that patient. Beyond this window, the result becomes useless. In cancer, for example, a primary biopsy should be reported in 48 hours or less based on the guidelines from US organizations.[4] Turnaround times in some LMIC laboratories have been noted to be, on average, 4 or more weeks, with some reports taking more than 6 months and others never being generated. To build an effective pathology laboratory, personnel, reagents and equipment, functioning facilities, and integration into the overall health plan and systems of the country are required. The good news is that there are many examples of functioning laboratories like this in HICs as well as some LMICs; thus, following those established examples and duplicating the result is clearly feasible. However, these existing laboratories were built over dozens of years with constantly evolving technologies (many of which are now legacy and redundant). As we tackle the laboratory build-outs in LMICs, we must always look to leapfrogging approaches that minimize the complexity of the laboratory system (and the network that supports it) while, in turn, maximizing patient outcomes.

Establishing an effective network of medical laboratories in a given LMIC of Africa is not enough to combat cancer. Clinicians in-country need to be trained to identify cancer; surgeons must be able to biopsy/remove lesions; oncologists must be able to act on a diagnosis; cadres of ancillary health workers must be created and put in place to support and care for patients. Reagents, equipment, and supplies must be in place for the system to function. One obvious question is, who will pay for all of this?

To answer that question, we must think about the population in a few segments. The first are the bottom billion, the poorest people on Earth who have little to no income. For these individuals, public health systems for care and treatment of cancer that are essentially free of charge must be in place (although minimum fees for entry to the system may be advisable in some settings). Imagine this: A small ship wrecks on an island with 10 people. Two lose everything they own and the rest have all their possessions. Is it not within the ethical and moral basis of humanity for the 8 to share with the two? The second segment of the population is the second and third billion who, unlike the poor, have income, although it is somewhat limited. Despite this limitation, these individuals can pay for a portion of their care and will do so willingly if that care is available, impactful, and timely. As we move up the segments, there is more disposable income and, thus, a personal desire for better (or the best) health care. A woman in the richest of these strata with stage II, estrogen-receptor-positive breast cancer is no different from a woman of the poorest with the same cancer. The treatment is the same. Accessing the treatment is the difference. As long as the two women receive the same treatment and have the same outcome, there is no ethical problem. If we charge the rich woman for sundries (a nicer room, gourmet food, luxury services like nail and hair care while in hospital), there is no ethical issue as treatment is still the same. If, however, we provide the rich woman with tamoxifen because she can pay for it and we do not give the poor woman tamoxifen because she cannot pay, we create an ethical dilemma that violates medical principles. Asking those with disposable income to pay and using the revenue to cover costs for the poor is the only solution to such a challenge. However, we must deal with the reality of an African country in this proposed payment structure. Let us return to the shipwreck and ask, what will these 8 with possessions of value spend that value on? There are no services available for anyone, so what good does money do? Simply put, if we build health care systems around cancer in any African country, the wealthy will access the system, infuse it with cash, and allow for the system to care for those without resources. It is most crucial that efforts for prevention and education about prevention of cancer be a component of this system and come from a government or private source.

SOLUTIONS FOR PERSONNEL SHORTAGES

One approach to deal with the challenge of personnel shortages is to send volunteer health care professionals into the areas to lend their expertise. There are many examples of this process, including the efforts of *Pathologists Overseas*, which has sent pathologists abroad for almost 2 decades, as well as focused programs, such as Human Resources for Health (in Rwanda and now Liberia), which includes on-site pathologists as part of the overall program to train staff. In Malawi, US- and European-based pathologists traveled to the University of Malawi College of Medicine from 2008 until 2016 to assist with surgical pathology sign-out and teaching. In 2013 and 2014, the American Society for Clinical Pathology (ASCP) sent delegations of volunteer cytotechnologists and pathologists to screen thousands of backlogged Pap smears. These professionals included a woman from Malawi, a man from Haiti, and a multicultural team from the United States. All of these examples are impactful at the time of the visit, but the true measure of value in sending volunteers is a sustainable result. What all of these programs have in common is the requirement that individuals in-country be trained well enough to sustain the work when the volunteers leave. In some countries, this may take a decade and, in others, only a few years. Regardless of the timeline, the impact of volunteers can be extremely useful if sustained to bridge a system from limited personnel to a full cadre. Outside of that construct, the use of volunteers is often of little long-term value. More importantly, volunteers have limited value if the field site does not have a functioning laboratory.

Another approach to meeting needs and building capacity is called twinning. In twinning, 2 organizations, one highly resourced and the other with identified needs, collaborate to meet the needs identified, expanding opportunities for both organizations. For example, the World Health Organization has established and implemented twinning partnerships between institutional health organizations and resource-limited countries that focus on shared learning and improving the services delivered. The Twinning Partnerships for Improvement's approach supports capacity building and reestablishing safe essential health services and encourages joint long-term efforts on strengthening the delivery of services.[5] For instance, the American International Health Alliance has established an office in Nigeria to support such partnership activities in this West African nation. It also manages partnerships in Botswana, Côte d'Ivoire, Ethiopia, Kenya, Mozambique, Namibia, Nigeria, South Africa, Tanzania, Uganda, and Zambia.[6] Partners in Health (PIH) establishes a local organization in each country where they work using a twin or partner of the US-based main organization, which ultimately is important for eventual autonomy. Local persons trained by PIH staff may move to other PIH sites, including in other countries, to train other local staff. The essential aspects of twinning are buy-in from both institutions to provide and accept the support, mutual exchange of knowledge and information, and a common, established goal for the sites.

It is important to separate true twinning from research collaboration. There are examples of excellent academic institutions from the United States and Europe building strong programs with foreign institutions centered on funded research programs, but there are also examples of strip-mining sites for samples and data with no capacity building. Entering a twinning partnership based on a single grant is very dangerous and, most would argue, impossible. Moreover, a twinning should be based on the needs of the local institution not the needs of the research design. To build health systems, twinning must be broader than a single disease or single modality. That said, as research collaboration continues to grow and expand in a given site, a threshold is reached, at which true twinning is the only natural way to proceed. Excellent examples of this include the University of North Carolina's program in Lilongwe with Kamuzu Central Hospital and the Uganda Cancer Institute collaboration with The Hutch in Seattle.

Individual twinnings can be most powerful and effective if they are part of a larger initiative. In October 2015, the White House Office of Science and Technology Policy issued a Call to Action for Cancer in Africa. It charged the ASCP with leading a cross-sector coalition, *Partners for Cancer Diagnosis and Treatment in Africa*, comprising industry, government, and nongovernmental organizations, to address the growing problem of cancer in Africa, citing diagnostics as a missing key component. Together, these globally respected organizations have pledged more than $150 million, with a 10-year commitment of infrastructure and in-kind resources to improve pathology services, principally through telepathology. The current participating or collaborating organizations include Partners in Health, the National Institutes of Health, the International Agency for Research on Cancer, the American Cancer Society, the Clinton Health Access Initiative, and industry leaders, such as Pfizer, Philips, Roche Diagnostics, Novartis, GE Healthcare, and Sakura Finetek. This coalition has committed to provide patients in underserved areas of sub-Saharan Africa and Haiti access to rapid cancer diagnostics and appropriate treatment.

PROGRESS AND LESSONS LEARNED

The authors have met with pathologists, clinicians, and leaders of individual sites and discussed their current laboratory needs in hopes of installing their telepathology solutions. It should come as no surprise that there is a range of laboratory functional status, from an empty room to a fully functioning laboratory, that desires state-of-the-art molecular diagnostics. The authors have expanded their focus to include ensuring that high-quality hematoxylin and eosin (H&E) slides and immunohistochemistry slides are available and will meet the needs of most patients. To this end, the authors have engaged in an equipment recruitment program to secure the main components of an anatomic pathology laboratory (tissue processors, embedding centers, microtomes, and staining systems) and the supporting components. The authors are working with industrial partners to create a reporting system based on synoptic reports that will allow for standardization across sites and measurement of the impact. The authors' major focus, however, remains the establishment of telepathology systems in-country. Telepathology will go a long way to assist in this effort, but it also needs financial support and volunteers to provide services. Successful telepathology requires systems that can handle heterogeneity in slide quality, focal plans, and specimen types and sizes; good Internet connectivity and a stable power source; reliable governmental support in logistical matters; and personnel with sufficient technical expertise to properly install and maintain the equipment.[7] Considering the ASCP's focus and role, it should be clear that no single partner can provide sufficient quantities of any one item to meet all of the needs. Moreover, multiple partners in each area (eg, treatment, imaging, and nursing) are needed to fill the massive gaps that exist to surmount the problem of cancer in Africa.

The first sites to receive telepathology have shown excellent initial progress. Under the guidance of the ASCP, Botswana implemented automated histopathology, whole-slide imaging, and cloud-based diagnostic systems. In October 2016, an enhanced automated histopathology and telepathology laboratory was officially opened (installed in March 2016) at the Butaro Center of Excellence for Cancer Care at the Butaro District Hospital in rural Rwanda. In Rwanda, the on-site pathologist has the technical staff scan every slide, which he or she then reads digitally from the computer; in short, the microscope is rarely used (a true leapfrogging technology). For challenging and complex cases, the pathologist clicks an icon, and the case is shared with a team of ASCP pathologists in the United States. To date, their turnaround time for the laboratory is approximately 69 hours for all cases (including cases with immunohistochemistry). New deployments to Uganda, Tanzania, Malawi, and Haiti are in progress. Upcoming implementation sites include Liberia, the Democratic Republic of Congo, Ghana, and Kenya.

The ASCP anticipates diagnostics will be delivered to hundreds of thousands of people, 75% of whom will be female. The ASCP will draw on its 8000 anatomic pathologist members to provide diagnostic services and its 91,000 laboratory professional members to provide support and training to laboratory professionals on the ground. This new initiative creates a new set of opportunities for the ASCP's pathologist members to be directly involved in combatting cancer on the front lines and more opportunities for their histotechnologists to support the project, both on the ground and virtually. To date, more than 600 pathologists have been recruited to review cases and are virtually deployed in teams of 15 assigned to specific countries covering the spectrum of surgical pathology. The ASCP is providing oversight and project management, coordinating partners, working with Ministries of Health, and building capacity through workforce-development initiatives. In addition, they remain the central hub for much-needed fundraising to drive the initiative forward by removing small and large financial obstacles while working diligently in parallel with local partners to create sustainable budgets moving forward.

Reflecting on this example initiative, it is clear that approaching cancer as a disease to be treated in a population cannot happen in a silo. If the authors chose to focus on ductal carcinoma of the breast, what would they do with the other several dozen tumors (both benign and malignant) of the breast? While they install anatomic pathology laboratories that perform, essentially, one test (the H&E slide) with thousands of results, how can they only justify reading those slides if they contain one specific cancer result? Thus, by choosing cancer and diagnostics, they are forced to bring along all the tools to identify patients with cancer, perform surgery, make the diagnosis, create a treatment plan, and support patients throughout the entire process. This system requires nursing and support staff every step of the way. Innumerable reagents and supplies must be available for the system to work. When the systems come online, patients of numerous economic strata will all need to access the care regardless of their ability to pay. If this system is of high quality and provides the best practices of care, utilization across these strata will result in an overall cost-neutral (or positive) system that can be sustained moving forward. Intact health systems addressing cancer diagnosis and treatment will save patients' lives and allow for expansion of the system to address additional noncommunicable diseases, which improves population health overall.

REFERENCES

1. American Cancer Society. Global cancer facts & figures. 2011. Available at: http://pressroom.cancer.org/releases?item=290. Accessed May 26, 2017.

2. Ferlay J, Soerjomataram I, Ervik M, et al. GLOBOCAN 2012 version 1.1, cancer incidence and mortality worldwide: IARC cancer base No. 11. Lyon (France):

INTERNATIONAL AGENCY FOR RESEARCH ON CANCER; 2014. Available at: http://globocan.iarc.fr. Accessed June 1, 2017.

3. American Cancer Society. Cervical cancer. Available at: https://www.cancer.org/cancer/cervical-cancer.html. Accessed September 15, 2017.

4. Alshieban S, Al-Surimi K. Reducing turnaround time of surgical pathology reports in pathology and laboratory medicine departments. BMJ Qual Improv Rep 2015; 4(1).

5. World Health Organization. Twinning partnerships for improvement: recovery partnership preparation package. Available at: http://www.who.int/csr/resources/publications/ebola/twinning-partnerships-package/en/. Published May 2016. Accessed May 30, 2017.

6. The American International Health Alliance. HIV/AIDS twinning center: Nigeria. Available at: http://www.aiha.com/our-projects/hivaids-twinning-center/nigeria/. Accessed May 30, 2017.

7. Fisher MK, Kayembe MK, Scheer AJ, et al. Establishing telepathology in Africa: lessons from Botswana. J Am Acad Dermatol 2011;64(5):986–7.

Voices from the Field

Interviews with Global Health Pathology Volunteers

Timothy K. Amukele, MD, PhD[a,b,*], Sarah Riley, PhD[c],
Merih T. Tesfazghi, PhD[d]

KEYWORDS

- Short-term medical mission • Volunteer • Pathology • Clinical laboratory
- Low-resource setting

KEY POINTS

- Most of the respondents were later in their life and careers. However, this trend may be due to the authors' selection bias.
- The primary motivation for involvement was personal reasons. Participation was largely via nongovernmental organizations, and volunteers stay in mission for many years.
- Most of the volunteer work was privately funded.
- The respondents' work resulted in peer-reviewed publications, abstracts, newsletters, and talks in grand rounds and meetings.

It is important to share the experiences of individuals who have been involved in volunteerism in pathology as a way to illuminate the *who*, *why*, and *how* of this uncommon experience. Medical missions, defined as "grass root, direct, medical service aid from wealthier countries to low and middle income countries,[1]" are an important part of how health care is provided in much of the world. One of the strongest structural drivers of the need for medical missions is the care gap between high-income and middle-income countries. The places in the world with the highest disease burdens are largely economically disadvantaged and also have the fewest physicians per capita.[2] However, there are many other drivers of missioning, including goodwill, interest in novel

Disclosure Statement: The authors have nothing to disclose.
[a] Department of Pathology, Johns Hopkins University School of Medicine, 600 North Wolfe Street/Carnegie 417, Baltimore, Maryland 21287, USA; [b] Clinical Core Laboratory at Infectious Diseases Institute, MU-JHU Research Collaboration, Makerere University-Johns Hopkins University, Mulago Hospital Complex, PO Box 22418, Kampala, Uganda; [c] Department of Pathology, Washington University School of Medicine, 660 S Euclid Avenue, St. Louis, MO 63110, USA; [d] Department of Pathology, Saint Louis University, St Louis, MO 63104, USA
* Corresponding author. Department of Pathology, Johns Hopkins University School of Medicine, 600 North Wolfe Street/Carnegie 417, Baltimore, MD 21287.
E-mail address: tamukel1@jhmi.edu

Clin Lab Med 38 (2018) 11–20
https://doi.org/10.1016/j.cll.2017.10.002   labmed.theclinics.com
0272-2712/18/© 2017 Elsevier Inc. All rights reserved.

cultures or disease states, an opportunity to educate, and so forth.[3–5] This care gap as well as the desire to help is not unique to any one specialty, but there is relatively very little written about volunteer work in pathology.

A review of the literature about medical missions shows that most (>80%) articles about medical missions are focused on surgical and then internal medicine interventions.[6] The largest survey to date of physicians involved in short-term medical missions shows the same surgical focus.[7] As a first step in closing the knowledge gap on pathology volunteering, the authors present narratives of a few pathologists who have participated in these missions as well as a brief overview of the work of Pathologists Overseas. Pathologists Overseas, founded in 1991 by Heinz Hoenecke, is the largest volunteer organization specifically focused on anatomic and clinical pathology. The article begins with a brief summary of the individual narratives grouped under the headings *who*, *why*, and *how*. The article closes with the full detailed narratives.

WHO

The profile that begins to emerge is both similar and different from that of medical volunteerism as a whole in key ways. In terms of similarities, the authors' respondents tend to be later in their careers and life spans. This finding is in keeping with previous studies that show that many volunteers who participate in short-term medical missions (STMMs) are at or close to the end of their formal working lives and are child free.[7,8] In addition, the involvement of those the authors interviewed tended to be long-term rather than short-term, also in keeping with trends seen in other studies of medical missions. A demographic profile of physicians captured from an online survey shows that 77% of participants in STMMs had participated in more than one trip.[5] In terms of differences, the experiences of the authors' cohort of respondents were more focused on capacity building rather than restricted to direct patient care. This finding is probably a characteristic of the work requirements of pathology itself, especially clinical pathology/laboratory medicine whereby samples have relatively short viability windows.

WHY

The motivations for the respondents varied widely but were largely personal, for example, new endeavors with a spouse after retirement, taking a year off during medical school, learning from a friend about a need in a foreign country, and so forth. This finding is in keeping with findings in other work exploring motivations for STMMs. Professional, demographic, and socioeconomic determinants seemed to be less of a motivator than personality and word-of-mouth recruitment by friends.[3]

HOW

How did the authors' interviewees get involved in medical missions? What was the length of their involvement? How was this involvement funded? Involvement in volunteering was largely through nongovernmental organizations (NGOs). Two of the 6 interviewees transitioned to working at least semi-independently afterward, but the introductory mechanism was an NGO. An NGO provides a mechanism for volunteering when there is not yet an established relationship between individuals or institutions and the sending and recipient countries. However, this can also be a bottle neck when the available NGOs are not well matched to the skills or interests of volunteers. For example, there are NGOs devoted to specific types of surgery (cleft palate, urology, and so forth), and this encourages the participation of volunteers with those skill sets. We do not yet have the same diversity of NGO options in pathology. The authors' interviewees also spent many years in medical missions. It is unclear if this reflects the authors' selection bias or the trends in pathology volunteerism; but if it indicates a true trend, it is quite a striking difference than what we see in medical missioning in general. A systematic review of articles about medical missions to low- and middle-income countries shows that 74% of the articles were about visits that lasted between 1 day and 4 weeks.[9] Finally, there are costs associated with volunteering abroad. These costs include direct costs, such as travel, as well as the opportunity cost for involvement in other fiscally productive activities. The authors' interviewees largely funded their work through private funds. This finding is in keeping with findings from studies focused on the economics of medical missions, which estimated that the total economic input for individual US physicians engaged in medical missions was more than $11,000.[1]

What is Your Name and Professional Role?

See **Table 1** for the question tool used to collect the narrative stories from volunteer pathologist interviewees.

Chris Hansen, MD
I am an Anatomic, Clinical and Histopathologist (AP/CP/HP) in private practice in Monterey, California. I am the laboratory medical director and work with 2 other pathologists in my group, with a pathology assistant.

Martin McCann, MD
I am a pathologist and practiced for more than 25 years in community hospitals in the United States. I served as an anatomic pathologist and cytopathologist in Dodoma, Tanzania from 2004 to 2015.

Merih Tesfazghi, PhD
I am a clinical chemistry fellow at Washington University Department of Pathology. I worked as a clinical laboratory scientist in Eritrea for several years, a country that benefited from several volunteering activities, such as Pathologists Overseas, Inc (PO).

Charles Marboe, MD
I am a professor of pathology and cell biology at Columbia University Medical Center and the residency program director.

Table 1	
Question tool used to collect the narrative stories from volunteer pathologist interviewees	
Identifier	What is your name and professional role?
Motivation and mechanism	How did you first get involved in volunteering? What were your motivations? What were the mechanisms for involvement, that is, who did you call or contact to get going?
Experience and nature of involvement	What is the nature of your participation in volunteerism (single vs multiple trips, single vs multiple sites, your role at the volunteer site)?
Funding	How has your volunteering been funded?
Academic or other output	Has your volunteer work resulted in an academic or nonacademic (blog, Web site, magazine) publication?

Jack Ladenson, PhD

My professional job is Oree M. Carroll and Lillian B. Ladenson, Professor of Clinical Chemistry at Washington University School of Medicine in St Louis, Missouri. Since the late 1990s, I have also been the director or codirector of clinical pathology programs at PO. PO was founded in 1991 by Dr Heinz Hoenecke. Its mission is to help improve pathology and clinical laboratory services in developing countries through the efforts of volunteer pathologists, technologists, and laboratory scientists.

Timothy Amukele, MD, PhD

I am the director of the clinical laboratories at Johns Hopkins Bayview Medical Center as well as the associate director of clinical pathology for PO.

How did You First Get Involved in Volunteering? What Were Your Motivations? What Were the Mechanisms for Involvement, that is, Who did You Call or Contact to Get Going?

Chris Hansen, MD

In 2006 to 2009, I was going through a divorce and decided to do something for my own peace of mind, so I answered an advertisement in a pathology journal about volunteering overseas in Ghana through PO, a nonprofit NGO.

Charles Marboe, MD

My interest in volunteering in sub-Saharan Africa started in medical school when I took a year off between the third and fourth years to work on a perinatal mortality project in Addis Ababa. This also stimulated a switch in my career interest from pediatrics to pathology.

Jack Ladenson, PhD

The nature of my participation in medical volunteer work has varied. For PO we (ie, Heinz Hoenecke, Victor Lee, Tim Amukele, Sarah Brown, or me) get a lead. After a little follow-up, a determination is made whether to visit the country to further evaluate the interest.

As far as I am aware, PO has performed 25 site visits and has established 12 projects. I was involved in all but Rwanda and Senegal. The first projects that PO got involved with were in anatomic pathology with heavy involvement by Heinz Hoenecke and Victor Lee. These projects involved Kenya (the first project), Nepal and Madagascar (with Frank Kiel), Ghana (with Tom Coppin and Barnes-Jewish pathology residents in AP/CP), St Lucia (with Harriet Fremland and CP with Susan Morin). I have visited all project sites except St Lucia.

Timothy Amukele, MD, PhD

I grew up in Nigeria until my teenage years, so even though I had spent most of my life and done all my training in the United States, I always had an appreciation for life outside the United States. I first got involved in volunteering abroad through PO during my residency training. Jack Ladenson and Mitch Scott had published a few articles detailing the impact of some of the work they were doing in Eritrea, and I was really attracted to how systematic their approach was. I mentioned this to my mentor Michael Astion, who introduced me to Jack. The rest is history.

What is the Nature of Your Participation in Volunteerism? (Single Versus Multiple Trips? Single Versus Multiple Sites? What did You do at the Volunteer Site?)

Chris Hansen, MD

I went to Ghana for 5 weeks in 2009, Malawi for 4 weeks in 2011 and 4 weeks in 2012, and Rwanda for 3 weeks each in 2014, 2015, and 2016. In Ghana I worked at Komfo Anokye Teaching Hospital, a 1000-bed hospital that I remember as having lost thier pathologists in 2005. The program supported volunteer pathologists for rotations that were at least a month long and overlapped with the previous and subsequent visiting pathologists. We saw about 30 current cases a day and signed out. We attended the tumor boards, and I gave pathology lectures to attending doctors of medicine (MDs) and training MDs. In Malawi at the time, there were no pathologists in training. On my first visit, there was a 6-month backlog of cases (several thousand) at the medical college in Blantyre, the commercial capital. I finished off about half of those cases in 2 weeks and then went to the main hospital in Lilongwe, the administrative capital, to read cases there (about 25/day). In Rwanda, the residency program was started in 2013 with about 4 residents per year. They graduate their first class in 2017. While there I read cases and taught the residents at the Central University Hospital in Kigali and King Faisal hospital in Kigali and read cases at Butaro (national cancer hospital). Each year I have covered a different topic (30 lectures on endocrine pathology in 2014, 25 lectures on gastrointestinal pathology in 2015, 20 lectures on immunostaining in 2016). For 2017, I have proposed facilitating having 2 Rwandan residents train at the University of California, Davis (UCD) for 2 months in molecular pathology (and first getting up to speed with the US system of medicine by shadowing me at my hospital for 2 weeks). Their rotation at UCD is scheduled for November and December of this year.

Martin McCann, MD

First volunteering motivations and nature of participation: My wife (a radiologist) and I retired from our practices in the United States in 1999. I took the Tropical Medicine Course led by Dr Robert (Bob) Gilman. To be certified by the American Society of Tropical Medicine, a 2-month course of field work was required. I did this in Lima Peru, doing fine-needle aspirations (FNAs) under the auspices of Dr Gilman's project in Lima. My time in Peru led to an interest in travel experiences. When my wife entered theology seminary to eventually become a priest in the Episcopal Church, I did multiple short-term medical mission trips to Haiti, Honduras, and the Dominican Republic. These trips were church sponsored, and I did general medicine. There are arguments for and against short-term medical missions; however, for me the experience was extremely rewarding and formative. I also did a couple of month-long visits to Kijabe Hospital, Kenya, where I participated as a surgical pathologist. (This site is sponsored by the World Medical Mission. They try to have 1 or 2 expatriate pathologists there to cover a large referral practice each month.) The overall experience for me was that I liked the patient contact of the short-term visits, but I felt more useful doing pathology. Fine-needle aspiration cytology filled this niche.

When my wife finished seminary in 2003, we volunteered with our mission agency of the Episcopal Church. We thought we would probably go someplace in the Caribbean or South America. Our mission director wanted missioners to Africa. Initially we went to Maseno, Kenya at a small hospital. I did general medical work as well as set up a tissue processor, microtome, and staining to do a small amount of surgical pathology. I did a few FNAs. This was also a good learning experience under a well-trained internist. I was not getting the amount of anatomic pathology I wanted, so while in Maseno we traveled around Tanzania where the mission director wanted more missionaries. The Bishop of the Diocese of Central Tanganyika was encouraging, and I set up a surgical pathology laboratory in a medical clinic there in Dodoma. My wife first taught at and later became director of communications at a local theological college. There are only about 18 pathologists in Tanzania, and they are located in Dar, Moshi, Mwanza, and Mbeya. There are none in the central region where Dodoma is.

I and an aide initially cut and stained incoming cases. Later I sponsored a histotechnologist to be trained at the Muhimbili National University in Dar es Salaam. I had on and off part-time workers. I was not so busy in the beginning, and I was able to teach medical technologists histopathology and clinical officers pathology. Gradually, referral cases and referrals for FNA grew in an exponential fashion. These referrals were mainly mission hospitals, as they seemed to have more upgraded surgical departments and a desire for evidence-based medicine.

Side note: There is a push-pull in every decision process. The encouragement (pull) of Dr Gilman to take his course and go to Peru was important to me. He said yes in an encouraging way. Our Bishop in Tanzania had the enthusiasm to bring both my wife and I to Dodoma for a long stay.

Merih Tesfazghi, PhD
Part of my experience in clinical laboratory science comes from my work at a national health laboratory in Eritrea as well as from my work at the Orotta School of Medicine. At the national health laboratory, I worked in different departments, mainly in the department of hematology. While working at these two institutes, I had the opportunity to interact with volunteer professionals that worked for the Asmara-Zurich twining project sponsored by the World Federation of Hemophilia, PO, and physicians from Cuba who helped sustain the first medical school in Eritrea.

I had participated in workshops organized by the volunteers, and I was involved in the establishment of new instruments and assays. At an institute level, I think their activities had great impact in modernizing the laboratory by helping the laboratory with acquiring new assays, new instruments, interfacing the instruments, introducing locally operational Laboratory Information System (LIS), providing overseas reference laboratories, enrolling laboratories in external quality assurance programs, as well as assisting in the establishment of the first-ever medical school in Eritrea. Their activities were both impactful and visionary. At a personal level, the greatest experience I gained from their activities was that I got inspired by the volunteers to grow like them. Most of the volunteers I encountered during my practice are now great friends and colleagues and have supported me in so many ways to achieving my goals this far.

Charles Marboe, MD
My interest in volunteering in sub-Saharan Africa started in medical school when I took a year off between the third and fourth years to work on a perinatal mortality project in Addis Ababa. This experience also stimulated a switch in my career interest from pediatrics to pathology.

Jack Ladenson, PhD
My role at the project sites has varied from support and cheerleading (Haiti, Malawi) to coordination, planning and recruiting, and funding. It has included helping to start one medical school (Eritrea) and sustain another (Zimbabwe). The key decisions are (1) whether to get involved; (2) what we want to accomplish; (3) volunteer on-site or periodically; and (4) assessment of people we would potentially work with, and so forth.

Timothy Amukele, MD, PhD
Since I started volunteering 9 years ago I have never stopped. Each hospital in each country is unique in terms of their capacity and what they need, but my goal in each

site has been to try to improve the systems rather than focusing on instrument donation. In particular, I have focused on establishing quality monitoring systems, for example, laboratory information systems and external quality assurance.

How has Your Volunteering Been Funded?

Chris Hansen, MD
PO and Partners in Health (PIH) are tax-deductible nonprofit organizations, so airfare, travel expenses, medical license costs, and so forth are tax deductible. My work partners have also offered me the option to alternatively submit my expenses to our corporation as a business expense. For the visiting residents, at my expense, I plan to cover their cost of housing when they live with me for 2 weeks and also when they are in Sacramento for 2 months.

Martin McCann, MD
The short-term missions were self-funded. I think the World Medical Mission (Kajabe, Kenya) can provide some funding if requested. While in Kenya and Tanzania, our church mission society provided medical insurance, a stipend of $1000 per month, and round trip flights every 3 years. (We came home to the United States each year.) We bought a car at our own expense. Housing is provided by the hosting diocese. Some church mission societies are much more reasonable and generous. An Atlanta church donated a hematology analyzer used in the medical clinic I was associated with. An anonymous donor bought a new tissue processor and embedding center for us. The original processor and microtomes were given by a hospital in Columbus, Georgia. I mention these because they were significant expenses and brought the laboratory up and running and carried it on. My charges covered my staff salaries, rent, and reagents. I did not (and as a missionary could not) take a salary.

Charles Marboe, MD
Travels to teach in Rwanda have been self-funded. Years ago, one other faculty member and I went to Gondar, Ethiopia to teach pathology; it was supported by our department chair because he was interested.

Jack Ladenson, PhD
The funding for my work has included some grants, US Agency for International Development (USAID), World Bank, and personal or corporate foundations but also funds at the Washington University, which were derived from licenses for tests developed in my research laboratory, for example, myoglobin, Creatinine Kinase-MB, troponin-I, as well as my own resources.

Timothy Amukele, MD, PhD
My travel and housing costs were covered by PO when I first started volunteering with them. Now I am affiliated with grant-funded programs in a few African countries, so much of my travel is supported by the grants.

Has Your Volunteer Work Resulted in an Academic or Nonacademic (Blog, Web Site, Magazine) Publication?

Chris Hansen, MD
My contribution was mentioned as an acknowledgment in an article in PlosOne, and there was an article in a UCD faculty publication.

Martin McCann, MD

We did a missionary newsletter to our church and supporters, but this would not be considered a publication. I did give a pathology grand rounds at Mount Saini Hospital in New York in February 2016.

Merih Tesfazghi, PhD

In August 2011, I accepted an invitation from George A. Fritsma (http://www.fritsmafactor.com) to write about the impact of PO's activities in Eritrea for the American Society for Clinical Laboratory Science's newsletter and was printed in January 2012.

Charles Marboe, MD

I have not published anything from this but have given a few visiting grand rounds on pathology in developing countries.

Jack Ladenson, PhD

The work of PO is described in the Washington University's newsletter, on PO's Web site, and peer-reviewed journals.[10–14]

Timothy Amukele, MD, PhD

My volunteer work has resulted in meeting abstracts and presentations but not a peer-reviewed publication yet, although the article is in preparation. I think that sharing our volunteer experiences is very important. That is how I got involved in doing this very rewarding work.

Other Shared Experiences?

Chris Hansen, MD

Besides the pathology work (reading cases, presenting at the tumor board, doing FNAs, and bone marrows) and teaching pathology residents, I also bring donated medical supplies on my visits. I was shocked on my first trip (Ghana) at the lack of basic medical supplies. Before each trip, I collect or purchase medical supplies and equipment for distribution. I am allowed two 50-lb bags on the flight, so I devote 35 lb to medical supplies. I am careful to only accept what I know will be used and to not take something that might be problematic (chemotherapy agents, toxic, and so forth). Most of what I take are what I call clinical kits, which include some or all of the following in each kit: stethoscope, sphygmomanometer, digital thermometer (C°), nonoutdated antibiotics, pregnancy tests (at least 250), glucose meter and test strips (at least 1000), urine dip sticks (250), sterile sutures, Tegaderm (3M, St Paul, MN), Steri-Strips (3M), reflex hammer, pen light, measuring tape, pregnancy wheel, wright peak flow meter, compact portable rechargeable nebulizer with

---

Box 1
Pathologists overseas: lessons learned

- You need someone local to work with and political acceptance.
- Set goals first, then select approach.
- Accept donated materials only if they are compatible with the goals.
- Keep things simple, but emphasize quality.
- Stay flexible; the unexpected will happen.
- Volunteers and companies of good will do exist.

Box 2
Funding acknowledgment

- Beckman-Coulter Foundation
- Pathologists overseas (many individual donors, and it is on Smile Amazon)
- USAID
- Washington University School of Medicine
- Wilding Foundation
- World Bank

---

albuterol, eye chart, and so forth. I try to bring some specialized supplies for specific clinics (fluorescein for eye clinic, bone marrow biopsy needles for heme, extra sutures for surgery, pediatric-size stethoscope, and blood pressure cuff for children). Besides the medical equipment, I also bring other supplies, such as deflated soccer balls and soccer cleats, which I hand out in small villages when traveling, always a big hit in Africa.

Jack Ladenson, PhD

I look at my volunteer career as helping capable people to help themselves, not too far removed from mentoring residents or fellows. The work itself is variable, but the process is similar to research in that one needs to assess where the project or field is (point A) and set a goal as to where you might want it to go (point B). I have never had a plan to get from A to B that did not have to be modified. I have also learned some general lessons (**Box 1**) and found that companies (**Boxes 2** and **3**) and people of good will (**Box 4**) exist and are the biggest asset. The lessons are as follows: (1) You need someone local to work with and political acceptance. (2) Set goals first, then select the approach. (3) Accept donated materials only if compatible with the goals. (4) Keep things simple, but emphasize quality. (5) Stay flexible; the unexpected will happen. (6) Volunteers and companies of good will do exist. It has been stimulating, rewarding, and fun; I have met people who have become lasting friends.

Box 3
Corporate donations to pathologists overseas projects

Beckman Coulter	Hematology analyzers and electrolyte analyzer
Becton Dickinson	Blood collection tubes
Comp Pro Med, Inc	Software for laboratory information system
Dade-Behring, Inc	Equipment
Life-Scan	Glucose meters
MAS	Quality control material
Mallinckrodt	Computers
Ortho	Blood bank reagents
Radiometer	Blood gas equipment
Roche: United States	Chemistry analyzer, technical support and training, highly discounted reagents
Sigma-Aldrich	Donated equipment
Washington University School of Medicine	Reference laboratory and books for medical school

---

Box 4
Volunteers for clinical pathology projects

Eritrea: 59 individuals of varied backgrounds and degrees; 6 were for periods of 3 months to 4 years

Bhutan: 28 individuals of varied backgrounds and degrees; 5 were for periods of 3 months to 1 year

---

REFERENCES

1. Caldron PH, Impens A, Pavlova M, et al. Economic assessment of US physician participation in short-term medical missions. Global Health 2016;12(1):45.
2. Scheffler RM, Liu JX, Kinfu Y, et al. Forecasting the global shortage of physicians: an economic- and needs-based approach. Bull World Health Organ 2008;86(7). 516–23B.
3. Caldron PH, Impens A, Pavlova M, et al. Why do they care? Narratives of physician volunteers on motivations for participation in short-term medical missions abroad. BMC Health Serv Res 2016;16:682.
4. Sykes KJ. Short-term medical service trips: a systematic review of the evidence. Am J Public Health 2014;104(7):e38–48.
5. Caldron PH, Impens A, Pavlova M, et al. Demographic profile of physician participants in short-term medical missions. BMC Health Serv Res 2016;16(1):682.
6. Wall LL, Arrowsmith SD, Lassey AT, et al. Humanitarian ventures or "fistula tourism?": the ethical perils of pelvic surgery in the developing world. Int Urogynecol J Pelvic Floor Dysfunct 2006;17(6):559–62.
7. Crump JA, Sugarman J. Ethical considerations for short-term experiences by trainees in global health. JAMA 2008;300(12):1456–8.
8. Bales K. Measuring the propensity to volunteer. Soc Pol Admin 1996;30(3): 206–26.
9. Martiniuk ALC, Manouchehrian M, Negin JA, et al. Brain gains: a literature review of medical missions to low and middle-income countries. BMC Health Serv Res 2012;12:134.
10. Available at: www.pathologistsoverseas.com. Accessed September 4, 2017.
11. Hoenecke H, Lee V, Roy I. Pathologists overseas: coordinating volunteer pathology services for 19 years. Arch Pathol Lab Med 2011;135:173–8. Available at: http://www.archivesofpathology.org/doi/pdf/10.1043/2008-0450-SOR1.1.
12. Ladenson JH, Scott MG, Klarkowski D, et al. Use of a major medical center clinical laboratory as a reference laboratory for a developing country: ordering patterns help set laboratory priorities. Clin Chem 2003;49:162–6. Available at: http://clinchem.aaccjnls.org/content/clinchem/49/1/162.full.pdf.
13. Windus DW, Ladenson JH, Merrins CK, et al. Impact of a multidisciplinary intervention for diabetes in Eritrea. Clin Chem 2007;53:1954–9. Available at: http://clinchem.aaccjnls.org/content/clinchem/53/11/1954.full.pdf.
14. Scott MG, Morin S, Hock KG, et al. Establishing a simple and sustainable quality assurance program and clinical chemistry services in Eritrea. Clin Chem 2007;53: 1945–53. Available at: http://clinchem.aaccjnls.org/content/clinchem/53/11/1945. full.pdf.

Global Health Pathology Research: Purpose and Funding

John S. Flanigan, MD*, Shannon L. Silkensen, PhD, Nicholas G. Wolf, BA

KEYWORDS

- Pathologist • Global health • Cancer research • Funders • Accurate diagnosis

KEY POINTS

- Pathologists are fundamentally positioned to contribute to basic biological knowledge, to increasing accurate and efficient diagnostics, to enhance cost-effective practice, and to shape health care policy.
- Scientific rationales for international research projects include the local preponderance of disease, rare genetic variants, and/or unique environmental exposures. Well-conducted research studies include performance indicators to monitor quality, efficiency, and impact. Peer reviewers expect a deliberate plan to accommodate the realities of conducting international research.
- Improved communications among researchers and funders will help generate the evidence needed to advance our understanding of human biology and improve the human condition.
- Pathologists should think strategically about how their investigations fit into a larger agenda to address the needs of the health system.

INTRODUCTION

Peer-reviewed research funding is highly competitive: it is incumbent on the investigators to demonstrate the value, relevance, and impact of their proposals. At present, the practice of both pathology and global health are evolving rapidly. Funders and investigators need to work together to define a well-designed, well-executed clinical research agenda that will generate a sustainable, powerful field of clinical research. Pathology clinical practice ranges from laboratory medicine to anatomic pathology, microbiology, transfusion medicine, and molecular diagnostics. In this era of precision medicine, diagnostic pathology plays a pivotal role in accrual to clinical trials. Areas of research include basic biological investigation through translation of current automated tests to new practice settings.

Disclosure Statement: All authors work for the National Cancer Institute.
Center for Global Health, National Cancer Institute, National Institutes of Health, 9609 Medical Center Drive, Rockville, MD 20850, USA
* Corresponding author.
E-mail address: John.Flanigan@nih.gov

Clin Lab Med 38 (2018) 21–35
https://doi.org/10.1016/j.cll.2017.10.003
0272-2712/18/Published by Elsevier Inc.

Pathologists become interested in global health for a variety of reasons, and perusal of the table of contents of this issue demonstrates their range of motivation. These motivations include altruistic volunteerism, education of the next generation of practitioners, sampling a comprehensive cross-section of human genetic diversity, and acquiring bio-specimens for basic research. Likewise, funders of global health have varying priorities. These priorities range from investigation of basic biology to scaling interventions that will reach the world's most disadvantaged citizens. It is beyond the scope of this article to debate the relative value of these underlying motivations; in fact, there is value in each of these approaches. The goal here is to improve communications among all interested parties to generate the evidence needed to advance our understanding of human biology and to improve the human condition.

The Center for Global Health[1] (CGH) of the National Cancer Institute[2] (NCI) at the National Institutes of Health[3] (NIH) was formed in 2011 to catalyze global cancer research. The CGH addresses the NCI's commitment to strengthen global cancer research, build a global cancer research community, and foster the translation of research results into practice. From the CGH's inception, pathology and laboratory medicine have played a pivotal role in global clinical research by contributing to an accurate diagnosis, monitoring the effects of therapy, and providing precise input into disease surveillance systems.[4] Over the past 5 years, the center has supported the intersection of pathology and global cancer research in many ways. The CGH has funded grants, contracts, and supplements to support new and enhanced diagnostic technologies. Additionally, the CGH has supported training the next generation of practitioners, hosted strategic planning sessions for pathology, and held workshops to increase the profile of pathology practice in low-resource settings.

This article summarizes the authors' experience to date and outlines future directions for pathology research. The NIH has a long history of working with the scientific community to generate funding announcements, and many of the 27 NIH institutes and centers pursue international projects. Peer reviewers use a well-defined set of criteria to work together to identify meritorious proposals.

- The first section discusses how the NIH's peer-review process applies to global health pathology research projects.
- The second section presents an illustrative sampling of NIH-funded projects with performance sites in low- and middle-income countries (LMICs) with 2 examples focused on cancer and anatomic pathology.
- The third section relates the research agenda to overarching strategic recommendations for enhancing global pathology.

APPLYING NATIONAL INSTITUTES OF HEALTH'S REVIEW CRITERIA TO GLOBAL PATHOLOGY RESEARCH

Performing research in international settings presents many opportunities for ingenuity. Access to facilities, equipment, communications, information technology, supplies, support staff, ethics review boards, demographic data, vital registration data, and baseline epidemiologic information can be challenging. Inclusive, intellectual partnerships among high-income country investigators and those working in local LMIC communities can not only address these challenges but can also refine and improve scientific hypotheses and assure relevance to local patient populations. For example, the CGH funded a partnership of Tanzanian and US investigators to document the high burden of esophageal cancer. Pathologists, epidemiologists, and clinicians worked together to elucidate geographic biological variation of esophageal cancer in East Africa. This collaboration has generated new hypotheses on disease causation.[5]

Many funders, including the NIH, have predominantly domestic mandates. Agency leaders ask the following: Why not do this study in your home setting? Experienced global health researchers must preempt this question. Credible rationales focus on the scientific question being asked. For example, is there a higher burden of an uncommon disease; are there rare genetic variants or environmental exposures that warrant conducting research outside the United States. Although social justice, humanitarian need, and interest in a foreign locale are all motivations for individual global health engagement, the NIH responds to clear, convincing, scientific rationale for working in any population, foreign or domestic. It is the responsibility of the investigator to effectively justify why the research project should be based at a foreign site. All NIH funding announcements include 5 major review criteria: significance, investigators, innovation, approach, and environment. Meritorious applicants weave their structured justification for working internationally into these established review criteria.

Significance

There must be a scientific premise driving the proposal. Testing the premise should lead to new scientific knowledge, new technical capacity, and/or impact clinical practice. It is important to relate the proposed study to the purpose of the funding opportunity described in the purpose and background sections of the funding opportunity announcement (FOA). **Table 1** highlights examples of significance statements from the NIH FOAs in various topic areas.

Please note that the aforementioned funding announcements involve broad areas of science. The following comments highlight how pathology fits into these topic areas.

Research training

The Fogarty International Center[11] is the major source of research training support for LMICs. Fogarty priorities have included medical education for primary practitioners, educators, and for both international and domestic junior researchers. To date, pathologist participation has been infrequent.

Research capacity

FOAs specifically addressing research capacity, such as Planning for Regional Centers Excellence in Non-Communicable Diseases in LMICs (RFA-CA-15-007),[7] are relatively uncommon. Although this announcement specifically mentions accurate diagnosis, most funding announcements address specific scientific questions.

Biological questions

Accurate tissue diagnosis is needed in many studies performed in global settings. Scientific reasons for studying populations in low-resource settings include variations in disease epidemiology by geography, population genetics, differing exposures, and risk factor burden. Sampling human genetic diversity enables investigators to study rare diseases and to identify new genetic drivers. Some investigations require patient populations naïve to current treatments or with higher burdens of advanced disease.

New technologies

There is interest in developing innovative, frugal technologies for diagnosing and monitoring diseases. Given the high performance of current pathology practice in the United States and a reluctance to streamline practice unless the highest standards of diagnostic accuracy can be met or exceeded, it is sometimes necessary to test new devices or strategies in lower-resource settings. Ethical considerations related to trials

Table 1
Significance statements from select National Institutes of Health funding opportunity announcements

FOA	Topic	Significance
PAR-16-279: Fogarty HIV Research Training Program for Low-and Middle-Income Country Institutions (D43)[6]	Research training	Over the years, some of the most important recent scientific advances in HIV/AIDS … have been facilitated through partnerships with LMIC scientists. Many of these partnerships have been supported by the FIC research training programs. Continued investment in training strengthens research at LMIC institutions and addresses the ongoing HIV epidemic. FIC research training programs are part of the solution to achieve an 'AIDS-Free Generation.'
RFA-CA-15-007: Planning for Regional Centers of Research Excellence in Non-communicable Diseases in Low and Middle Income Countries[7]	Research capacity	Many region of the world have untapped potential and research capabilities. To develop a plan that will coordinate the basic, translational, clinical, and population science research for Non-Communicable Diseases (NCDs) in these regions will generate the evidence needed to advance our understanding of human biology.
PAR-15-093: Basic Cancer Research in Cancer Health Disparities (R01)[8]	Biological questions	These research project grants will support innovative studies designed to investigate biological/genetic bases of cancer disparities
RFA-CA-15-001: Cancer Detection, Diagnosis, and Treatment Technologies for Global Health (UH2/UH3)[9]	New technologies	To conduct projects that adapt, apply, and validate existing or emerging technologies into a new generation of user-friendly, low-cost devices. To develop assays that are clinically comparable to currently used technologies for imaging, in vitro detection/diagnosis, prevention or treatment of cancers in humans living in LMICs.
PAR-16-238: Dissemination and Implementation Research in Health (R01)[10]	Health systems, scalability of intervention, and program science	To identify, develop, test, evaluate and/or refine strategies to disseminate and implement evidence-based practices (eg, behavioral interventions; prevention, early detection, diagnostic, treatment and disease management interventions; quality improvement programs) into public health, clinical practice, and community settings.

in LMICs are addressed in good clinical practice guidelines, and there is a growing experience in performing trials in these settings.[12] An example of this type of program is the NCI program Cancer Detection, Diagnosis, and Treatment Technologies for Global Health (UH2/UH3) (RFA-CA-15-001).[9]

Health systems, scalability of interventions, and program science

International policy makers need data to establish norms and standards. Some funders concentrate on bringing interventions to scale for underserved populations. Demonstrated best practices are needed by all parties interested in advancing global health. Evidence is needed on cost-effectiveness, affordability, integration of systems, and improving communication and coordination of effort in both research and clinical care. Funders concentrating on scaling programs are reluctant to invest in extensive research data acquisition. Well-conducted research studies can indicate a narrower set of key performance indicators of quality, process indicators to monitor efficiency, and, most importantly, metrics to assess the impact of the outcome. Implementation science research is a systematic tool to assess multidimensional interventions and can be a highly effective way to translate scientific evidence into practice (**Fig. 1**). Pathologists can play a key role in designing systems and assessing the impact in this field.

Investigators

Principal investigators, collaborators, and other researchers must have the skills, knowledge, and resources necessary to carry out the proposed research project.[13] Pathologists most often contribute to basic science research by developing and

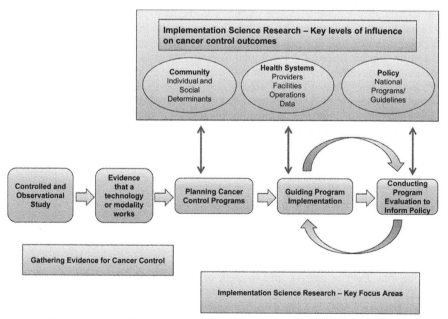

Fig. 1. Getting from scientific evidence to public health practice: role of implementation science research. (*From* Sivaram S, Sanchez MA, Rimer BK, et al. Implementation science in cancer prevention and control: a framework for research and programs in low and middle-income countries. Cancer Epidemiol Biomarkers Prev 2014;23(11):2278; with permission.)

applying leading-edge technology to diagnostics[14] and by joining a team of investigators with complementary expertise. Successful clinical research projects are aligned with other medical services and ongoing patient care.

Team science is clearly a trend in the performance of research. Working across geography, cultures, and economic resources adds an additional dimension to team work. Inclusion of experienced global health practitioners on the research team improves the likelihood of successful research project completion. Furthermore, these investigators are familiar with the scientific needs of the local community and have earned the trust of the local population. Pairing investigators from LMICs with those from greater-resourced universities is increasingly prevalent. It can be an explicit requirement, such as in the NCI Regional Center of Research Excellence Program,[7] or it can often be part of the training mission of the academic partners.[15] Fulfilling partnerships between paired investigators are built on clear, agreed on, upfront expectations of the benefit, such as publications, presentations, and future collaborative grant applications.[16] Furthermore, mutually fulfilling partnerships include clear delineations of budgetary and other in-kind resource control.[16] Full participation of international investigators enables research to advance more quickly and is to the long-term advantage of all.

A clearly reasoned approach to leadership, governance, and organizational structure is a crucial element of peer review for complex projects. Study sections reviewing global health projects are particularly careful to look for evidence of the scientific productivity among the proposed partners. Meritorious applications specify realistic governance structures, including strategies for dealing with the differing expectations of coinvestigators.

Innovation

Meritorious applications challenge current paradigms in research or practice. In the authors' experience, grading innovation in global health FOAs has been challenging for peer reviewers and reaching consensus has engendered some debate. Proposals based on performance of current pathology techniques in new settings are not sufficiently innovative. Global health pathology research must include making new connections and applying novel solutions to existing problems. Applying current methodology to an LMIC setting in and of itself is insufficient. Innovation related to new techniques or instrumentation may be apparent to reviewers, but innovation based on translating known interventions to new settings must be clearly justified by the applicant. The Center for Translational Science at the National Heart, Lung, and Blood Institute[17] addresses these issues in implementation science by sponsoring workshops and has released a translational science FOA, T4 Translational Research Capacity Building Initiative in Low Income Countries (U24) (RFA-HL-17-003).[18] Again, this support is relatively uncommon.

Approach

Addressing potential problems, proposing alternative strategies, and offering benchmarks of success are all required elements of successful applications, domestic or international. Peer reviewers and funders are attentive to the pitfalls of working abroad and expect a premeditated plan to deal with not only scientifically warranted adjustments but also the realities of logistics, politics, and the environment on research programs. The anticipated duration of a research project influences risk assessment of possible delays. Such delays need to be weighed when measuring the duration of the project, current financing, and the anticipated start of follow-on programs.

Environment

The environment includes both scientific and physical resources favoring success. Institutional support, partnership strengths, and access to facilities are usual elements. Importantly, unique features of the scientific environment, including subject populations and collaborative partnerships, can be emphasized. The NCI's Regional Centers of Research Excellence RFA announcement included several cues investigators should consider when preparing applications with international components. These prompts include the following:

- Will the scientific environment in which the work will be done contribute to the probability of success?
- Are the institutional support, equipment, and other physical resources available to the investigators adequate for the project proposed?
- Will the project benefit from unique features of the scientific environment, subject populations, or collaborative arrangements?
- How will the institutional support contribute to the success of the RCRE planning grant?[7]

Additionally, the NCI-designated Cancer Centers Program is a signature program of the US NCI. The physical space supported by these centers is described here:

Physical space

Centers are more successful in establishing an identity if they have a distinct physical location. Not all members of the cancer center need be physically located in facilities controlled exclusively by the center; however, the location of members across program areas (basic laboratory; clinical; and prevention, control, and population-based science) in close physical proximity enhances shared use of resources and facilitates scientific interactions. Even if proximity is impossible, center-shared resources and other services should still be reasonably accessible to all members, including consortium members.

In your application, briefly describe the physical facilities dedicated to cancer research, center-shared resources, and administration. Indicate how the center facilitates access to shared resources and other services (ie, clinical protocol and data management). Discuss any plans for expansion.[19]

Having reviewed scoring methodology, the second section reviews a sample of currently funded NIH research.

LANDSCAPE OF NATIONAL INSTITUTES OF HEALTH–FUNDED GLOBAL PATHOLOGY RESEARCH IN LOW- AND MIDDLE-INCOME COUNTRIES
Overview of Global Health Programs and Partnerships

As reviewed in the previous section, there are many reasons for US universities to expand their portfolios and conduct research in LMICs. Establishing efficient, equitable, and sustainable partnerships with international institutions is essential to the production of the best science in LMICs.[4] In 2016, the Center for Strategic and International Studies (CSIS) conducted a study of the global health partnerships of 82 North American Universities and 44 international partnering institutions. The goal of this study was to examine the benefits and characteristics of successful partnerships.[20] Their data demonstrate that, in general, these partnerships were mutually beneficial, and that most partnerships had an equitable arrangement. The largest perceived benefits were seen in education and research. Collaborations among research institutions were the most frequently reported activity among North American universities and international partners.

Academic twinning programs provide a 2-way transfer of expertise and skill. For example, when pediatric oncologists in low-resource and high-resource settings are twinned, these teams of committed health care professionals are perfectly poised to develop and implement locally appropriate treatment protocols. Furthermore, all patients have an increased access to treatment. Working together, implementation of locally appropriate protocols and an increased access to care contribute to an overall increase in childhood cancer survival rates.[21]

For international institutions, the partnerships were less successful with respect to health impact, policy development, and advocacy. The data show some unevenness around decision-making, lack of bidirectional funding, and publication authorship. In general, the study found that global health partnerships are perceived as beneficial for both North American universities and international institutions.

According to the CSIS survey, funding was one of the most important factors for program success. Research funding can come from many different types of organizations, such as universities, government, nongovernmental organizations, private donors, or foundations. A strength of NIH funding is explicit guidance for budget allocation among investigators and institutions. This alignment of budget, roles, and responsibility allows for transparency and accuracy of task ownership. The survey found that international research agencies, such as the NIH, were the second most important source of funding for international institutions and were deemed a very important or essential source of funding by most North American universities (**Fig. 2**). Next the authors examine this relationship in more detail by analyzing the contents of the NIH's research portfolio in cancer and anatomic pathology.

Portfolio Analysis of National Institutes of Health–Funded Cancer Research in Low- and Middle-Income Countries

The mission of the US NCI is to coordinate the National Cancer Program. This program conducts and supports research, training, health information dissemination, and other cancer-related programs. It provides research grants and cooperative agreements to coordinate and support research projects conducted by universities, hospitals, research foundations, and businesses throughout this country and abroad. To enhance survival and improve patients' quality of life requires evidence-based clinical protocols, and the NCI is one of the largest funders of evidence-based clinical research. To illustrate the contribution one dedicated funder can make, the authors examined the NCI's investment in global cancer research over time.

Fig. 3 shows a comprehensive analysis of the NCI-supported extramural research portfolio between fiscal year (FY) 2008 and FY 2014. Importantly, the total number of NCI-supported extramural cancer research projects both domestically and in LMICs remains relatively constant.

The NIH uses 3 main grant mechanisms to implement its scientific agenda: training, research, and cooperative agreement.

- NIH training grants provide the protected time and research budget for postdoctoral, postmedical, and early stage faculty members to develop into independent investigators.
- NIH research grants support a discrete, specified, circumscribed project.
- NIH cooperative agreements support discrete research projects that are conducted between extramural and intramural NIH researchers and program staff.

The sophistication of the research question, the local environment, and the scientific maturity of the investigators all contribute to the choice of the grant mechanism. **Fig. 4**

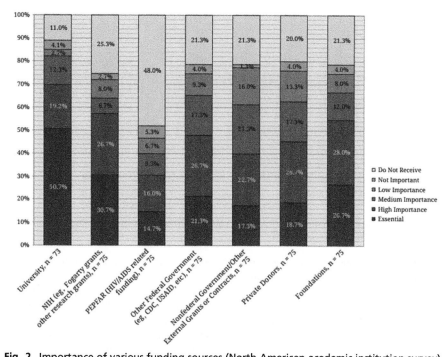

Fig. 2. Importance of various funding sources (North American academic institution survey). CDC, Centers for Disease Control and Prevention; HIV, human immunodeficiency virus; PEPFAR, President's Emergency Plan For AIDS Relief; USAID, United States Agency for International Development. (*From* Muir JA, Farley J, Osterman A, et al. Global Health Programs and Partnerships: Evidence of Mutual Benefit and Equity. Center for Strategic and International Studies. March 2016. Available at: https://csis-prod.s3.amazonaws.com/s3fs-public/publication/160315_Muir_GlobalHealthPrograms_Web.pdf; with permission.)

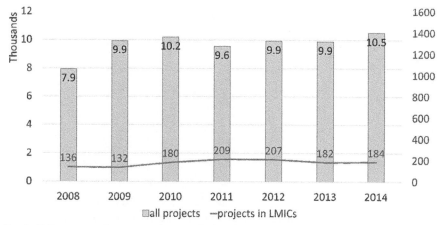

Fig. 3. NCI-supported extramural research, fiscal year 2008 to 2014.

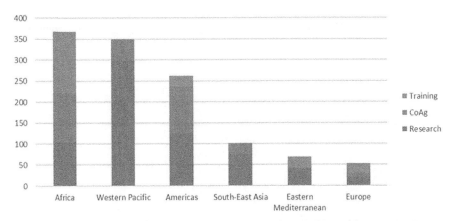

Fig. 4. NCI-supported extramural research projects by the World Health Organization region. CoAg, cooperative agreement.

shows the distribution of NCI-supported extramural cancer research projects by the World Health Organization (WHO) region.

An example of research conducted as part of a training grant in Africa was a project conducted by Dr Akwi Asombang, a gastroenterology Fogarty fellow from the Washington University School of Medicine. Fogarty Fellows and Scholars[22] are carefully chosen participants invited to conduct yearlong research projects in LMICs. During Dr Asombang's fellowship in Zambia, she demonstrated that eating fruits and vegetables year-round was protective against gastric cancer. She documented this observation by measuring urinary isoprostanes, which are biomarkers of oxidative stress.[23]

Research grants addressing specific cancers are a recurring source of global health support when the distribution of malignant neoplasms is not uniform across the country or region. Some diseases, such as virally induced cancers, have geographic and environmentally associated incidence patterns. **Fig. 5** shows the distribution of the

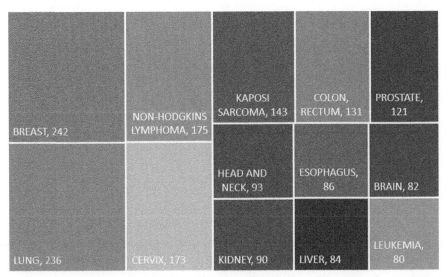

Fig. 5. NCI-supported extramural research by anatomic organ site for LMICs for FY 2008 to 2014; projects can be coded for more than one organ site.

NCI-supported extramural research programs in LMICs by anatomic organ site for FY 2008 to 2014. Research topics include contributions from environmental exposures, infectious agents, and unknown biological variables. As pathologists join global research teams, their expertise in diagnosis and staging will ensure that accurate data are available to advance our understanding of human biology.

Portfolio Analysis of National Cancer Institute Pathology Research in Low- and Middle-Income Countries

The NCI supports a modest program of pathology-related research specific to LMICs. In 2017, the NCI anticipates supporting approximately 35 pathology-related cancer research projects. These grants run the gamut from etiologic studies of gastric cancer to culturally appropriate screening and diagnosis cervical cancer screening programs. **Fig. 6** shows the distribution of projects by research area.

The distribution of projects shows that there are opportunities to engage in research currently, especially as a member of an investigational team. One of the NCI-supported research projects was designed to improve the pathologic diagnosis capabilities of lymphoproliferative disorders at Kamuzu Central Hospital in Lilongwe, Malawi.[24] Through this joint research project, investigators discovered a high concordance between real-time diagnoses in Malawi and final diagnoses in the United States. This high concordance rate demonstrates the value that strong, local pathology services provide to real-time clinical care and research in LMICs. In the next section, the authors discuss how these scientific pursuits help to meet the overarching strategic goals for strengthening global pathology.

CHALLENGING PATHOLOGISTS TO THINK STRATEGICALLY

All research occurs within a system of scientific investigation, teaching, and patient care delivery. Given the complexity of pathology systems and the many points for improvement suggested in this issue, it is important to relate any proposed investment of time, talent, and funds in research to the needs of the larger system. In May of 2016, the NCI convened a group of international experts in pathology and global health to outline a strategy for supporting pathology. At the time, many organizations were engaging in international initiatives in research, clinical instruction, communication,

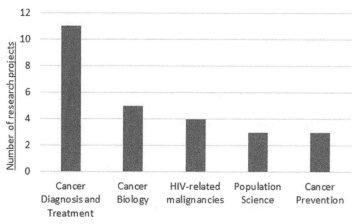

Fig. 6. NCI-supported research related to pathology in 2017, by research area. HIV, human immunodeficiency virus.

and telepathology. Building on years of advocacy, the first ever article on pathology in *Disease Control Priorities, Third Edition*[25] was in preparation; the WHO, in Geneva, was preparing *Priority Medical Devices for Cancer Management*,[26] including equipment standards for pathology laboratories; the International Committee on Cancer Reporting was increasing the availability of evidence-based synoptic reporting[27]; the NCI had funded several new contracts and grants specific to pathology in LMICs. The experts' recommendations fell into broad categories. They are summarized next with remarks pertinent to the research agenda.

Leadership

Historically, high-impact medical institutions from high-income countries have developed a triad of research, teaching, and clinical care. The concentration of medical skills, scientific investigation, and a significant number of trainees has led to increased system productivity. Internationally, medical schools are often smaller with fewer faculty members and a limited research capacity. An engaged research community can strengthen these institutions; as discussed, pathology is a key component of research and quality care.

Advocacy

Specific to pathology, evidence of improved clinical outcome related to accurate diagnosis and careful patient laboratory monitoring is needed. Pathology and laboratory medicine are longstanding foundational elements of medical practice in the United States and Europe and many components predate rigorous cost-effectiveness analysis. The introduction of *best buy* medical interventions in developing countries as guided by the WHO and international funders requires more specific data on patient impact and cost-related epidemiologic measures, such as disability-adjusted life years.[28] Beyond documenting an economic case for current pathology practice, investigating pathways to streamline diagnoses and to measure the relationship between precision and efficiency are of interest to clinicians, public health practitioners, and policy makers in both high-resource settings as well as LMICs.

Training and Education

Producing more investigators and scientifically prepared clinicians is of immediate importance to pathologists. Research in optimizing workforce development is an area of applied research widely appreciated in the global health community. An important part of systems research is identifying efficiencies in task shifting, task sharing, and supporting optimal performance of practitioners who depend on data generated by pathologist and clinical laboratories.

Quality Assurance and Communication

Improving access to data both for research and clinical care is an area of interest in all settings, independent of income. Standardizing descriptive language, establishing interoperability of databases, and making information accessible to clinicians, investigators, and policy makers is a shared priority. Including performance improvement in data management at the level of laboratory information systems, clinical medical records, and surveillance systems, such as cancer registries, offers opportunities to demonstrate the key role of pathologists in collaborative endeavors.

Technology Development and Translation

The Affordable Cancer Technology program for LMICs[29] is the largest funded portfolio within the Center for Global Health, NCI. The point-of-care technologies, such as molecular diagnosis using lateral flow devices and rapid evolution of genomic precision medicine, are alluring areas for investigators hoping to bring new tools to address LMIC disease burden. The involvement of experienced pathologists in developing and implementing these tools in clinical practice is self-evident.

Experienced pathologists, especially those with field experience in lower-resource settings, also remind us "to look before you leapfrog" (Modupe Kuti, personal communications, 2015) because new technology can have unintended consequences and translation to new practice environments and new populations is often more challenging than predicted by the prototyping experience. Pathologists have an important role both as investigators and clinical practitioners in validating new technologies and judging their suitability to local practice needs. The combination of technical expertise and clinical judgment is paramount in guiding changes in practice; involvement in all phases of technology development and translation to human use is perhaps the greatest responsibility of a pathologist.

SUMMARY: PATHOLOGISTS AND THE PATH TO AN ERA OF ACCURATE DIAGNOSIS AND EVIDENCE BASED CARE IN LOW- AND MIDDLE-INCOME COUNTRIES

Pathologists have made great progress in educating investigators, clinicians, and patients on the importance of correct diagnosis and monitoring data. Given the complexity of modern research and care, the demand for accuracy will only increase. Pathologists are fundamentally positioned to contribute to basic biological knowledge, to increasing accurate and efficient diagnostics, to enhance cost-effective practice, and to shape health care policy. The opportunities found in the developing world should be regarded as new windows to formulate provocative questions and to address the burden of disease for all the world's population. Innovative research by pathologists can add to progress in global health by embedding accurate diagnosis and precise laboratory monitoring as a cornerstone of scientific research and practice.

REFERENCES

1. NCI Center for Global Health (CGH). National Cancer Institute. 2017. Available at: https://www.cancer.gov/about-nci/organization/cgh. Accessed June 13, 2017.
2. Comprehensive cancer information. National Cancer Institute. 2017. Available at: https://www.cancer.gov/. Accessed June 13, 2017.
3. National Institutes of Health (NIH). National Institutes of Health (NIH). 2017. Available at: https://www.nih.gov/. Accessed June 13, 2017.
4. Varmus H, Trimble EL. Integrating cancer control into global health. Sci Transl Med 2011;3(101):101cm128.
5. Mmbaga EJ, Deardorff KV, Mushi B, et al. Characteristics of esophageal cancer cases in Tanzania. Journal of Global Oncology 2017. [Epub ahead of print].
6. PAR-16-279: Fogarty HIV research training program for low-and middle-income country institutions (D43). National Institute of Health grants. 2017. Available at: https://grants.nih.gov/grants/guide/pa-files/PAR-16-279.html. Accessed June 13, 2017.
7. RFA-CA-15-1007: planning for regional centers of research excellence in non-communicable diseases in low and middle income countries (P20). National Institute of Health grants. 2017. Available at: https://grants.nih.gov/grants/guide/rfa-files/RFA-CA-15-007.html. Accessed June 13, 2017.
8. PAR-15-093: basic cancer research in cancer health disparities (R01). National Institute of Health grants. 2017. Available at: https://grants.nih.gov/grants/guide/pa-files/PAR-15-093.html. Accessed June 13, 2017.

9. RFA-CA-15-1001: cancer detection, diagnosis, and treatment technologies for global health (UH2/UH3). National Institute of Health grants. 2017. Available at: https://grants.nih.gov/grants/guide/rfa-files/RFA-CA-15-001.html. Accessed June 13, 2017.

10. PAR-16-238: dissemination and implementation research in health (R01). National Institute of Health grants. 2017. Available at: https://grants.nih.gov/grants/guide/pa-files/PAR-16-238.html. Accessed June 13, 2017.

11. Fogarty International Center. Fogarty International Center. 2017. Available at: http://www.fic.nih.gov. Accessed June 13, 2017.

12. MacLeod SM, Knoppert DC, Stanton-Jean M, et al. Pediatric clinical drug trials in low-income countries: key ethical issues. Paediatr Drugs 2015;17(1):83–90.

13. NCI grant activity codes/mechanisms. National Cancer Institute: Division of Extramural Affairs. 2017. Available at: https://deainfo.nci.nih.gov/flash/awards.htm#R01. Accessed June 13, 2017.

14. Laboratory of pathology | Center for Cancer Research. National Cancer Institute: Center for Cancer Research. 2017. Available at: https://ccr.cancer.gov/Laboratory-of-Pathology. Accessed June 13, 2017.

15. Koplan JP, Baggett RL. The Emory Global Health Institute: developing partnerships to improve health through research, training, and service. Acad Med 2008;83(2):128–33.

16. Dean L, Njelesani J, Smith H, et al. Promoting sustainable research partnerships: a mixed-method evaluation of a United Kingdom–Africa capacity strengthening award scheme. Health Res Policy Syst 2015;13:81.

17. Center for Translation Research and Implementation Science (CTRIS) - NHLBI, NIH. National Heart, Lung, and Blood Institute. 2017. Available at: http://www.nhlbi.nih.gov/about/org/ctris. Accessed June 13, 2017.

18. RFA-HL-17-1003: T4 Translation research capacity building initiative in low income countries (TREIN) (U24). National Institute of Health Grants. 2017. Available at: https://grants.nih.gov/grants/guide/rfa-files/RFA-HL-17-003.html. Accessed June 13, 2017.

19. PAR-17-095: Cancer Center Support Grants (CCSGs) for NCI-designated cancer centers (P30). National Institute of Health Grants. 2017. Available at: https://grants.nih.gov/grants/guide/pa-files/PAR-17-095.html. Accessed June 13, 2017.

20. Muir JA, Farley J, Osterman A, et al. Global health programs and partnerships: evidence of mutual benefit and equity. A report of the CSIS Global Health Policy Center. 2016. Available at: https://csis-prod.s3.amazonaws.com/s3fs-public/publication/160315_Muir_GlobalHealthPrograms_Web.pdf. Accessed June 6, 2017.

21. Hopkins J, Burns E, Eden T. International twinning partnerships: an effective method of improving diagnosis, treatment and care for children with cancer in low-middle income countries. J Cancer Policy 2013;1(1):e8–19.

22. Global health program for fellows and scholars - Fogarty International Center @ NIH. Fogarty International Center. 2017. Available at: https://www.fic.nih.gov/Programs/pages/scholars-fellows-global-health.aspx. Accessed June 13, 2017.

23. Asombang AW, Kayamba V, Mwanza-Lisulo M, et al. Gastric cancer in Zambian adults: a prospective case-control study that assessed dietary intake and antioxidant status by using urinary isoprostane excretion. Am J Clin Nutr 2013;97(5):1029–35.

24. Montgomery ND, Liomba NG, Kampani C, et al. Accurate real-time diagnosis of lymphoproliferative disorders in Malawi through clinicopathologic

teleconferences a model for pathology services in sub-Saharan Africa. Am J Clin Pathol 2016;146(4):423–30.

25. Fleming KA, Naidoo M, Wilson M, et al. An essential pathology package for low- and middle-income countries. Am J Clin Pathol 2017;147(1):15–32.

26. WHO list of priority medical devices for cancer management. Geneva (Switzerland): World Health Organization; 2017. Licence: CC BY-NC-SA 3.0 IGO.

27. Ellis DW, Srigley J. Does standardised structured reporting contribute to quality in diagnostic pathology? The importance of evidence-based datasets. Virchows Arch 2016;468(1):51–9.

28. Global Burden of Disease Cancer Collaboration. Global, regional, and national cancer incidence, mortality, years of life lost, years lived with disability, and disability-adjusted life-years for 32 cancer groups, 1990 to 2015: a systematic analysis for the global burden of disease study. JAMA Oncol 2017;3(4):524–48.

29. First cohort of ACTs enters second phase. National Cancer Institute. 2017. Available at: https://www.cancer.gov/about-nci/organization/cgh/blog/2017/acts-transition. Accessed June 14, 2017.

Training the Next Generation of African Pathologists

Ann Marie Nelson, MD[a,b,*], Martin Hale, MB ChB, FCPath (Anat) SA[c],
Mohenou Isidore Jean-Marie Diomande, MD, FWACP[d],
Quentin Eichbaum, MD, PhD, MPH, NNHC, JD[e],
Yawale Iliyasu, MBBS, MD, FMCPath(Nig), FICS, MIAC, IFCAP, FCPath(ECSA)[f],
Raphael M. Kalengayi, MD, MMedSC, SpPath, PhD[g],
Belson Rugwizangoga, MD, MMed(Path)[h], Shahin Sayed, MMed(Path)[i]

KEYWORDS

- Global health • Pathology • Training • Accreditation • Quality

KEY POINTS

- Access to and availability of health care depend on adequate, well-trained health care providers.
- The current state of pathology workforce and training faces challenges to recruitment and retention of staff, development of standards and credentialing, and reliable funding.
- The cost of training is paid by the trainee in several countries and, coupled with poor salaries, creates a significant barrier to recruitment and retention of good trainees.
- Government salaries are often inadequate, forcing trained physicians and technical staff to seek employment in the private sector or to emigrate to countries with better opportunities.

Continued

Disclosure Statement: The authors have nothing to disclose.
[a] Department of Pathology, Duke University School of Medicine, Durham, NC 27710, USA; [b] InPaLa Consulting, 1330 Floral Street NorthWest, Washington, DC 20012, USA; [c] Department of Anatomical Pathology, National Health Laboratory Service, University of the Witwatersrand, 7 York Road, Parktown, Johannesburg, 2193, South Africa; [d] UFR Sciences Médicales, Université Félix Houphouët-Boigny, 01 BP V166, Abidjan 01, Côte d'Ivoire; [e] Department of Pathology, Microbiology and Immunology, Vanderbilt University Medical Center, The Vanderbilt Clinic, 4511C, Nashville, TN 37232, USA; [f] Department of Pathology, College of Medical Sciences, Ahmadu Bello University, Samaru, Zaria, Kaduna State 810001, Nigeria; [g] Department of Pathology, University of Kinshasa, Kinshasa 11, Democratic Republic of Congo; [h] University of Rwanda School of Medicine and Pharmacy, Avenue d'Armee, PO Box 3286, Kigali, Rwanda; [i] Department of Pathology, Aga Khan University Hospital, 3rd Parklands Avenue, P.O.Box 30270, Post code 00100, Nairobi, Kenya
* Corresponding author. InPaLa Consulting, 1330 Floral Street NorthWest, Washington, DC 20012.
E-mail address: amnpath62@gmail.com

Clin Lab Med 38 (2018) 37–51
https://doi.org/10.1016/j.cll.2017.10.004
0272-2712/18/© 2017 Elsevier Inc. All rights reserved.

labmed.theclinics.com

Continued

- These case studies demonstrate features required for successful training: a reliable funding source, adequate numbers of qualified teachers, access to training material and procedures, and opportunities for meaningful work and advanced training.
- Creation of regional colleges of pathology holds the promise of more uniform training standards, the ability to share workforce between countries, and the ability to advocate for better funding and for national health plans that include pathology and laboratory diagnoses.

INTRODUCTION

Quality patient care should be the goal of health care systems at all levels and in all settings. Pathology and laboratory medicine have been the missing links in global health programs that have been developed and implemented over the past few decades. For example, disease and cause of death data based on clinical impression or verbal autopsies reflect the basic demographics of the population or the disease category, but may not recognize the actual condition, whether an infection or a noncommunicable disease.[1,2] The double burden of communicable and noncommunicable diseases makes histologic diagnosis and more complex clinical laboratory capability a priority. With the introduction of precise therapy, the need for a precise diagnosis is critical.

Although no clear guidance has been issued from international health organizations indicating the number of pathologists (anatomic and clinical) required per capita for adequate health care, the number in low- and middle-income countries (LMIC) is clearly insufficient. Because the current workforce is so overburdened, the quality of a pathologist's professional performance is likely to suffer. Exacerbating the staffing shortage is a concomitant scarcity of trained laboratory technologists, histotechnologists, and cytotechnologists.[3] Beyond insufficient personnel, pathologists in many developing countries have little or no access to current, relevant medical literature or to continuing education programs. In addition, infrastructural support is either lacking or poorly maintained, further contributing to poor professional performance.

In this article, the authors focus on African training activity (primarily anatomic pathology) with several case studies; address challenges; and discuss current efforts to create regional standards.

HISTORICAL PERSPECTIVES

Postgraduate training in pathology was formally established in South Africa by the South African Institute for Medical Research (SAIMR) in the late 1940s with a 3-year postgraduate fellowship in Clinical Pathology, later extended to 4 years. Many graduates of this program went on to become heads of departments of pathology at other universities in South Africa. Because of limited postgraduate training positions, several of these graduates pursued specialty training overseas in countries such as the United Kingdom; the Diploma in Clinical Pathology from the Hammersmith Hospital was a revered qualification.[4] Many of the illustrious names in the history of pathology in South Africa and Rhodesia (now Zimbabwe) obtained this qualification, going on to establish postgraduate training programs of their own, the fruits of which continue to this day.

With the passage of time, countries in Southern Africa established their own postgraduate qualifications and examining bodies. South Africa was the first of these, with the Colleges of Medicine of South Africa in 1954, the College of Pathologists being part of this structure. In addition, universities created the Master of Medicine (MMed) degree, with both the College fellowship and university degrees offering these in the individual disciplines of pathology. The MMed concept has extended to other universities in Botswana, Zimbabwe, Zambia, and East Africa.

The University College Ibadan, Nigeria commenced clinical teaching in October of 1957, the same year the Faculty of Medicine was formed and the University Teaching Hospital was opened. Professor G.M. Edington was named chairman of the Department of Pathology in 1960 and started training Nigerian pathologists, while Uganda started pathology training at Makerere University in 1960s.

The Catholic University of Lovanium in the Belgian Congo was founded in 1954, followed in 1956 by a Faculty of Medicine and a Hospital (Cliniques Universitaires de Léopolville) with the Department of Anatomical Pathology starting in 1959. After independence in 1960, the country became the Democratic Republic of Congo (DRC), and Leopoldville was renamed Kinshasa. In 1965, the University became known as the Lovanium University of Kinshasa (UNIKIN) and the Teaching Hospital, Cliniques Universitaires de Kinshasa.

In 1972, Lovanium University was nationalized and renamed the UNIKIN. Between 1968 and 1976, a Congolese medical doctor was sent to Belgium for pathology training and obtained his PhD. Professor R.M. Kalengayi returned to UNIKIN to establish a diagnostic service as well as undergraduate and postgraduate training in pathology.

APECSA (Association of Pathologists of East, Central, and Southern Africa) was established in November 1990 in order to improve communication with organizations interested in pathology education and to coordinate activities within the region. The Society was formed based on the recommendations of a survey on medical training conducted in 1985 by Professor M.S.R. Hutt. Professor Hutt and Professor Sebastian Lucas (UK) specifically looked at diagnostic and training capacity in pathology at medical schools within East Africa, including the number of histopathologists, clinical pathologists, and trained technical staff.[5,6] In order to update this information and reassess pathology capacity on the continent, some of the original APECSA members together with InPaLa, an international group of pathologists associated with the International Academy of Pathology, developed an on-line survey (see later discussion).

As described above, the medical education programs in Africa were established within public universities and hospitals. The same is true today. The challenge of poverty and emerging economic classes creates the need for a vast public health system, which includes pathology and laboratory services for those who cannot afford private health care. Most of the population in most countries in this region seeks care in public institutions. South Africa and Kenya have expanding numbers of private hospitals and medical specialists to accommodate the health care needs of those who can afford care. Many other countries have private laboratories, often in the capital or other major cities, that charge fee-for-service to both private and public practitioners because many university and public hospitals do not have access to equipment and reagents to perform diagnostic tests. Patients with adequate financial resources often travel to other countries for specialized diagnosis and care.

PATHOLOGY TRAINING IN SUB-SAHARAN AFRICA

Data on training are taken from the survey of pathology capacity in sub-Saharan Africa that was conducted between 2011 and 2014. The information requested included numbers of pathologists and technicians, training positions, workload and workflow, infrastructure, and availability of cancer care.[3,7] The data were organized by region (East, West, Southern, and Francophone Africa; **Box 1**). Missing information was gathered through the end of 2015 via extensive additional e-mails and one-on-one discussions with working pathologists and clinicians in Africa. Medical school data were obtained from the sub-Saharan Africa Medical Schools Study (SAMSS.org). Complete survey data with interactive details on pathology capacity in Africa can be found at the African Strategies for Advancing Pathology (ASAP)[8] Web site (pathogyinafrica.org).

Although there are currently pathology training programs in 25 countries (**Fig 1**), the rate of training is not sufficient for the needs of the regions. From conversations, it can be estimated that less than 1% of medical graduates opt for training in pathology, but there are no reliable data. Factors that hamper recruitment of trainees and retention of profession staff include poor salaries compared with other specialties, such as surgery and medicine; inadequate provision of laboratory facilities and supplies; and limited opportunities for continuing education. All these lead to lack of job satisfaction. The need to seek additional salary through the private sector further depletes the public workforce.[9]

Data Summary by Region

Southern Africa: 7 countries
South Africa accounts for nearly one-third of all pathologists in Africa with 285 anatomic pathologists and 75 trainees (Case Study 1). Zimbabwe has 5 pathologists and 2 trainees. Botswana employs 6 pathologists from other countries and currently has 5 national trainees; Namibia also uses a foreign work force of 5 pathologists. There are 3 pathologists in Madagascar, but none in Swaziland or Lesotho.

Francophone sub-Saharan Africa: 18 Countries
At the time of the survey, there were 83 pathologists in 15 countries. Since that time, Guinea and Benin have each added 2 pathologists on site. The DRC (Case Study 2) and Côte d'Ivoire (Case Study 3) have the most, but still fall significantly below 1 per million population. (Rwanda is the only country in the region that has improved the number of pathologists per million people, but now affiliates with Anglophone East Africa [Case Study 6]).

Eleven countries have a total of 53 pathologists in training in the region. In most programs, the cost is paid by the trainee. Chad sends residents to other African countries for training; Burundi had to cancel their program because of a lack of funds.

Lusophone Africa: 4 countries
Guinea Bissau and Cape Verde are included in the Francophone countries but have no public-sector pathologists. Angola has 12 pathologists and 4 trainees. Mozambique currently has 8 pathologists and 4 trainees.

Anglophone sub-Saharan West Africa: 5 countries
Nigeria has 150 pathologists and 20 training programs for Anatomic Pathology with greater than 200 trainees in 5-year programs that are paid for by the government (Case Study 4). Ghana has 30 pathologists (3 of whom are Nigerian) and 2 training programs with 5 trainees. Liberia, Sierra Leone, and Gambia had no pathologists at the time of the survey.

Anglophone East Africa: 9 countries
Seven countries have a total of 178 pathologists. Kenya has the most with 60 (25% in private practice). The University of Nairobi has greater than 20 trainees, including a few international participants from other countries in the region. Tuition is required, but the

Box 1
Countries of sub-Saharan Africa by region, as discussed in the survey

Francophone Africa

Benin
Burkina Faso
Burundi
Cape Verde
Cameroon
Chad
Côte d'Ivoire
Central African Republic
Democratic Republic of Congo
Gabon
Guinea
Guinea-Bissau
Mali
Mauritania
Niger
Senegal
Republic of Congo
Rwanda[a]
Togo

West Africa: Anglophone

Ghana
Nigeria
Gambia
Liberia
Sierra Leone

East Africa

Ethiopia
Kenya
Malawi
South Sudan
Tanzania
Uganda
Zambia

Southern Africa

Angola
Botswana
Lesotho
Madagascar
Mozambique
Namibia
South Africa
Swaziland
Zimbabwe

[a] Now associates with East Africa.

Pathology Trainees By Region

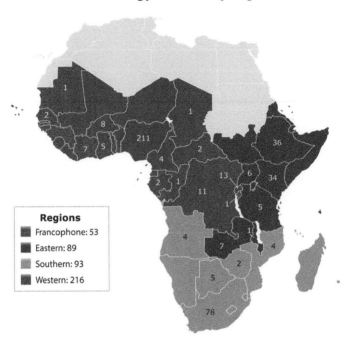

Fig. 1. Map of sub-Saharan Africa showing number of residents in countries of each region (data are from 2015 and differ from some information in the case studies). (*Data from* December 2015 based on African Strategies for Advancing Pathology Survey.)

Kenyan government pays for those employed by the Ministry of Health. Aga Khan now has a training program with 4 residents per year whose tuition is paid by the institution (Case Study 5).

Uganda lists 24 pathologists, but not all work in surgical pathology and some are working in other countries. They have 6 slots for training, but students must pay their own tuition, and trainees from other countries fill several of the positions. Tanzania has 22 pathologists with 5 trainees; Malawi, 9 pathologists and 1 trainee, and Zambia, 6 pathologists with 7 trainees. Ethiopia had only 1 pathologist in 1990, and now has 55 with 36 trainees. South Sudan did have 2 pathologists, but the health system functions poorly because of the civil war. The authors have no data on Djibouti or Somalia.

STRATEGIES AND RECOMMENDATIONS MOVING FORWARD

What approaches should be considered in expanding the pathology workforce? What are the essential factors required for success?

Case Studies

Five of the case reports detail training programs in each of the regions and were chosen to demonstrate successes and challenges in the training programs (Appendix 1). The first 4 are in large government medical schools and hospitals. South African medical education systems are the oldest and have well-developed standards of training and accreditation. DRC and Côte d'Ivoire were the first in Francophone Africa. Amado Bello in Nigeria was created in order to expand medical care and training to northern

Nigeria. Unlike the first 4, Aga Khan is a private health and hospital system that developed postgraduate training to fill clinical needs and is adding a medical school. Each of these programs serves as a source of trained pathologists for the rest of the country as well as the region.

The final case study for Rwanda is included to describe what is required to start, de novo, a pathology training program and to demonstrate challenges to building and sustaining a quality education that is an integral part of a functional health system.

Challenges for Medical Training in Low-Resource Settings of Africa

Regional harmonization of curricula and certification

Medical education in low-resource settings faces unique challenges but also presents specific opportunities. The landmark *Lancet* report of 2010 on "Health Professionals for a New Century" by Frenk and colleagues[10] emphasized the importance of linking health education curricula to local health needs and contexts.

The approach to pathology education is arduous given the continent's severe shortages of qualified pathology professionals and education facilities, the establishment of Economic Community of West African States (ECOWAS), College of Pathology of East, Central, and Southern Africa (COPECSA), and the South African pathology standards, as well as the efforts toward stepwise accreditation for pathology laboratories are highly laudable moves in the right direction, and the efforts of these bodies should be strongly supported. Development of local standards of assessment and accreditation is important for sustainability of pathology education on the continent and ultimately serves the interests of faculty recruitment and retention. The brain drain of pathology professionals, not only to HICs but also to the private sector within African countries, detracts from the much-needed educational efforts for training and capacity building of pathologists on the continent. This issue clearly requires urgent attention.

Finally, because pathology as a discipline asks fundamental questions pertaining to the scientific basis of disease, the issue arises of how much support should be given to research. Students drawn to pathology are curious about pathogenesis and may wish to undertake research. If resources were not limited, the answer to this question would be a simple "yes." However, in settings of limited resources providing such opportunities presents a nettlesome dilemma because it may both enhance faculty retention in academic pathology departments and also siphon away financial resources needed for education and training of increased numbers of diagnostic anatomic and clinical pathologists. Any research partnerships should include agreements to avoid this problem.

National and regional collaboration on requirements is necessary to assure a more uniform content and quality of education and to assess competence of trainees. South Africa developed training and accreditation standards more than 50 years ago. The ECOWAS recently developed and came to a consensus on a harmonized curriculum. The COPECSA has formulated a curriculum that will soon be approved (Appendix 2)

Quality assurance and the role of technical staff

Pathology and laboratory medicine are disciplines that require reliable and reproducible results. Specimen handling from procurement to fixation, processing, and staining/testing must meet standards to assure accurate interpretation, making it essential to have qualified, trained personnel in the laboratories. It is critical that full cognizance is given to meeting accepted accreditation standards, be it in the teaching and training environment or in the clinical practice setting.

Further data

Additional data are needed to formulate guidelines on establishing or modifying pathology training programs, to determine what is required for sustainability, and to monitor and evaluate impact. The American Society for Clinical Pathology (ASCP) is working on an updated survey by country and by individual institutions that will provide greater detail on current staffing and training as well as national strategies, funding, partners, and other factors related to training outcomes. It is important that the data are kept as current as possible in order to reflect improvement and identify areas of need.

SUMMARY

The ever-increasing demands of medical care, brought about by population growth, complexity and depth of medical investigation, the looming era of personalized medicine, and therapy require fully functional, integrated pathology that is not an add-on to health care but stands at the center of the health care delivery process.[11,12]

Although this may be seen as an impossible task, with the right approach, departments of pathology can be rebuilt, but requires strong, focused leadership from within the specialty accompanied by financial and institutional support for a sustained period of time. As these departments grow, develop critical mass, and become self-sustaining, they can be used to extend and support other training platforms, either by using a "hub-and-spoke" concept or by setting up "twinning program", whichever is most suitable. Unfortunately, all too often, support begins to wane as administrators seek to control budgets; soft targets such as teaching platforms, particularly successful ones, are the first to feel the squeeze, and it is only a matter of time before the impetus is lost. External partnerships provide valuable transfer of knowledge and technology, subspecialty training, and mentoring, but these are short- to mid-term solutions.[2]

Pathology is accustomed to some degree of relegation the world over, but this is exacerbated in LMIC. If this hard-won pathology education is to be used to the fullest, it is essential that there is political buy-in accompanied by local ownership and support so that health care can be delivered to those who desperately need it. The evidence presented in this article suggests that the tide may be turning, and the ripples of change need to be supported by the international community to turn this into a tsunami.

ACKNOWLEDGMENTS

Drs Ephata Kaaya, Zahir Moloo, and Robert Lukande and Ms Diane Sterchi provided information on training. Mr Jack Chirieleison created the graphics.

REFERENCES

1. Fligner CL, Murray J, Roberts DJ. Synergism of verbal autopsy and diagnostic pathology autopsy for improved accuracy of mortality data. Popul Health Metr 2011;9:25.
2. Carlson JW, Lyon E, Walton D, et al. Partners in pathology: a collaborative model to bring pathology to resource poor settings. Am J Surg Pathol 2010;34:118–23.
3. Nelson AM, Milner DA, Rebbeck TR, et al. Africa: pathology in the sub-Sahara. In: Boyle P, Ngoma T, Sullivan R, et al, editors. The state of oncology in Africa 2015. Lyon (France): iPRI Scientific Publication; 2016.
4. Mills A. A pathologist remembers. Memories of childhood and later life. Bloomington (IN): AuthorHouse UK Ltd; 2013. 1663 Liberty Drive.

5. Hutt MS, Spencer H. Histopathology services for developing countries. Br Med J 1982;285:1327.
6. Lucas SB. Report on pathology in sub-Saharan Africa. Inaugural Meeting of Association of Pathologists of East, Central and Southern Africa (APECSA). Dar es Salaam 1990 (includes data from study by Prof MRS Hutt).
7. Nelson AM, Milner DA, Rebbeck TR, et al. Oncologic care and pathology resources in Africa: survey and recommendations. J Clin Oncol 2016;34:20–6.
8. African Strategies for Advancing Pathology Group Members. Quality pathology and laboratory diagnostic services are key to improving global health outcomes. Am J Clin Pathol 2015;143:325–8.
9. Kaschula ROC. The practice of pathology in Africa. Arch Pathol Lab Med 2013; 137:752–5.
10. Frenk J, Chen L, Bhutta ZA, et al. Health professionals for a new century: transforming education to strengthen health systems in an interdependent world. Lancet 2010;376(9756):1923–58.
11. Robboy SJ, Weintraub S, Horvath AE, et al. Pathologist workforce in the United States: I. Development of a predictive model to examine factors influencing supply. Arch Pathol Lab Med 2013;137:1723–32.
12. Bainbridge S, Cake R, Meredith M, et al. Testing times to come: an evaluation of pathology capacity across the UK. Report of Cancer Research UK. 2016. Available at: https://www.cancerresearchuk.org/sites/.../testing_times_to_come_nov_16_cruk.pdf. Accessed June 7, 2017.
13. Available at: http://www.health.uct.ac.za/fhs/about/history. Accessed June 4, 2017.
14. Marais Malan. In quest of health: the South African institute for medical research 1912-1973. Johannesburg (South Africa): Lowry Publishers; 1988.
15. Available at: http://isystems.hpcsa.co.za/iregister/RegisterSearch.aspx. Accessed June 7, 2017.
16. Available at: http://cs2016.statssa.gov.za/. Accessed June 7, 2017.
17. Available at: http://www.gov.za/ABOUT-SA/HEALTH#sefako. Accessed June 7, 2017.

APPENDIX 1: CASE STUDIES OF CURRENT TRAINING MODELS
Case Study 1: South Africa by Martin Hale

In order to gain specialist registration with the Health Professions Council of South Africa (HPCSA), a 4-year training period in one of the pathology disciplines at an accredited institution is required, terminating with a single exit examination in the discipline concerned convened by the College of Pathologists. Often the training period is extended, particularly in Anatomical Pathology consequent to its extensive knowledge base, with most trainees writing the specialist examination after 5 years.

Medical education in Southern Africa had its beginnings with the establishment of medical schools in the region, the first at the University of Cape Town, the faculty being established in 1912.[13] This was followed soon after by the establishment of the SAIMR, also in 1912. The SAIMR was from its early days closely associated with, and indeed played an instrumental role in, establishing a medical school within the University College, later to become the University of the Witwatersrand.[14] This close association continues to the present day, paving the way for the creation of the concept of joint posts between the SAIMR and the University of the Witwatersrand, with the School of Pathology being formalized between the 2 institutions in 1970. This allowed full integration of the teaching, research, and service responsibilities. Although this arrangement at times creates elements of disagreement and friction between the parties concerned, there is no doubt that it is on the whole beneficial to all and is a model that should be considered for implementation in other LMICs, bringing with it economies and efficiencies not seen with divided models.

The training of anatomic pathologists in South Africa is a joint responsibility of the universities and the National Health Laboratory Service, the universities comprising Sefako Makgatho University of Health Sciences, University of Pretoria, University of the Witwatersrand, University of KwaZulu-Natal, University of the Free State, Walter Sisulu University, Stellenbosch University, and the University of Cape Town. Training includes the full spectrum of anatomic pathology inclusive of immunohistochemistry, electron microscopy, and molecular pathology. Currently, there are 114 registrar posts recognized by the HPCSA, with only 75 occupied, a situation that requires immediate attention. Indeed, the number of funded registrar posts needs to be significantly increased over and above these to meet existing and future health care needs.

In common with the rest of the world, there is an acute shortage of anatomic pathologists practicing in South Africa, with the number registered being 285, although review shows that this includes retired professionals and those practicing outside the country, between them, probably accounting for approximately 50 to 100 of these.[15]

The current population of South Africa is 55.6 million, of which 8.8 million have private health insurance.[16,17] Compounding the limited number of anatomic pathologists is the knowledge that the majority by far are in the private sector serving approximately 8.8 million lives, with approximately 50 anatomic pathologists in the public sector providing care to 80% of the population (44.5 million). This results in ratios of pathologists to the population cared for in the public sector that are very similar to countries in East Africa.[9]

Case Study 2: Democratic Republic of the Congo by Rafael Kalengayi

Since 1976, 27 pathologists have been trained with 8 attaining a PhD in the DRC or abroad; 5 of the 8 are practicing and teaching pathology in the DRC. Of the remaining 22, 13 are practicing in-country and 6 are scattered across the world (United States, Europe, Japan, and sub-Saharan Africa).

Currently, there are 12 laboratories in the DRC, with 8 of these in Kinshasa and one each in Kimpese, Lubumbashi, Bukavu, and Goma staffed by 8, 2, 3, 2, and 1 pathologists, respectively. Postgraduate training takes place in 2 sites, Kinshasa and Lubumbashi, the former currently having 20 residents (the number has increased since 2014).

Case Study 3: Cote d'Ivoire by Isidore Diomande

The Faculty of Medicine of Abidjan, created in 1966, is part of the University Felix Houphouet-Boigny of Cocody-Abidjan. It has 3 teaching hospitals, 2 of which have Anatomic and Clinical Pathology (Cocody and Treichville). Cocody has a workload of 4000 specimens per year (2/3 Anatomical Pathology [AP], 1/3 Clinical Pathology [CP]), while Treichville receives 5000 to 6000 specimens (2/3 AP, 1/3 CP). Cocody Hospital has 4 pathologists and 5 histotechnicians; Treichville Hospital has 5 pathologists and 2 histotechnicians. Automated immunohistochemistry has been available since 2013, consequent to a partnership between Roche Laboratory and the Ivorian Government to support the diagnosis and treatment of breast cancer, the predominant cancer in women. Mammography, including core breast biopsies, Her2, ER, and PR testing, are routinely used; Roche subsidizes the cost of chemotherapy.

Teaching in anatomic pathology started in 1970 with Professor Robert Loubière from France, seconded by 2 Ivorian assistants (Prof E. Marcel and the late Prof D. Akribi) and 2 French assistants. Since 1980, the training staff is exclusively composed of Ivorians. The specialty training program started in 1991 with trainees from Cote d'Ivoire, Burkina Faso, Mali, Congo Brazzaville, Central Africa Republic, Mauritania, Senegal, Togo, and Chad. To date, 22 pathologists have been trained. Foreign pathologists have returned to their countries, and Ivorians are practicing in Abidjan and Bouake.

The training program encompasses 4 years and includes a limited rotation and a research component for the preparation of a dissertation. Ivorian trainees are charged an annual tuition fee of 1150 USD while their international counterparts pay 1700 USD per annum.

Case Study 4: Nigeria by Yawale Ilyasu

Ahmadu Bello University (A.B.U.), located in Zaria and the first university in North Western Nigeria, was founded in 1962. It has 2 campuses, the Samaru main campus, which includes the Faculty of Medicine among others, and the Congo campus, which hosts the faculties of Administration and Law. The Faculty of Medicine has a large medical program with its own teaching hospital, the A.B.U. Teaching Hospital (ABUTH, Zaria), one of the largest hospitals in Nigeria and Africa.

The Department of Pathology (Morbid Anatomy/Anatomic Pathology) was established in 1972 and is the pioneer department of the other 3 clinical pathology departments in A.B.U./ABUTH, Zaria. The department has a dual role of training and clinical laboratory diagnostic services carried out by 13 pathologists, 9 resident pathologists, laboratory technicians, and the secretarial staff. The other 3 clinical pathology departments have 23 fellows, including 11 hematologists, 7 medical microbiologists, and 5 chemical pathologists and several laboratory technicians and secretarial staff.

The department's academic programs, in addition to residency training in Pathology, which began in 1979, include training of medical students of A.B.U. and other undergraduate students of Pharmacy and Nursing Sciences and postgraduate master and doctorate degrees in Pathology (Clinical Laboratory Management).

Annually, the department processes and reports on 3500 histopathologic specimens, 2000 cytopathologic slides, performs variable numbers of postmortem examinations, and hosts clinicopathologic meetings with the surgeons. Residents in pathology rotate to each pathology department for a period of 3 months. In addition, those in anatomic pathology undertake an additional 6 months doing autopsy pathology in centers such as Ibadan, Oyo State, and Lagos, in the southern part of the country, where there is better exposure.

In the last 5 years, the Department of Anatomic Pathology has produced 14 fellows of both the National Postgraduate Medical College of Nigeria and the West African College of Physicians: 4 were retained, 2 are post–fellowship residents, 4 are in other teaching hospitals, 3 are in various federal medical centers, and 1 is in a specialist hospital. The clinical pathology departments produced 22 fellows in the same period: 10 in hematology and blood transfusion, 7 in medical microbiology, and 5 in chemical pathology.

Case Study 5: Aga Khan, Kenya by Shahin Sayed

The Aga Khan University (AKU) is an international university, which was chartered in Pakistan in 1983. In East Africa, AKU comprises the School of Nursing, the Medical College, the University Hospital, and an Institute of Educational Development. The University (East Africa) has been offering Masters Programs in Internal Medicine, Surgery, Diagnostic Radiology, Pediatrics, Anesthesia, Anatomical Pathology, and Clinical Pathology since 2006. All programs are approved by the Commission for Higher Education and the Medical Practitioners and Dentists Board of Kenya. The undergraduate program in Medicine and Surgery will begin in 2020.

There is an acute shortage of medical specialists and subspecialists within the East African region and especially in pathology. The AP and the CP programs at AKU were established in response to national and regional priorities, there being only one other training program in Pathology (AP/CP combined) offered by the University of Nairobi.

The programs in AP and CP are each 4 years in duration. Currently, there are 8 residents in each program (2 per year); however, there is an allowance for supernumerary positions (one in CP and one in AP). A total of 7 full-time faculty in AP and 8 full-time subspecialty faculty in CP oversee the program. In addition, a part-time faculty is in charge of the forensic pathology teaching. The eligibility criteria for residency include an undergraduate degree in Medicine recognized by the Kenya Medical and Dentist's Board of Kenya and the passing of a vigorous residency interview process at AKU.

Since the inception in 2006, there have been 15 AP and 13 CP graduates from the program, all of whom have been absorbed within Kenya and Tanzania. Three of the former residents have undergone further subspecialty training (Pediatric Pathology at the University of Cape Town, Molecular Pathology at Glasgow University, and Renal Pathology at the University of Toronto). In addition, 2 of the alumni (currently faculty in the Department of Pathology and Laboratory Medicine at AKU, Nairobi) have recently enrolled in a PhD program at the University of Stellenbosch in Cape Town, South Africa.

Residents in AP are exposed to more than 20,000 surgical cases annually and 15,000 gynecologic and nongynecologic cytology cases. There is a well-established automated immunohistochemistry platform offering a broad panel of antibodies. The Clinical Pathology section of the laboratory provides a repertoire of 800 tests and runs 3.2 million analyses per year, providing ample opportunities for hands-on experience. Transfusion medicine uses gel technology and a platelet apheresis program. Molecular pathology investigations are available for infectious diseases together with BCR-ABL for chronic myelogenous leukemia.

A research component and the completion of a MMed thesis form part of the eligibility criteria for the final-year examinations. At the end of 4 years and successfully meeting the eligibility criteria, residents sit University qualifying examinations for the MMed in Anatomic Pathology and MMed in Clinical Pathology, respectively.

Case Study 6: Establishing a Pathology Residency in Rwanda by Belson Rugwizangogo

The Republic of Rwanda's Vision 2050 and the Sustainable Developments Goals highlight the importance of high-quality health care services, qualified and skilled staff across the health system, and access including histologic diagnosis by an anatomic pathologist, universally considered the gold standard, to guide further therapeutic options in many diseases, but especially cancer.

To support this, the Government of Rwanda approved the MMed in Anatomic Pathology at the University of Rwanda College of Medicine and Health Sciences (UR/CMHS) School of Medicine, starting in the academic year 2013/2014. Before this, the 3 pathologists chosen to set up and coordinate the training were sent for residency in Tanzania, Kenya, and China.

The MMed Anatomic Pathology residency is a 4-year program enthusiastically welcomed by the partners in the health system and oversubscribed for the posts available. The residents receive stipends and tuition fees from the Ministry of Health of Rwanda. **Table A1** shows the number of the residents enrolled in this program since its launch in October 2013.

Table A1
Enrollment of residents in the Master of Medicine anatomic pathology program

Academic Year	Number of Residents		
	Men	Women	Totals
2013–2014	5	1	6
2014–2015	2	1	3
2015–2016	3[a]	1	4[a]
2016–2017	2	2	4
Total	10[a]	5	17[a]

[a] Two enrolled residents have suspended the studies for personal concerns; therefore, the current number of residents is 15.

A training program is well designed with an objective assessment of knowledge and skills, and consequently, some trainees may be required to repeat a year (**Table A2**), with the first group graduating in 2017.

Table A2
Residents in the Master of Medicine anatomic pathology program, academic year 2016-2017

Class	Number of Residents		
	Men	Women	Totals
I	2	2	4
II	1	1	2
III	3	1	4
IV	4	1	5
Total	10	5	15

Initially, the University of Rwanda relied on visiting lecturers working for other institutions in Rwanda and faculty from partner institutions abroad to deliver the curriculum. Participating partner institutions include US Institutions (USI) through the Partners in Health (PIH), ASCP, and the Human Resources for Health[2] to provide superspecialists to teach different courses in the different modules, whereas other contents are covered by local UR/CMHS staff, visiting staff, and staff of the hospitals in which the pathology residents rotate.

The current (2017) contribution of the USI faculty is estimated to be 96 credits of the 240 credits in the program (40.0%). Year 3 residents are required to undertake rotations (observership) in Molecular Pathology/Diagnostics Laboratories abroad, because this is not available in the East-African Region. These rotations are performed in the USI.

The future of Pathology Services in Rwanda depends on the sustainable development of the Pathology Residency in the country producing highly skilled and knowledgeable graduates that are retained in the system.

Career development plans for existing and prospective teaching staff are being developed in partnership with PIH and ASCP, for Anatomic Pathologists, Clinical Pathologists, Laboratory Scientists, and the residents, focusing on mentorship, research, teaching, and clinical service with the aim to build a Pathology residency program that will serve as a center of excellence in the East and Central African Region. The graduates will be deployed to different hospitals and teaching institutions in Rwanda by a joint committee of the Ministry of Health and the University of Rwanda. The objective of this career development plan is to have, within the next 7 years, well-trained staff that owns the Pathology Residency Program in Rwanda in all aspects of its mission. The expectation is to have by 2024: 24 medical staff with professional fellowships in various Pathology subspecializations (including 4 postdoctoral fellowships), 9 PhDs, and 41 laboratory scientists. This process has already started with one pathologist already pursuing a Fellowship in Nephropathology in Boston, Massachusetts.

APPENDIX 2

ECOWAS (Francophone, Anglophone, and Lusophone Countries of West Africa)

In 2003, the ECOWAS authorized free circulation and installation of medical specialists throughout the region, which created a heightened need to ensure a uniform level of skills across health care sectors. The harmonization process began under the supervision of the West African Health Organization (WAHO), with the creation of an Experts Committee (EC), composed of the directors of all medical specialized training programs. In addition, a Steering Committee (SC) was created that consisted of the deans of the medical schools, the representatives of the anglophone colleges (West African College of Surgeons, West African College of Physicians, National Postgraduate Medical College of Nigeria, and Ghana College of Physicians and Surgeons), the universities and other higher education institutions in the region, and a representative of the African and Malagasy Council for Higher Education. Workshops were organized to facilitate the harmonization of programs in both francophone and anglophone countries, and the recommendations made by the EC were subsequently validated by the SC. Consensus has been achieved on denomination of the qualification, duration of study, faculty required, academic governance, admission criteria, curricula, teaching methods, and infrastructure.

Although there are certainly disadvantages to the process, the harmonization of training programs is the most effective method of regional integration. Harmonizing training programs has facilitated recognition of diplomas throughout the ECOWAS region and has led to the free circulation and exchange of medical professionals, trainees, and trainers in the ECOWAS region.

Obstacles had to be overcome. These obstacles included language (French, English, and Portuguese are spoken in the ECOWAS region); faculties were requested to teach the different languages in their programs. WAHO supervised this process and continues sponsoring the exchange of language specialists for 1 to 3 months in the region. Second, for some, harmonizing training programs proved to be financially prohibitive ($300,000). The process is also lengthy, and to date, only Burkina Faso has created a Diploma of Specialized Study in ACP. Accreditation of programs and institutions is overseen by the Regional Council for Education and Training of Health Professionals created by the Council of Ministers of Health.

College of Pathologists of East, Central, and Southern Africa

Established in 2010 at the APECSA meeting in Kampala, Uganda, the COPECSA was formed to develop leadership and promote regional excellence in the practice of pathology and to be responsible for maintaining standards through training, examinations, and professional development. Currently, COPECSA has a representation of 120 pathologists across Africa, specifically, Burundi, Eritrea, Ethiopia, Kenya, Malawi, Mauritius, Nigeria, Republic of South Africa, Rwanda, Republic of Tanzania, The Seychelles, Uganda, Zambia, and Zimbabwe.

One of the strategic goals of the College is to harmonize pathology training in member countries. A comprehensive curriculum in Anatomical Pathology, General

Pathology, and Clinical Pathology has been developed to serve as a regional guide. Through its various partnerships, COPECSA has been engaged in several training projects. The College partnered with the Royal College of Pathologists (UK), The British Division of the International Academy of Pathology, Aga Khan University Hospital Nairobi, Stellenbosch University, and the East Central and Southern Africa (ECSA) Health Community on the *Lab Skills Africa* program. This program was designed to improve the quality of pathology and laboratory medicine across 20 laboratories in Kenya, Uganda, Tanzania, Zambia, and Zimbabwe using integrated skills training, knowledge transfer, leadership development, and mentoring; it served a combined population of 110 million people with 1.7 million tests (HIV, rapid malaria, peripheral blood film, hemoglobin/hematocrit estimation, urinalysis, and tuberculosis) and provided training and mentoring to 100 pathologists, biomedical scientists, laboratory technologists, and technicians.

In 2016, COPECSA, in partnership with the University of Colorado Cancer Center and ASAP, was the recipient of a National Cancer Institute PAR 15-155 initiative, which evaluated the best approaches to training anatomic pathologists and senior residents in ECSA. This program engaged 17 pathology departments and trained 52 pathologists and senior residents in institutions from Zimbabwe, Kenya, Uganda, Tanzania, Zambia, Rwanda, Burundi, Malawi, Madagascar, Mozambique, and Botswana.

In partnership with the International Academy of Cytology, a total of 27 practicing pathologists from the region trained in image-guided fine-needle aspiration biopsy during a tutorial in Nairobi.

From Access to Collaboration

Four African Pathologists Profile Their Use of the Internet and Social Media

Julia Royall, BA, MA[a],*,
Micongwe Moses Isyagi, BDS, MMed, FCPath(ECSA)[b],
Yawale Iliyasu, MBBS, MD, FMCPath(Nig), FICS, MIAC, IFCAP, FCPath(ECSA)[c],
Robert Lukande, MBChB, MMed, FCPath(ECSA)[d],
Edda Vuhahula, DDS, PhD, FCPath[e]

KEYWORDS

- Internet • Social media • Telepathology • Pathology • Africa

KEY POINTS

- African pathologists use the Internet and social media in sub-Saharan Africa to communicate and collaborate with colleagues in the region and globally; to update knowledge and for continuing professional development; and to have positive effect on health, quality assurance, and safety because they can easily seek second opinions and share cases.
- The challenges include the cost of Internet service to individuals and institutions, fluctuations and unreliability of power, and lack of access to reliable sources of vetted information.
- Understanding and aiding colleagues in their technical constraints is to the benefit of pathologists globally.

Something new is happening on our planet. It is true that technological progress in modern times has linked people together like a complex nervous system. The means of travel are numerous and the communication is instantaneous. We are joined together like cells of a single body. But this body, as yet, has no soul.
Antoine de Saint-Exupery, 1939-1944 in Wartime Writings

Disclosure: All authors declare no relationship to any commercial company with direct financial interest in the subject matter or materials discussed in the article or with a company making a competing product.
[a] Office of International Programs, US National Library of Medicine, National Institutes of Health, 6361 Highway 26, Dubois, WY 82513, USA; [b] Legacy Specialty Clinics, 134, KK 3 Road, Kigali, Rwanda; [c] Department of Pathology, Faculty of Medicine, Ahmadu Bello University, Zaria, Kaduna State, Nigeria; [d] Department of Pathology, College of Health Sciences, Makerere University, Mulago Hill Road, Room B24 Pathology Building, Kampala, Uganda; [e] Department of Pathology, Muhimbili University of Health and Allied Sciences (MUHAS), Dar es Salaam, Tanzania
* Corresponding author.
E-mail address: julia.royall@gmail.com

INTRODUCTION

In the early 1990s, the nascent Internet was enhanced by the World Wide Web to become a critical tool for scientific research and collaboration around the world. This tool was just as important in sub-Saharan Africa (SSA) as anywhere else, and perhaps even more so. In SSA, outside organizations initiated efforts to leapfrog aging telephone systems of copper wire directly into the invisible digital world, all in the service of health and medicine.

A small non-governmental organization called SatelLife pioneered HealthNet in SSA in 1990.[1] HealthNet comprised a single satellite, no larger than a stack of medical journals, ground stations that featured a ham radio connected to a computer via a terminal node controller, and send-and-receive antennae. In this rudimentary system, messages in ASCI (American Standard Code for Information Interchange) text were picked up and delivered via a low earth orbit satellite. One pathology image could easily have consumed nearly all available space, because the satellite carried only 16 MB.

From this modest beginning, telecommunications rapidly developed on the African continent from 1990 to the present with users across SSA quickly adopting digital communications solutions. They have used cellular and smartphone technologies to overcome the connection challenges of landlines and replaced them with a digital web of communication access.[2] In doing so, they have greatly expanded the communication network on the continent. In addition, African research sites have been able to experiment with bandwidth strong enough to support African researchers as they joined their colleagues in the international scientific community.[2]

In SSA there is approximately 1 pathologist for every 10 million people. Pathologists are not evenly distributed on the continent, as shown in **Fig. 1**, which provides an overview of where pathology resources are needed most and where there is an oversupply.[3] As elsewhere in the world, pathologists tend to be concentrated in major urban centers close to large teaching institutions where professional and career growth opportunities exist.[4]

In SSA, under ordinary circumstances, the turnaround time for receiving anatomic pathology results can be from 3 days to 12 months using ordinary mail. Access to the Internet, and importantly to social media, has changed this in some locations. The pooling of diagnostic resources and personnel has begun to improve the scope and quality of pathology services. It is now possible for pathologists to share clinical, cytologic, and histologic images for diagnoses and second opinions quickly and easily. Access to the Internet enables lone pathologists to practice with confidence because they can easily consult with colleagues. High-end techniques in pathology do exist in SSA but they are out of reach in many locations. However, using simple staining techniques and cheap digital images transmitted over the Internet, waiting times for biopsy diagnosis can be greatly reduced in low-resource settings.

New electronic tools have now been introduced at every level of health care and research in Africa. Some have proved useful and cost-effective, especially those supported by African ingenuity and buy-in. Some others, as everywhere else, have tended toward unsustainable gadgetry.

Pathologists have joined their colleagues in the conversation about the use of the Internet, but the particular image-based needs (for transmission and sharing) of anatomic pathologists, combined with their scarcity as a profession in SSA, have presented special challenges vis a vis infrastructure. Nonanatomic pathology laboratory data can be transmitted easily because the quantity of data is small; thus, even with a minimum of Internet access, clinical laboratory results (microbiology, chemistry, hematology, and transfusion medicine) can be transmitted in a timely fashion. Online

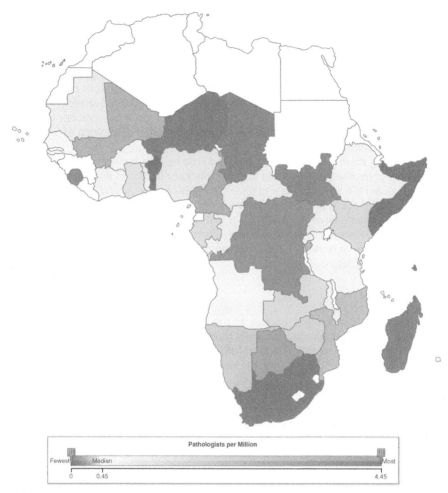

Fig. 1. Distribution of pathologists in SSA. (*From* Number of pathologists per million population in Africa. Available at: http://maptest.pathologyinafrica.org/resources/surveydata/maps/maps/map.php?type=n_path%7Cmin-max%7C1%7C1%7C1%7CNumber+of+pathologists+per+million+population. Accessed May 16, 2017.)

health-related networks outside of anatomic pathology share and transmit non–anatomic pathology laboratory information easily because the preimage processing needs are a lot less than for anatomic pathology, making telepathology a more appropriate technology for the practice of cytopathology and hematopathology.

The use of information technology and social media by African pathologists in support of better diagnoses is a story best told by the pathologists themselves. This article discusses 4 African pathologists and presents their voices as they talk about their work, their use of Internet and Web-based tools, and how they cope with the challenges of adopting these remarkable new opportunities in their unique situations. African countries are among the last to receive complete Internet access, and the access challenges described by the pathologists in this article are similar to those in rural areas and other low-income and middle-income countries (LMICs) around the world.

The pathologists interviewed for this article are members of African Strategies for Advancing Pathology (ASAP) (www.pathologyinafrica.org), which includes individuals from SSA, the United States, the United Kingdom, and Europe. All members have experience working in Africa, and have expertise and interest in histopathology, cyto-pathology, medical microbiology, hematology and hematopathology, infectious disease pathology, information management, public health advocacy, public health policy, health systems, laboratory management, and process improvement. Although those interviewed are in anatomic pathology/histopathology, they consider that their experiences also are relevant to and can be applied in other disciplines of pathology and laboratory medicine.

The pathologists in this article comment in response to a survey that queried each on their use of Internet/social media in their laboratory practices and communication with colleagues, the advantages and disadvantages of Internet and social media use and examples of each, and challenges they encounter in their daily practices. Each was asked for examples of how their use of Internet and social media made a quantifiable difference in laboratory outcomes and patient treatment. They also spoke to cost and power issues. In addition, each was encouraged to imagine and describe their laboratories of the future.

YAWALE ILIYASU

Yawale Iliyasu is Associate Professor in the Department of Pathology at his alma mater, Ahmadu Bello University Faculty of Medicine in Nigeria. He is a fellow of the National Postgraduate Medical College of Nigeria in Pathology, International College of Surgeons (Surgical Pathology), International Academy of Cytology, and is an International Fellow of the College of American Pathologists. Dr Iliyasu was the first pathologist produced by Nigeria's medical corps; previously the pathologists serving the country's military were from India and Pakistan. He served as a medical officer in the Nigerian Army for 29 years, and was the Chief Consultant Histopathologist of the Nigerian Army from 1994 to 2010. He was a founder of the College of Pathologists of East, Central, and Southern Africa (COPECSA) and a member of the Sub-Saharan Lymphoma Consortium. His areas of interest are lymphomas and colorectal carcinogenesis.

Yawale Iliyasu: Every week, as President of the West African Division of the International Academy of Pathology, I use the Internet to send pathology review articles to our members across the West African subregion. In addition, we have online access to the *Archives of Pathology & Laboratory Medicine* and 7 other journals, courtesy of Friends of Africa, a US and Canadian Academy of Pathology (USCAP) initiative. These journals are sent to more than 70 institutions in SSA. They are downloaded on CDs and stored in the departmental library; the CDs serve as backup when the journals cannot be reviewed online because of poor Internet connectivity.

We first used the Internet for e-mails, to write to colleagues, send articles, consult with colleagues in other hospitals, and send histology reports, sometimes saving us 4 or 5 hours of driving.

Social Media for Interaction and Collaboration

GoToMeeting

GoToMeeting (GTM) [https://www.gotomeeting.com] is used to send slides and get second opinions from our international collaborators. We bring in other local pathologists for dermatopathology, making sure individual pathologists have installed the free

GTM software and are used to it. Using GTM, we can discuss cases among ourselves and receive immediate feedback.

Skype

We use Skype for question-and-answer sessions with our colleagues in the United Kingdom who visit us in person twice a year. We also discuss specific cases using Skype.

WhatsApp

We use WhatsApp, a free messaging app available for Android and other smartphones. With Yahoo's Histopathology Service [https://histologistics.com/tag/yahoo/] we reach all the pathologists in West Africa. We discuss cases and look at images using iPhone or any smartphone, e-mailing images and even sending video using WhatsApp or Twitter. We are very motivated to use these tools.

Facebook

We use Facebook for announcements and WhatsApp when we want interaction. These tools have made a huge difference in the diagnosis and treatment of patients. We do local and international consultations. We have 300 pathologists in Nigeria, with 12 pathologists in our department. Unlike other African countries, Nigeria has a very strong pathology base. We use the tools available to enable us to make good diagnoses.

Challenges

Of course, we have challenges: Bandwidth giving us high resolution is expensive. Even though we wish for high resolution, we do not have it yet. We use what we have. We are still capable of getting diagnoses on most cases, using the present tools, despite all the challenges.

Sometimes the network is down, so we wait. We have tried having multiple providers; perhaps 2, 3, or 4 networks so that, if one fails, we can use another. Occasionally, there are power cuts, but we have generators.

Telemedicine/telepathology is a very effective tool that can be used to send images to our foreign collaborators for consultations. However, telepathology should be combined with the training of African pathologists.

Collaborations

African pathologists rarely send out infectious and tropical pathology cases to our colleagues in Europe and America. We in Nigeria do this on a daily basis and have acquired a lot of experience over the years. Pathologists in Europe and America wishing to specialize in infectious/tropical pathology need to spend some time in Africa and other tropical countries to widen their experience.

One of the major problems with international collaboration is that our international partners sometimes bring projects that have minimal impact on the health of our population. The projects are conceived abroad with little or no input by African pathologists who serve only as provider of "raw materials."

Laboratory of the Future

The laboratory of my dreams is one that is fully equipped, with an uninterrupted power supply and Internet facility.

MICONGWE MOSES ISYAGI

Moses Isyagi is Senior Lecturer and Head of Department of Maxillofacial Surgery and Pathology at the School of Dentistry in the College of Medicine and Health Sciences at the University of Rwanda. A Fellow of the COPECSA, Dr Isyagi completed his post-graduate training in pathology and graduated from Makerere University in 2007 and obtained his fellowship in 2016. His major interests are head and neck pathology, tele-pathology, and automated diagnostic pathology.

Dr Isyagi has been associated with Makerere University, Uganda Cancer Institute, and the Kigali Health Institute and is currently working with the University of Rwanda College of Medicine and Health Sciences, where he is actively involved in teaching of oral pathology and medicine as well as providing pathology support services to the college biomedical laboratory service.

Moses Isyagi: The Internet and social media have enabled me to become more aware of patient needs and expectations, especially now that patients search the Web to explore symptoms or treatment options and often want to confirm information they have gathered on the Internet. In addition, Internet and social media enable me to follow up symptoms and treatment as well as to communicate with colleagues to obtain additional information regarding patient care. These tools have enabled communication of laboratory results to treating physicians at a faster rate, especially given that pathology results are still being typed out in the typing pool.

Internet Use

I first started using the Internet in 1995 (via SatelLife's HealthNet)[1] to obtain current medical information for use in my undergraduate studies and later in my postgraduate studies. My first use of the Internet was exciting; I realized that I was now exposed to an ocean of knowledge and information that was previously out of reach to me and went beyond what the standard reference textbooks could offer. Information could be accessed almost immediately when needed. The Internet removed the need to go to the library to search for information in printed media; information could be acces-sible at point of care or in the laboratory. In practice, I have used the Internet for con-sultations regarding difficult cases as well as for ordinary dental patient and pathology consultations.

Unlike that found in the library, information on the Web is from a variety of sources. Unlike a reference text book, whose authors are known authorities on a subject, infor-mation on the Internet requires critical review to determine its authenticity and valid-ity.[5] Because information is readily accessible and may be needed urgently, lack of time or patience may lead a clinician to overlook the need for this critical analysis. The information overload from a plethora of sites providing similar content compounds the problem.

Because I find viewing multiple tabs distracting, I often limit my searches to defined search criteria and specific known peer-reviewed sites, comparing the information with that in standard reference text books or review articles to confirm authenticity and validity of content.

Social Media

I first used social media in 2007 when I was introduced to Facebook. Facebook made it possible for me to get in touch with friends and family without having to spend so much on postage and calls. I like using social media, because it enables me to get in touch immediately with an individual or groups of people and receive almost imme-diate feedback. I like the feeling of being connected and in touch.

On the other hand, social media can sometimes be an unwelcome distraction at work because of the amount of trivia it carries.

I usually use social media for initial clinical or pathology consultations when junior colleagues in remote hospitals have a case they want to discuss. The use of social media enables me to understand the essentials of the case in advance. Social media offers additional advantages, including cost savings compared with phone calls and the ability to share images in a discussion or a consultation with a colleague.

Social media and the Internet provide certain cost advantages in terms of communication compared with phone calls and normal mail. For instance, a 1-hour Skype call can cost less than $1.00 using a mobile Internet connection on a smartphone, and this can include document and image transfer. The average cost for of a 1-GB bundle is less than $1.00.

Confidentiality and Security

Confidentiality and security on social media are major concerns in the field of health. As a rule, I rely on cropped images and a brief summary. No patient identifier information is included in the text. If more detailed information is to be shared, then I make a direct phone call or use a password-locked PDF document (the password is shared with the receiver by SMS or a separate e-mail.) For pathology consultations, I work with specific consultants who are registered with their professional councils. Opinions from discussion platforms are reviewed, and I carry professional responsibility for accepting or rejecting an opinion and incorporating it in biopsy reports signed out by me.

Laboratory of the Future

The laboratory of the future is built around a telepathology platform in which all diagnoses are automated. The pathologist uses software based on decision-making algorithms. Slide readings are via a virtual microscope at hospitals where the laboratory technologist prepares the slides. The pathologist can read the slides from any location, and an automated diagnosis can be generated for later confirmation. This system can address challenges in countries where pathologists are in short supply but Internet access is readily available.

ROBERT LUKANDE

Robert Lukande is an anatomic pathologist in the Department of Pathology, College of Health Sciences at Makerere University in Uganda, where he teaches, conducts research, and provides consultation. He attended Makerere University Medical School for his undergraduate and specialist training. In addition to his medical training, he has a postgraduate qualification in computer science. Dr Lukande is passionate about extending the reach and changing the perception of pathology and laboratory medicine in SSA through embracing new technology-supported approaches. His primary focus is on autopsy pathology.

Dr Lukande is President of the Association of Pathologists of East, Central, and Southern Africa (APECSA) from 2014 to 2018. He is keen on promoting pathology leadership and mentorship in the subregion, and he is a USCAP international ambassador. Regarding the latter, he sees his charge as being to communicate with pathologists-in-training, engaging their interest and participation.

Internet Access

Robert Lukande: I first used the Internet to perform a literature search for my research proposal on evaluating the diagnosis of Burkitt lymphoma and the role of immunohistochemistry staining, and later for writing my thesis on the same. As an academic pathologist, I continued to use the Internet in writing my research articles. If clinicians are to remain relevant and current in their practices, the Internet is an unavoidable tool.

Searching on the Web is fast, convenient, and opens many doors, through the various links, to massive amounts of information available in online journals, but it is still expensive and not readily available in this part of the world. The speed of connectivity is still slow and the connection intermittent. To cope with the drawbacks, I invest in buying bundles for connectivity from the telephone companies here in Uganda. (I invest an average of US$50 per month to stay connected even when I am out of the office.)

Social Media

I first started using social media as a tool for keeping in touch with friends via Facebook. Later, I found many professional pathology organizations on Facebook and Twitter. Through them, I have been connected to relevant and current information vital for practice and research.

Social media is a fast way to contact particular persons of interest. Social media provides current information and is easily available; however, because it depends on Internet connectivity, it shares the same drawbacks of high cost and intermittent availability.

The positive difference that Internet and social media have made in laboratory outcomes is obvious. We can easily access SOPs (standard operating procedures), protocols, and recommendations, which assists with standardizing report writing in the department, grossing techniques, and staying current with new stains (particularly immunohistochemistry).

Access to Internet and social media has made a huge difference in how I treat patients. I am current in my practice and recommendations, and my patients are the ultimate beneficiaries of this knowledge.

Of course, accurate and quicker diagnoses translate to better outcomes in reducing mortality and morbidity. However, the impact is still low because of the scarcity of pathologists and their low use within the health system. In this part of the world, pathologists have not been stretched to their full potential in the health system because of a lack of laboratory infrastructure and understanding of the potential of pathology and its impact on patient outcomes.

I use the Internet to read expert opinions and recommendations from professional societies. I then download the current recommendations for Pap smear testing, for example, directing patients as to when they should come in for the next Pap smear. This information or recommendation forms part of the cervical Pap smear report, so that patients always know what to do next when they receive their pathology report.

Laboratory of the Future

My laboratory of the future is one with unlimited and uninterrupted 24/7 Internet connectivity. Staying connected is the door that opens to the world of knowledge in this knowledge-based era. Knowledge is the key ingredient that distinguishes progressing societies from stagnant ones.

EDDA VUHAHULA

Edda Vuhahula is on the faculty of the Department of Pathology at Muhimbili University of Health and Allied Sciences (MUHAS) in Dar es Salaam, Tanzania. After graduation from MUHAS in 1985, she received a PhD in Pathology from Hiroshima University in 1995 and the Fellowship of COPECSA in 2010. Concentrating on molecular pathology, she has held postdoctoral fellowships at Adelaide University in Australia and at the Gade Institute of Pathology in Norway. Her research and clinical interests are in head and neck pathology and melanoma.

Dr Vuhahula has held various leadership positions in laboratory medicine pathology organizations, including APECSA, East Africa Division of the International Academy of Pathology (EADIAP), COPECSA, and Head of Department of Pathology at MUHAS.

She has been addressing the problems of quality in histopathology in East Africa since 2008. With support from the British Division of the International Academy of Pathology (BDIAP), she has organized several basic training sessions for histotechnicians and pathologists in East Africa and neighboring countries.

Note Dr Vuhahula's mention of prepaid air time. Although most in the academic world of high-resource settings have unlimited data plans paid for monthly, most of their African counterparts rely on purchased credits for their cell phones.

Dr Vuhahula: We have access to several journals, especially on surgical pathology and cytology, and use the Internet to access others. The most useful to me are those that explore diagnostic challenges in cytology and surgical pathology as well as experimental pathology. Quality assurance is an interesting issue, and we prescribe electronic material for quality assessment. For the past few years, access to many paper-based journals has ceased. However, teaching materials, scientific research references, as well as diagnostic surgical pathology descriptions (including color images) are accessible free via the Internet. These resources are very useful to practicing pathologists and academicians to keep updated and provide appropriate information for clinical decisions.

Internet Access

We use Internet and social media in our daily laboratory practice:

- Internet and other social media are mainly used for communication among pathologists and laboratory technical staff as well as clinicians.
- When we encounter a condition that is difficult to diagnose or rare, we are able to access information via the Internet.
- Social media such as WhatsApp are commonly used by all staff for communication.
- Discussion groups on the Internet are mainly used to get information on difficult and rare conditions for diagnostic purposes but also for communication among pathologists, technical staff, and clinicians. Laboratory workers can easily communicate through WhatsApp.

Computers and Internet services came to our laboratory about 15 years ago. Initially, it was not easy to use the Internet and the Web because most of us were not conversant in their use, but, with time, training, and more exposure, we found it to be a very useful tool for retrieving diagnostic information, obtaining information and literature reviews for research, and preparing teaching materials.

Getting current information at minimum cost is a benefit; however, there are drawbacks, including lack of knowledge on how to access the information, lack of availability of computers, and frequent local power outages. To remedy the first of these, my university's library conducts short training sessions for university staff and residents (who also work in the hospital laboratory) on how to access relevant, peer-reviewed information. Each department has 1 or more shared computers. Most of the staff, especially the academics, have laptops or iPads.

The issue of power failure is beyond our department's mandate; normally, we send a report to the university about the problem and wait for a solution.

Social Media Access

My first use of social media was with WhatsApp, a quick and easy application that uses a mobile phone. I continued to use it because I can communicate with a whole group with the same interests at once and get a response quickly. It is fairly cheap,

I can communicate from wherever I am, and power is not an issue after the phone has been charged. The challenges in using WhatsApp include the expense, because it does require prepaid air time, which is unaffordable to ordinary laboratory technical staff. In addition, the information obtained may not be accurate, and the group may not be able to respond quickly to a specific need. If my phone does not have enough air time, I know I will read what the group has said when I am able to buy air time; I just wait. To determine whether the information received via WhatsApp is accurate, I usually check other reliable sources. In a situation in which no one is responding to an inquiry, I normally Google or use other search engines to find the information.

For example, I had histologic findings that I could not interpret. Using WhatsApp, I described the morphologic features and performed a differential diagnosis with my colleagues. They provided their opinions and suggested ancillary tests to be performed. The rapid response from my colleagues made my search by Internet more focused.

With access to Internet and social media, we have almost a paperless laboratory, but the difficulty comes when there is no power. Recently, we had a teleconference and the technology failed us. As a result, we missed the meeting and kept about 20 colleagues waiting for an hour. When technology fails, we either do not participate fully in discussion, because we must communicate in writing, or we miss the teleconference completely. Often the problem comes from the computer software not having been updated.

However, when all is working, we can give clinicians rapid results to give to their patients. When we receive a patient specimen, the details are entered in a system, so that a laboratory technician can see that we have a specimen in the laboratory. A pathologist gives it a gross examination and marks sections for processing by a laboratory histotechnologist. On completion, the laboratory scientist submits the processed slides to the pathologist for reporting. Once the results are ready and typed, the clinician can access them by computer in the ward or clinic and plan for treatment. A signed paper report follows later.

Laboratory of the Future

My laboratory of the future will have no power problems! There will be enough computers and mobile phones for all to electronically access patients' specimen information from wherever they are. There will be policies and software in place to protect the confidentiality of the patients as well as discussions among laboratory professions and clinicians made through the Internet and social media. This laboratory of the future will have a budget for all of these functions and will operate 24/7.

SUMMARY

There is no doubt that the shared practice of pathology via the Internet holds great potential for SSA and the work of pathologists.

In August 2006, Dr Isyagi set out to show how even a slow Internet connection could provide an accessible channel for transmission of pathology results between rural and referral hospitals. With funding from the US National Library of Medicine, he piloted a static telepathology proof of concept in Uganda. His objective was to examine the potential for telepathology to address unmet pathology needs in LMICs. Using simple stains, digital imagery, and the Internet, he found that biopsy waiting time in rural settings could be decreased greatly.[6] The proof of concept involved making touch imprint smears from routine lymph node biopsy samples at a rural hospital in a Burkitt lymphoma–endemic area of Uganda. The smear slides were stained with hematoxylin-eosin and examined. Images of the slides were then captured using a 1.3-megapixel digital photomicroscopy camera. Next, images and medical history summary were e-mailed to a pathologist 600 km away for comment on quality of image and possible diagnosis. The time interval between sending the image and receiving the response was noted.

Within an hour, response and feedback on how to improve the imaging were received. All the specimens were identified as nonspecific chronic inflammation, not Burkitt lymphoma. Diagnosis was confirmed by subsequent pathologic sectioning and staining. All participants thought that this was a better method for handling biopsy specimens from remote settings.[6]

Although there are numerous high-tech solutions in pathology, they are not accessible to many LMICs. Dr Isyagi showed that easy staining techniques, cheap digital imaging, and a rudimentary Internet connection can greatly reduce the biopsy diagnosis waiting time in low-resource settings in Africa.[7]

Various telepathology initiatives in SSA have been described in the literature. These initiatives range from proof of concept to full telepathology services to multinational collaborative platforms.[8–11] These efforts face challenges on many levels, from technical to professional to legal, but they also have important implications well beyond Africa.

Telepathology

Telepathology is defined as the practice of pathology at a distance by visualizing an image on a video monitor rather than viewing a specimen directly through a microscope.[12] In order to be fully effective, telepathology services require efficient and effective laboratory facilities that can produce slides meeting the requirements for quality digital photomicrographs. In turn, in order to produce images of diagnostic value to pathologists, laboratory staff need to have competencies in slide and tissue processing as well as photomicrography.

In SSA, Internet connectivity varies within countries and even within regions in particular countries. Means of connectivity range from mobile phone, modems, or cable, the bandwidths of which are also variable. Therefore, in order to succeed, investment in telepathology infrastructure needs to take into consideration the available Internet capacity.

From a pathologist standpoint, the transition from microscope slide–based examination to digital photomicrograph image examination can pose interpretation challenges. Quality assurance and control may require concordance studies between the interpretation of digital and analog slides. Dr Deo Ruhangaza began working in Butaro District Hospital in Rwanda in March 2016 and reviews and signs out all of his cases digitally with a whole-slide scanner. Such a transition is not only possible but is efficient and allows easy sharing of consultations. Medicolegal responsibility for the diagnoses needs to be clearly defined within collaborating groups. It may become necessary to reach agreements on medicolegal standards.

In contrast, there are great advantages to promoting the use of telepathology, and not only for physicians in Africa. As telepathology takes root in SSA there is the potential to create pooled digital archives for research and teaching purposes as well as for cross-referencing. Rare conditions can now be accessed easily on these databases and the true incidence of such conditions clarified. SSA also offers an opportunity to contribute to the data pool of image-based case studies focusing on conditions that are now rare in the developed world, as well as images from patients who have emerging diseases of interest to pathologists worldwide.

As a teaching tool, telepathology archives offer a repository for postgraduate training and continuing professional development, as well as quality assurance initiatives with regard to image quality, diagnosis, and standardization of practice.

Pathology in Africa faces numerous challenges: scarce human resources, poor infrastructure, low financing/funding, and an ever-increasing burden of work in a field in which opportunities for recognition and full use of clinicians' skills are not common. These factors limit the quality of health care (especially vis a vis safety and outcomes of patient care) as well as the growth and progression of the discipline and practice.

However, amid these challenges, telepathology brings the hope of availability of consultation, collaboration, increased productivity, and quality of health care. All these translate to a vibrant and relevant field for pathologists and clinicians that could attract more trainees as well as retain existing pathologists. The success and impact of these professionals will be informed by increased and sustainable funding for Internet infrastructure development from partners (government, academic institutions, development agencies, and foundations). The Internet will open many more important doors for pathology, of which telepathology is but the one that we can envision now.

In the past, telepathology often had a north-south unidirectional flow; however, it also can be bidirectional: south-north and south-south. Further, it may be the south-south collaboration of pathologists in SSA that will change the face of Africa as these clinicians take their seat at the global table of science and medicine. Dr Andrew Githeko, a senior scientist in Kenya, describes the early installation in 1999 of enhanced Internet at the CDC-KEMRI (Kenya Medical Research Institute) site in

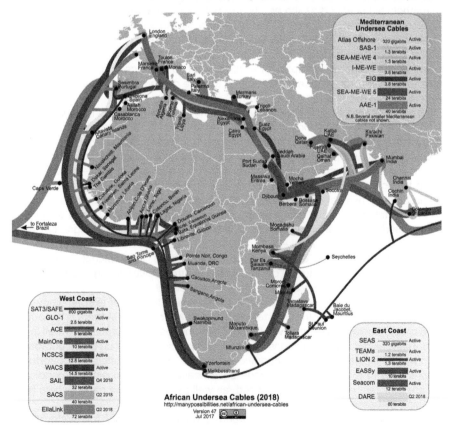

Fig. 2. African undersea cables. (*From* Song S. African undersea cables. Available at: https://www.flickr.com/photos/ssong/35774979346/sizes/l. 2017. Accessed August 2, 2017.)

western Kenya: "Our communication system at Kisian is as good as those in the US and Europe. More importantly, we are a part. We manage projects, some set in Maryland, some set in [the] UK. We forward mail to each other, we plan, we agree and disagree. We are a part. It is not one man writing a letter, giving instructions. There is a difference here. It's a completely different way of communicating!"[13]

If **Fig. 1** is a snapshot of the paucity of pathologists in SSA, **Fig. 2** might well represent the possibility as the undersea cables of the connected world move inexorably up and down the coasts of Africa, reaching inland via fiber optic to create electronic highways for commerce as well as medicine and science.

The capacity of the Internet has grown to serve researchers and clinicians in SSA, but its application continues to be constrained by issues of service cost and power unreliability. However, pathologists understand that they can realize their collective strength in communicating and collaborating with colleagues in the region and around the world, in using electronic tools to support their local, regional, and international colleagues in education and continuing professional development, standardization of practice, and worldwide collaboration. In an era of globalization, understanding and aiding colleagues in their challenges is to the benefit of pathologists everywhere.

ACKNOWLEDGMENTS

Yawale Iliyasu, Edda Vuhahula, Robert Lukande, and Moses Isyagi contributed interviews. Drs Isyagi and Lukande also contributed to the rest of the article. Thanks to science editor Lois Wingerson; Jack Chirieleison for mapping application; Ann Nelson and African Strategies for Advancing Pathology (ASAP); Donald A.B. Lindberg, MD; US National Library of Medicine; and the Fogarty International Center at the National Institutes of Health.

REFERENCES

1. Groves T. SatelLife: getting relevant information to the developing world. BMJ 1996; 313(7072):1606–9. Available at: http://www.ncbi.nlm.nih.gov/pubmed/8991004. Accessed May 16, 2017.
2. Royall J, van Schayk I, Bennett M, et al. Crossing the digital divide: the contribution of information technology to the professional performance of malaria researchers in Africa. Afr Health Sci 2005;5(3):246–54.
3. Number of pathologists per million population in Africa. Available at: http://maptest. pathologyinafrica.org/resources/surveydata/maps/maps/map.php?type=n_path %7Cmin-max%7C1%7C1%7C1%7CNumber+of+pathologists+per+million+ population. Accessed May 16, 2017.
4. Adesina A, Chumba D, Nelson AM, et al. Improvement of pathology in sub-Saharan Africa. Lancet Oncol 2013;14(4):e152–7.
5. Asemi A. Information searching habits of internet users: a case study on the Medical Sciences University of Isfahan, Iran. Webology 2005;2(Number 1). Available at: http://www.webology.org/2005/v2n1/a10.html. Accessed May 16, 2017.
6. Static telepathology in a rural African hospital setting: a pilot experience by Makerere University Faculty of Medicine. CATAI2008-QUALITY CONTROL.BIOBANKING. Available at: http://juliaroyall.com/wp-content/uploads/2007/12/munabi-xvi_ winter_proceed.pdf; https://www.google.rw/search?q=Ian+Munabi%2C+Moses+ Isyagi%2C+Julia+Royall+and+Nelson+Sewankambo.+Static+Telepathology+ in+a+rural+African+hospital+setting%3A+a+pilot+experience+by+Makerere+ University+Faculty+of+Medicine.+CATAI2008-QUALITY+CONTROL.BIOBANKIN. Accessed May 16, 2017.

7. Wamala D, Katamba A, Dworak O. Feasibility and diagnostic accuracy of Internet-based dynamic telepathology between Uganda and Germany. J Telemed Telecare 2011;17(5):222–5.

8. Gimbel DC, Sohani AR, Busarla SVP, et al. A static-image telepathology system for dermatopathology consultation in East Africa: the Massachusetts General Hospital experience. J Am Acad Dermatol 2012;67(5):997–1007.

9. Weinstein RS, Graham AR, Lian F, et al. Reconciliation of diverse telepathology system designs. Historic issues and implications for emerging markets and new applications. APMIS 2012;120(4):256–75.

10. Sohani AR, Sohani MA. Static digital telepathology: a model for diagnostic and educational support to pathologists in the developing world. Anal Cell Pathol 2012;35(1):25–30.

11. Raphael M, Leoncini L, Ilunga J, et al. Telepathology in hematopathology: experience in francophone Africa. Asia Pac J Clin Oncol 2014;10:67.

12. Weinstein RS, Bloom KJ, Rozek LS. Telepathology. Long-distance diagnosis. Am J Clin Pathol 1989;91(4 Suppl 1):S39–42. Available at: http://www.ncbi.nlm.nih.gov/pubmed/2929514. Accessed May 16, 2017.

13. Royall J. Faces of change. Am J Public Health 2005;95(4):559–61.

Pathology-Based Research in Africa

Maria P. Lemos, PhD, MPH[a], Terrie E. Taylor, DO[b,c],
Suzanne M. McGoldrick, MD, MPH[d], Malcolm E. Molyneux, MD, FRCP[e],
Manoj Menon, MD, MPH[f,g,h], Steve Kussick, MD, PhD[i], Nonhlanhla N. Mkhize, PhD[j,k],
Neil A. Martinson, MBBCh, MPH[l,m], Andrea Stritmatter, BA, HTL (ASCP)[n],
Julie Randolph-Habecker, PhD[n,*]

KEYWORDS

- Pathology • Histopathology • HIV/AIDS • Malaria • Cancer • Burkitt lymphoma
- Infectious disease

KEY POINTS

- There is an increasing role for pathology data in understanding disease in low-income and middle-income areas.
- Active collaboration with African partners is critical for the success of a study.
- There is a need to build pathology and histopathology infrastructure in low-income and middle-income areas to support research.
- The capacity to perform complex techniques, such as multicolor immunofluorescence, flow cytometry, in situ hybridization, and digital pathology, needs to be added to research and clinical settings in Africa.

Disclosure Statement: The authors have nothing to disclose.
[a] Fred Hutchinson Cancer Research Center, 1100 Fairview Avenue N, E4-203, Seattle, WA 98101, USA; [b] College of Osteopathic Medicine, Michigan State University, East Lansing, MI, USA; [c] Blantyre Malaria Project, University of Malawi College of Medicine, Blantyre, Malawi; [d] Seattle Genetics, Seattle Children's Hospital, Fred Hutchinson Cancer Research Center, 21823 30th Dr SE, Bothell, WA 98021, USA; [e] Liverpool School of Tropical Medicine, Pembroke Place, Liverpool L35QA, UK; [f] Vaccine and Infectious Disease Division, Fred Hutchinson Cancer Research Center, 1100 Fairview Avenue, M1-B140, Seattle, WA 98109, USA; [g] Clinical Research Division, Fred Hutchinson Cancer Research Center, 1100 Fairview Avenue, M1-B140, Seattle, WA 98109, USA; [h] Department of Medicine, University of Washington, 1100 Fairview Avenue, M1-B140, Seattle, WA 98109, USA; [i] PhenoPath Laboratories, 551 North 34th Street #100, Seattle, WA 98103, USA; [j] Centre for HIV and STIs, National Institute for Communicable Diseases (NICD), National Health Laboratory Service (NHLS), Johannesburg, South Africa; [k] Faculty of Health Sciences, University of the Witwatersrand, Johannesburg, South Africa; [l] Perinatal HIV Research Unit (PHRU), MRC Soweto Matlosana Collaborating Centre for HIV/AIDS and TB, University of the Witwatersrand, Johannesburg, South Africa; [m] Johns Hopkins University, Center for Tuberculosis Research, Baltimore, MD, USA; [n] Pacific Northwest University of Health Sciences, 200 University Parkway, Room BHH 423, Yakima, WA 98901, USA
* Corresponding author.
E-mail address: j.habecker@focushisto.com

Clin Lab Med 38 (2018) 67–90
https://doi.org/10.1016/j.cll.2017.10.006
0272-2712/18/© 2017 Elsevier Inc. All rights reserved.

INTRODUCTION

The combination of the climate, the socioeconomic and geopolitical landscape, and history of colonialism has created many challenges for the continent of Africa, including a pronounced burden of disease. The African HIV epidemic is paramount, with South Africa leading the world with the largest number of people living with HIV/AIDS.[1] There are increasing efforts to provide access to prevention and treatment, yet there is no cure and approximately a third of new infections are seen in young people ages 15 to 24.[2]

In addition to HIV, older disease like tuberculosis (TB) and malaria have also had severe impacts on families, communities, and the economic development of countries in Africa. In the case of malaria, public health efforts, including insecticide-treated mosquito nets, indoor residual spraying, and access to diagnostic testing and treatment, have led to a decrease in infection and mortality.[3] Although malaria is no longer the leading cause of death in children in sub-Saharan Africa (SSA), chronic malarial infections, infections with other viruses and parasites, and malnutrition can lead to long-term health effects.

As mortality attributable to communicable diseases continues to fall in resource-limited settings, cancer has become responsible for an increasing burden of morbidity and mortality, with an estimated 17.5 million cases diagnosed in 2015 and approximately 9 million deaths. Cancer is now likely responsible for a greater death toll than HIV, malaria, and TB combined and responsible for approximately 15% of all deaths globally.[4–7] Given population growth, aging, and lifestyle factors (eg, tobacco use), the cumulative burden and mortality rates attributed to cancer are expected to increase in the next 20 years globally and resource-limited regions will be disproportionately affected.[4,8]

In light of the disease burden present in Africa, it makes sense to conduct pathology research efforts there. Pathology research in Africa provides insight into the following:

1. TB, malaria, HIV, and cancer are important globally, not just in Africa. They account for significant mortality/morbidity in developing countries too.
2. It is an ideal place to understand pathologic features of diseases that have unique comorbidities, TB-HIV infection being a classic inter-relationship.
3. It is important to characterize and define treatments for disease states that are diagnosed later than in other parts of the world.
4. Research is an important and successful method to create economic growth, private and government partnerships, and build capacity and infrastructure.
5. In the globalized world, a high burden of infectious disease anywhere increases transmission everywhere.

This article presents 3 research efforts that have used different aspects of pathology to dissect a facet of disease. From them, the challenges can be seen but also the opportunities as global efforts move forward.

CHALLENGES TO THE USE OF PATHOLOGY FOR THE STUDY OF FATAL MALARIA IN MALAWI, 1996 TO 2010
Studies in the Pathogenesis of Severe Malaria

For first 20 years after independence in 1964, the Life President of Malawi forbade medical research: "I don't want my people being treated as guinea-pigs," he said. With the early recognition of HIV-AIDS in Malawi in 1984 and the acceleration of the epidemic during subsequent years, the need for research was increasingly appreciated. Malawi's first medical school, the College of Medicine, graduated its first doctors in 1992, and research became an accepted function of this new institution. A National Health Science Research Committee (NHSRC) was formed to assess national research proposals, and the College of Medicine Research Ethics Committee (COMREC) was then developed to attend to proposals emanating from the College.

The Ministry of Health recognized the importance of malaria as a leading cause of morbidity in children, and in 1982 the new National Malaria Control Programme introduced country-wide first-line therapy with oral chloroquine for febrile illness presumed to be malaria. The Ministry of Health also recognized the burden of mortality from complicated malaria, especially the encephalopathic form cerebral malaria, with its fatality rate of 20% to 30% despite treatment, and highlighted it as a top research priority.

The NHSRC approved a proposal in 1987 for a clinical study of children admitted to hospital with coma attributed to malaria. At the time, little was known regarding the clinical features and pathogenesis of this clinical syndrome. Several findings, including the importance of hypoglycemia and acidosis, emerged and routines for the precise recording of clinical and laboratory data in unconscious children were developed.[8,9] It soon became clear that, without access to brain tissue, many conclusions about intracerebral pathophysiology remained speculative. This was particularly the case in malaria, a disease in which parasites are known to sequester in deep tissues to complete their maturation and replication.

Forensic autopsies had been allowed within the constitution of the Republic, which mandated hospital autopsies for "unexplained deaths," although few practitioners knew of this law, and it was rarely carried out owing to the scarcity of pathologists. It was in this context that an additional proposal was approved in 1995, for a study to perform autopsies on children dying with malarial coma. Several requirements were stipulated by COMREC:

- The appropriate parent/s or guardian/s must give consent.
- The explanation of the procedure, and the request for consent, must be delivered by a Malawian member of staff in the local language of the guardian/s.
- After sampling, organs must be replaced in the body.
- Autopsy must be performed with minimum delay.

Obtaining Consent

Before embarking on the study, the first of its kind for the study of pediatric cerebral malaria, the researchers were advised against using focus groups to assess the attitudes of parents and guardians in the general pediatric wards to the concept of autopsy. If the scenario set before a focus group actually came to pass, the organizers of the discussion would be culpable. Instead, discussions were broached with the clinical team and responses were diverse. Many stated that they would refuse autopsy under any circumstances, whereas others indicated that they could approve if certain reasons prevailed. Common objections to autopsy included

- Distaste for the idea
- Beliefs/suspicions about the misuse or selling of body parts
- Concern about delay — the compelling tradition being that funeral and burial should take place quickly after death
- The need to view the body (at least the face) unmutilated
- "It's not going to help — it's too late."

Reasons put forward for possible acceptance of autopsy were

- A wish to know the cause of death (which might dispel suspicions of witchcraft)
- A hope to prevent further deaths in the family/community
- Willingness to contribute to medical knowledge

Guided by understandings about sensitivities gained in the preliminary discussions, consent forms in were prepared both in English and Chichewa, and these were approved by COMREC.

Conducting the Study: Operational Aspects

The aim of the study was to examine in detail the pathology of fatal pediatric malaria to address several hypotheses concerning its pathogenesis. The procedure required collecting samples from numerous tissues, including many specified sites within the brain (**Fig. 1**). Because the brain had to be returned to the skull before returning the body to the family, the brain had to be dissected and sampled in the mortuary, as part of the autopsy procedure.

To study microvasculature, smears of most tissues on slides were obtained. Samples were fixed in neutral buffered formalin for routine hematoxylin-eosin (H&E) staining, in glutaraldehyde for electron microscopy, in optimal cutting temperature (OCT) compound followed by liquid nitrogen for immunohistochemistry (IHC), and in RNA*later*, followed by liquid nitrogen for expression analyses. Samples flash frozen in liquid nitrogen in the mortuary were later transferred to a $-20°C$ freezer for long-term storage. One coronal brain section was preserved, intact, in neutral buffered formalin. This section, as well as the dorsal and ventral surfaces of the intact brain, were photographed, using a photo stand, in the mortuary. In the early years, a film camera was used; eventually digital methods were implemented. The need for different sectioning and staining methods called for a variety of containers and preservatives. It was necessary to have trays prepared and labeled in advance, sufficient to provide for the next few autopsies.

In the event of the death of a study patient, the first constraint to autopsy was obtaining the consent of the right guardian/s, without unseemly haste. Often the guardian who was present believed she/he could not take responsibility for giving approval. Ascertaining and then finding the decision maker in each family was the critical first step; occasionally, this took too long or proved impossible.

If consent was achieved, the next hurdle was assembling the team (mortuary technicians, clinical assistants, investigators, and at least 1 pathologist). Because autopsies were infrequent and because the timing was unpredictable, the composition of the team varied considerably over the course of the study. **Fig. 2** shows an example of a body prior to autopsy.

On completion of the autopsy, the body had to be made as presentable as possible, with a shroud and coffin, and transport home was made available for the body and for closest relatives and guardians.

The correct documentation and appropriate storage of samples were crucially important. The precarious electricity supply necessitated reliable back-up generators, and liquid nitrogen or dry shippers had to be dependably replenished and maintained.

Conducting the Study — Ethical Aspects

Researchers were concerned that some guardians might feel compelled to give their consent for autopsy. For this reason, a Malawian on the team was responsible for pursuing consent. The request was best given by a nurse or clinician who had been involved with the detailed management of the patient during life and who was thus known to and trusted by the guardian. Sometimes provision of a coffin and/or transport home might afford an undue inducement: to counter this, postautopsy provisions were not mentioned until after the guardian/s had decided whether or not to give consent.

The statistics of consenting to the autopsy of children in this study suggest that guardians exercised their freedom to decline the procedure. Over the period of the pathology study, 2147 patients with cerebral malaria were enrolled into the overarching clinical study; of these, 368 died and autopsy was requested from guardians of 325; requests were made when performance of an autopsy was deemed manageable. Of these 325 requests for consent to autopsy, consent was given in 103, a consent rate of 31.7%. This compares favorably to other pediatric autopsy series, in which acceptance rates ranged from 3.6% to 19%.[10–12]

Reasons given by guardians for consenting to autopsy were similar to those identified in initial discussion with the clinical team: a wish to know the cause of death, a hope that others in the family could be spared a similar fate, and a wish that the death could benefit future generations. It became obvious that a factor contributing to agreement was that the clinical team was perceived to have clearly worked hard to try to save the child's life.

Reasons given for declining were also similar to the former findings, but operational reasons were in greater prominence — especially the need to proceed quickly with the funeral and burial, which may have to take place at a distance from the hospital.

Feedback about the findings of the autopsy was provided as soon as possible to the guardians or parents. Sometimes this could be done immediately; more often it was helpful to wait a few days during which initial laboratory results on sampled tissues could become available, and the results could inform the feedback at an appointment arranged with the family. Guardians almost always seemed to appreciate being able to discuss a child's illness and sometimes to know that there was an explanation other than witchcraft.

Special Considerations

As the study progressed, the presentation of retinopathy was both diagnostic and prognostic in cerebral malaria.[13] To know how this abnormality might relate to events in the brain at a histopathologic level, it became important to obtain eyes at autopsy. Replacement with glass eyes minimized disfigurement of the face. This extension to the autopsy was permitted by COMREC and added to the consent process. When the collaborating ophthalmologist sought ethical approval at one of her academic affiliates outside of Malawi, it was denied; this generated an interesting and illuminating discussion about the ethical jurisdictions of local (vs remote) research ethics committees.[14]

When many full autopsies had eventually been conducted, additional questions relating to some localized tissues could be addressed with limited postmortem sampling; these did not require the autopsy team or the presence of a pathologist. For example, samples of cerebral frontal lobe tissue (supraorbital route)[15] and of subcutaneous tissue were readily obtained by needle aspiration,[16] involving minimal expenditure of time and causing little or no disfigurement.

An extensive and prolonged study of this kind provided an important opportunity for both local and international trainees to acquire skills in clinical assessment and management, documentation, storage and analysis of data, and histopathologic and ultrastructural techniques. Such training was a necessary and valuable component of the whole program.

Value and Limitations of Autopsy

It was essential to have detailed prospective documentation of all possible clinical and laboratory information about each patient, so that pathologic findings could be set in

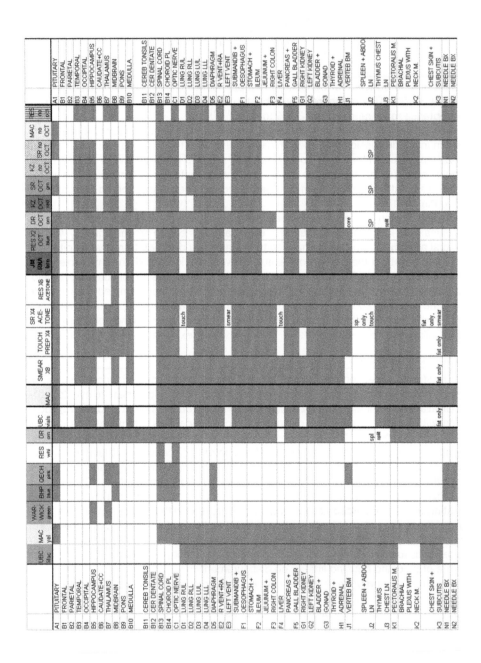

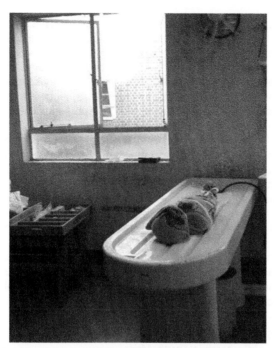

Fig. 2. A body prior to autopsy, wrapped in a traditional shroud (a local chitenge) on the plinth of the mortuary at the Queen Elizabeth Central Hospital in Blantyre, Malawi.

the fullest possible clinical context. Nevertheless, the limitations of autopsy are clear, including (1) samples represent a single point in time, the time of death; (2) some delay is inevitable between the moment of death and the obtaining of tissues, during which further changes may occur; (3) an association of features may be demonstrated but not whether that association is causal; and (4) the process of autopsy may itself alter the findings.

An example of the latter in this study was in the search for evidence that death in cerebral malaria may be due to raised intracranial pressure and cerebral herniation. Although signs of raised pressure were common at autopsy, significant herniation was found only occasionally. When antemortem MRI became available, herniation was common and was associated with a fatal outcome, but it was reversible in survivors.[17] It became clear that removal of the calvarium at autopsy allowed the macroscopic features of herniation to resolve so that they could not be detected when the base of the brain was examined. These findings have provided a basis for imminent clinical studies to test the hypothesis that preventing cerebral swelling or its consequences may reduce the case fatality of cerebral malaria in children.

◄──

Fig. 1. Sampling protocol for autopsies performed for the study of clinicopathologic correlates of fatal cerebral malaria. Organs are listed by row. The first 7 columns on the left represent samples destined for formalin fixation and paraffin embedding. Two samples were preserved for electron microscopy. Tissue smears and touch preps were each prepared using 2 different approaches (air fixation and acetone fixation). Frozen samples (9 right-most columns) were processed for expression analyses (in RNA*later*), IHC (in OCT), or were flash frozen.

Findings in Brief

Autopsies have led to several new insights into the pathogenesis of the most commonly fatal form of severe *Plasmodium falciparum* malaria. They demonstrated that not all patients dying with coma and parasitemia died of malaria and that retinopathy identified during life could distinguish malaria deaths from others.[18] Autopsies showed that in cerebral malaria, parasites sequester in multiple tissues as well as the brain,[19] and genetic analysis of parasites indicated a narrower range of parasite clonality — in both peripheral blood and all tissues — in fatal disease than in uncomplicated infections. At sequestration sites throughout the body there is commonly deposition of fibrin and accumulation of platelets within microvessels,[20] associated with a loss of endothelial protein C receptors.[21] The study confirmed clinical evidence that severe hepatic, pulmonary, and renal damage is not an important feature of fatal malaria in children.[22] Autopsies proved the common presence of cerebral swelling in fatal malaria, although it took antemortem MRI to quantify intracranial pressure and to demonstrate cerebral herniation, features associated with a fatal outcome.[23]

Although histopathology has both benefits and limitations, in the context of clinical, laboratory, and radiological assessments it may allow the development of hypotheses testable in life. Further studies may contribute to progress against this major cause of death in African children.

CONSIDERATIONS FOR PATHOLOGY ENDPOINTS IN HIV STUDIES IN SOUTH AFRICA
HIV and HIV Clinical Research in South Africa

South Africa has the largest HIV epidemic in the world and the largest antiretroviral treatment program.[1,24] Voluntary medical male circumcision (VMMC), provision of pre-exposure prophylaxis for special populations, educational programs, and widespread distribution of condoms have reduced new HIV infections, but young women remain at extreme risk of acquiring HIV.[1,24]

Because South Africa continues to have high HIV incidence and also has a well developed infrastructure, it has also become a leading site for HIV vaccine research studies, with informed/mobilized communities who participate in disrupting the HIV epidemic and strong support from international collaborations.[25,26] Such HIV research efforts have begun to incorporate pathology approaches in clinical research and have most recently even incorporated the use of IHC/immunofluorescence (IF) microscopy endpoints into some clinical studies.

Usefulness of Pathology Approaches and Immunohistochemistry/ Immunofluorescence Microscopy in HIV Clinical Studies

Because a majority of HIV infections in South Africa and the world occur via sexual transmission,[27] it is important to determine how the mucosal environment can facilitate or prevent the establishment of HIV infection. This is highlighted by the fact that immune defenses in the genital/mucosal compartment are often compartmentalized.[28–33] IHC/IF approaches are uniquely suited to characterize the localization and distribution of responses at sites of HIV exposure.

HIV prevention strategies may also need to balance priming of a potent immune response with minimizing inflammation at mucosal sites, because inflammation may contribute to increased HIV transmission.[34,35] In this context, pathology tools are capable of assessing clinical and subclinical inflammation in these tissues and can support safety assessments in vaccine trials.[33] This may be especially important in Africa, because inflammation at the mucosal/genital compartments can be greater in individuals at risk of HIV[36,37] and some studies have indicated that local inflammation can affect the efficacy of interventions.[38–40]

Pathology approaches are also important in informing public health decisions regarding HIV care. Studies demonstrating that treatable infections, such as TB and cryptococcal disease, are common autopsy findings in HIV-associated mortality[41,42] have promoted screening and treatment programs for HIV-infected individuals aiming to reduce mortality and to improve TB control.

Pathology approaches, especially IHC/IF, do not, however, have the throughput or sensitivity of other approaches and thus are unlikely to become assays used in large and complex observational studies. They also are not included in HIV prevention efficacy studies, where intact mucosal surfaces are essential to estimate an intervention's activity. Therefore, most pathology approaches to date have been introduced in small phase I studies and cohort analysis.

Tissue Sample Collections in South Africa

In high HIV prevalence settings, VMMC provides men with a cost-effective intervention that achieves a 53% to 66% reduction in the risk of infection.[43–47] In only 6 years, South Africa aims to circumcise 4.3 million men and reach 80% circumcision prevalence among men ages 15 to 49.[1] The scaling up of VMMC provides unique opportunities to access discarded tissue from circumcisions, which under normal circumstances would be incinerated. Because most of the men circumcised are under 25 and have been tested for HIV, such tissue affords the opportunity to characterize HIV target cells in the foreskin as well as the barriers that reduce infections in heterosexual men.

Various programs have planned pathology approaches to study discarded tissue from VMMC. For example, the Male Mucosal Study funded by the European & Developing Countries Clinical Trials Partnership focused on collecting formalin-fixed foreskin samples from young men 14 to 25 years of age obtained from VMMCs at Kwazulu-Natal Edendale Hospital and WhizzKids. A collaborative project among the University of Cape Town, North Western University, University College London, and the Karolinska Institute plans to characterize the immune targets of HIV infection as well as increase understanding of the effect of sexually transmitted infections on HIV susceptibility. Using IF microscopy, this group evaluated keratin thickness of inner and outer foreskin as a measure of barrier functions in adolescents.[48]

A collaboration between the Khula Ndoda Circumcision Clinic, managed by the Perinatal HIV Research Unit at the Chris Hani Baragwanath Academic Hospital in Soweto; the Fred Hutchinson Cancer Research Center (FHCRC); and the National Institute of Communicable Diseases has operationalized the collection of fresh foreskin tissue for explant culture. With the support of the Collaboration for AIDS Vaccine Discovery from the Bill & Melinda Gates Foundation, they conducted studies of antibody transudation in foreskin explants of HIV-negative men by IF. They demonstrated that antibody first diffuses freely into dermal compartments of the foreskin (**Fig. 3**), and it is later captured by cells that localize it into epithelial compartments.

In addition to tissue studies of the male foreskin, the gastrointestinal and female genital tract mucosae are also important sites of HIV transmission that need to be assessed in countries with high HIV incidence. Small biopsies of these mucosal tissues can be collected by specialized clinicians but may require a collaborative effort among several specialists, presenting large operational challenges. The Cape Town assay controls mucosal protocol was established among the Desmond Tutu HIV Foundation Clinical Trials Unit at Groote Schuur Hospital, the University of Cape Town gastroenterology, obstetrics and gynecology departments at the Groote Schuur Hospital, and the Cape Town HVTN Immunology Laboratory. Since opening in 2014,

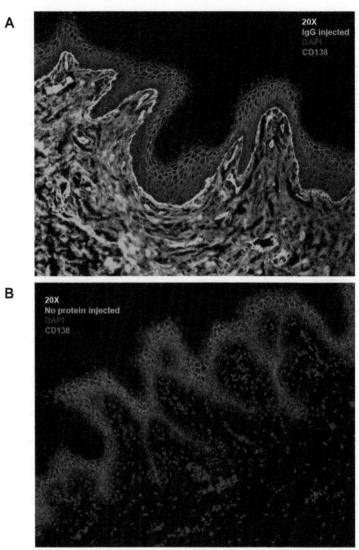

Fig. 3. Within 2 hours of culture, injected IgG accumulates at the basal membrane of the epidermis in foreskin explants. Within 6 hours of collection, foreskin tissue explants from 3 men undergoing VMMC were sectioned, injected with antibodies (human IgG-Ax647), and cultured for 2 hours to observe the areas of antibody diffusion (*A*). Control samples received no antibody in their injection or antibodies conjugated to another fluorochrome (*B*). Samples were fixed in formalin for 24 hours and rinsed in water 3 times, rehydrated in 2 baths of 10% sucrose in 1× phosphate-buffered saline (PBS), followed by 3 baths of 1× PBS, and embedded in OCT. After sectioning of the slides, samples were stained with anti-CD138 stain and biotin-conjugated goat antimouse IgG1 F(ab')2 and avidin–Alexa Fluor 568 (*pseudocolored red*). All slides were counterstained with DAPI.

the protocol has collected colonic (n = 18) as well as vaginal and cervical tissue samples (n = 12) from healthy volunteers with low HIV risk, because collections may increase HIV risk while healing.

It has been proposed that clinical trial volunteers might be less willing to donate biopsy samples, and that participant retention might be affected by this kind of invasive sampling. Although rectal biopsies are painless (because there are no pain receptors in the colon mucosa), anoscope insertion can be embarrassing and invasive. Cervical and vaginal biopsies can cause discomfort, although many female participants have experienced vaginal and cervical clinical procedures for cervical cancer prevention and management, such as speculum insertion and Papanicolaou smears. To assess acceptability and tolerance of repeated biopsy collections in healthy, low-risk volunteers from the rectum, vagina, and cervix, the US National Institute of Allergy and Infectious Diseases funded the HIV Vaccine Trials Network (HVTN 116) (clinicaltrials.gov identifier NCT02797171). The study opened in February 2017 and plans to enroll 110 men and women with low HIV risk in 4 United States cities and in Cape Town.

Fixation and Embedding

Formalin fixation provides great morphologic preservation and long-term stability of the tissue after paraffin embedding. Such a technique was used in the Male Mucosal Study successfully, to measure the thickness if the foreskin epithelial barrier.[47]

One limitation to processing of formalin fixed samples in South Africa, however, is securing a pure supply of ethanol without methanol contamination, which is essential for proper dehydration of formalin-fixed samples previous to embedding. Methanol contamination can impair many IHC/IF antigens, and most commercial pathology laboratories in the country perform ethanol/methanol or methanol-based dehydration procedures for H&E stains. One alcohol-free fixation/embedding procedure is presented in **Figs. 3** and **4**, developed as part of the Collaboration for AIDS Vaccine Discovery project in Johannesburg.

Freezing of fresh tissue samples in OCT compound is also possible, but requires −80°C storage, access to liquid nitrogen, and methyl butane for freezing, with their associated logistical considerations. For example, HVTN 116 includes embedding of rectal, vaginal, and cervical biopsies in OCT compound in Cape Town. The goal is to study the localization of infused broadly neutralizing antibodies, VRC01 and VRC01-LS, in mucosal and genital surfaces.

Immunohistochemical Staining and Image Analysis

For clinical trial purposes, sample sectioning, IHC staining, imaging, and pathology analysis require more support. Many of the supplies for IHC need to be imported, and the supply chain can be slow. Several large public hospitals have their own pathology services, but they are understaffed and may not have both hematology and solid organ expertise or capacity to evaluate clinical trial samples. There are at least 2 commercial pathology services certified by the South African National Accreditation System and the International Organization for Standardization 15189 standard, with operational capacity in Cape Town, Johannesburg, Durban, and Pretoria.

HVTN 116 involves sample collections, embedding of biopsies and ex vivo explant assays in South Africa. To ensure comparability with US-collected samples, however, IHC assays will be conducted at a single laboratory in the United States, where anti-idiotypic staining will be used to identify the location of infused monoclonal antibodies VRC01 and VRC01-LS in tissues. If a successful validation of the preservation and embedding techniques in South Africa is demonstrated in this phase I study, further training of local staff might allow conducting the assay endpoint locally.

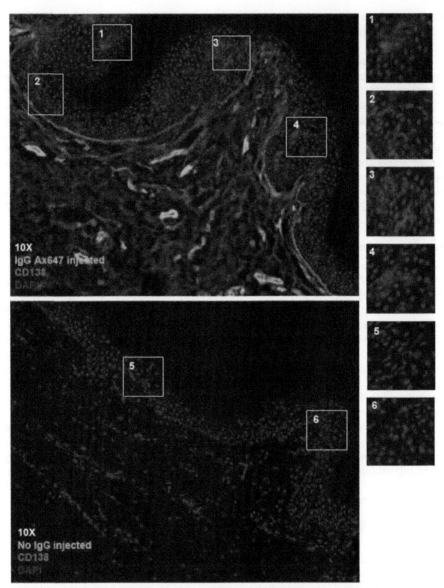

Fig. 4. Within 24 hours of foreskin explant culture, injected IgG can be identified in epithelial cells. Within 6 hours of collection, foreskin tissue explants from 3 men undergoing VMMC was sectioned, injected with antibodies (human IgG-Ax647), and cultured for 24 hours to observe the areas of antibody diffusion. Control samples received no antibody in their injection, or antibodies conjugated to another fluorochrome. Samples were stained as indicated in **Fig. 3**. CD138 was lost from the explant's epithelium at long incubation times (24 hours), suggesting some ex vivo modifications. IgG deposited at epithelial basal membrane and dermis, with sparse cells.

Summary

In South Africa, HIV clinical studies have recently introduced some pathology endpoints into cohort studies and phase I trials. Pathology approaches provide a unique ability to define immune response locations within the mucosa and to characterize subclinical inflammatory responses potentially induced by an intervention. South Africa is developing strong collaborations to support the collection, processing, embedding, sectioning, and staining of IHC samples. So far, pathology approaches have been instrumental for the study of TB-HIV comorbidities and the characterization of foreskin barrier functions and antibody transudation. Results of these approaches in the study of preventive approaches within the female reproductive track and the colon will be available to the public in upcoming years.

ONCOLOGY IN LOW-RESOURCE SETTINGS IN AFRICA
Burden of Cancers in Adults and Children in Low-income and Middle-income Countries

Among LMIC including Africa, Asia (excluding Japan), Latin America and the Caribbean, Melanesia, Micronesia, and Polynesia, the leading causes of cancer among women are breast, cervical, and lung; breast cancer is the leading cause of cancer-related death among women in these regions, followed by lung cancer and cervical cancer. Among men, lung cancer, liver cancer, and stomach cancer are the leading causes of cancer and cancer-related death in developing nations. Unfortunately, the outcomes remain poor for most patients with cancer in resource-limited countries, with case fatality rates inversely correlated with economic development.[4,49] This disparity is in large part due to a weak or nonexistent oncology health care infrastructure that results in both delays to diagnosis and subsequent treatment. As a result, most patients present with advanced disease with limited access to effective cancer-directed therapy.[50,51]

Although cancer is comparably rare in children, making up approximately 2% of all worldwide cancer diagnoses, a majority of childhood cancers sufferers (80%) live in low-income and middle-income countries (LMICs). Children with cancers living in resource-rich countries have excellent outcomes, with average 5-year survival of approximately 80%.[51–53] This contrasts to the overall survival of children with cancers in low-income countries, where it is often as low as 10% to 30%.[51,54,55]

The incidence of different childhood cancers seems to vary between more affluent countries and LMICs.[5,8] For example, acute lymphoblastic leukemia and brain tumors are the most common childhood cancers in the United States and Europe; however, Burkitt lymphoma (BL), Wilms tumor, and Kaposi sarcoma are more common in SSA.[4,55] The increased incidences of BL and Kaposi sarcoma in SSA are linked to higher incidences of or earlier infection with Epstein-Barr virus (EBV) and/or HIV.[56,57] It is still unclear if there is a true difference in incidence for acute lymphoblastic leukemia and brain tumors, or if children with these cancers are misdiagnosed and/or never reach a cancer treatment centers.

There are many reasons why outcomes are inferior in LMICs: lack of access to cancer treatment centers, inability to give appropriate intensive treatment due to lack of supportive care and unavailable drugs, and treatment abandonment, to name a few.[52,54] How inaccuracies in pathology diagnosis have an impact on survival is difficult to study in the setting of limited resources, due to inadequate data capturing and high rates of loss to follow-up and treatment abandonment. The treatments for different childhood cancers vary significantly, however; therefore, incorrect diagnoses would have an impact on the survival of children with cancers. For example, BL, lymphoblastic lymphoma, and rhabdomyosarcoma can present in similar ways and appear as small round blue cells on H&E staining. The treatment of each of these childhood cancers is very different in intensity, length of treatment, and treatment modalities.

Challenges to Pathologic Diagnosis in Low-income and Middle-income Countries

Appropriate treatment of cancers requires correct diagnosis, resulting from the careful integration of a pathologist's findings in the tissue with the overall clinical setting. Because resources for appropriate tissue procurement, tissue processing, and pathologic interpretation are all limited in LMICs,[58–63] there is an increased risk of incorrect diagnosis in such countries compared with those in which these resources are available.

Challenges to tissue procurement include the frequent utilization of inexpensive fine-needle aspiration, in which the tissue is disaggregated, in place of slightly more expensive core needle biopsies or significantly more expensive operating room–based excisions, in which the complex architecture of the tissue is retained. For solid tumors, in which the individual cancer cells usually look entirely different from their benign counterparts, the microscopic evaluation of inexpensive fine-needle aspirations can often provide strong support for a malignant diagnosis. In contrast, for tumors of hematopoietic origin (so-called liquid tumors), the individual benign and malignant cells often look similar, such that evaluation of the growth pattern of these cells, in the context of the overall architecture of the intact tissue, is often critical for distinguishing benign from malignant processes.

Even when adequate starting tissue is obtained in LMICs for diagnosis, significant tissue-processing challenges often exist. In most pathology laboratories in both LMICs and more affluent settings, the substrate for a large majority of pathologic diagnoses is formalin-fixed, paraffin-embedded tissue (FFPE), which is microscopically evaluated by a pathologist on glass slides. The requirements for adequate tissue processing, routine sectioning, and staining are substantial and include specialized equipment, trained staff, and access to consumables and reagents. Unfortunately, compared with their counterparts in more affluent areas, pathology laboratories in LMICs experience higher rates of poor-quality fixation, embedding, and/or sectioning that limit the ability of the pathologist to visualize the cells of interest under the microscope.

In addition to suboptimal tissue procurement or processing, a third major challenge in LMIC pathology is the frequent reliance on routine, inexpensive, H&E staining rather than more definitive techniques to make cancer diagnoses. As understanding of the biology of specific cancers has increased, so has understanding of potential high-yield therapeutic targets that vary between the different cancer types; the ever-increasing cell type-specific nature of modern cancer therapy now requires exact knowledge of the tumor cell type to enable optimal therapy. Although H&E histology is usually sufficient to distinguish benign from malignant cells in adequately fixed and processed tissue, it is often not sufficient to determine the exact tumor cell type among malignancies, particularly for metastatic cancers identified in secondary locations, such as lymph node, liver, lung, and brain. For example, the so-called small blue round cell tumors are a family of very different tumor cell types requiring different therapies, which nonetheless look similar on H&E-stained sections. In such cases, more expensive and/or complex ancillary techniques, such as IHC, as shown in **Fig. 5**, are usually required to facilitate the definitive identification of tumor cell type. Many pathology laboratories in LMICs lack the resources to perform IHC and, therefore, run a much greater risk of misclassifying tumors compared with laboratories in which IHC is performed.

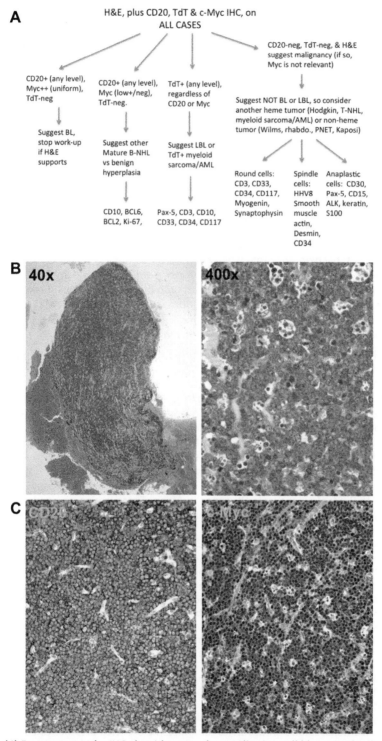

Fig. 5. (A) Demonstrates the IHC algorithm tested on pediatric small blue round cell tumors from SSA. Because BL is the most common pediatric malignancy in SSA, the initial round of

A fourth major challenge to accurate diagnosis and prognosis is the lack of standard genetic and/or molecular diagnostic techniques, including fluorescence in situ hybridization, chromogenic in situ hybridization, polymerase chain reaction, and cytogenetics. Like IHC, genetic and/or molecular techniques help establish diagnosis and/or prognosis and are becoming more and more established in non-LMIC areas; in contrast, few LMIC pathology laboratories have access to these techniques.

Finally, for particularly aggressive hematopoietic cancers in which immediate diagnosis and initiation of therapy are critical for patient survival (eg, acute leukemia and high-grade lymphoma), even good-quality histology, IHC, and molecular diagnostics may not be adequate for optimal patient care. In such cases in which rapid and accurate diagnosis is required, multiparametric flow cytometry (MFC) on nonfixed tissue is currently without equal (**Fig. 6**). Ironically, despite that many LMICs already have MFC infrastructure to allow T-cell subset monitoring in HIV-infected patients, this technology has not been adequately leveraged to aid in the diagnosis of aggressive hematopoietic cancers in LMICs.

The consequence of these challenges to the entire process of pathology in LMICs is an unacceptably high error rate when diagnostic accuracy is rigorously studied. The example of BL diagnosis will be used to propose a streamlined, cost-effective, manual IHC algorithm plus a robust MFC assay that both offer high diagnostic sensitivity and specificity and should be relatively straightforward to implement in LMICs.

Streamlining of Burkitt Lymphoma Diagnosis in Uganda

The FHCRC and the Uganda Cancer Institute (UCI) have had a decade-long partnership with the goal of studying infectious disease–related cancers, like Kaposi sarcoma (human herpesvirus [HHV] 8), cervical cancer (human papillomavirus strains), and Burkitt lymphoma (BL) (EBV). By studying the infectious agents and their role in oncogenesis, investigators hope to find new preventative and treatment modalities that can be applied to patients living in low-resource settings.

EBV was the first human virus known to cause cancer and is associated with BL, nasopharyngeal carcinoma, and certain stomach cancers. How EBV causes any of these cancers remains unclear and is the subject of ongoing research. The role EBV plays in the pathogenesis of endemic BL is particularly interesting because it is found in 90% to 95% of all endemic BL cases in Africa. There is also an overlap between areas where malaria is endemic and areas with high rates of BL.[64] This interplay of

---

IHC was targeted to BL and included antibodies to CD20, TdT, and c-MYC. When these 3 stains did not confirm BL, several second-tier IHC combinations were performed, according to the details of the algorithm. The application of this algorithm to approximately 65 pediatric small blue round cell tumor cases suggested that TdT IHC is expendable for reliable diagnosis of BL, allowing this diagnosis to be made with near certainty with only 3 slides: H&E, CD20, and c-MYC IHC. (*B*) Shows low-power (40×) and high-power (400×) views of a representative, very small, 2 mm to 3 mm in oral biopsy from a pediatric BL patient in the patient series. The 40× view shows an atypical diffuse lymphoid infiltrate, which at 400× has the characteristic appearance of BL, including medium-sized tumor cells and a starry sky appearance. Importantly, using only CD20 and c-MYC IHC (*C*), the diagnosis of BL can be rendered with approximately 100% sensitivity and specificity: the uniform CD20 supports a mature B-cell process, whereas the uniform strong c-Myc protein expression strongly suggests the c-MYC gene–containing chromosome 8 translocation characteristic of eBL. Additional studies on this series confirmed the expected presence of EBV infection (positive EBER-1 in situ hybridization) and the expected absence of lymphoblastic differentiation (negative TdT IHC).

A

TUBE	FITC	PE	PE-TR	PE-Cy5	PE-Cy7
1	KAPPA / CD8	LAMBDA / CD4	CD45	CD3	CD20
2	CD5	CD10	CD45	CD34	CD19
3	CD38	CD7	CD45	CD56	CD33
4	CD15	CD117	CD45	CD14	HLA-DR

B

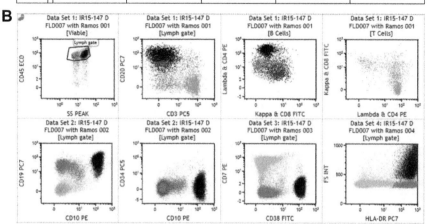

Fig. 6. (*A*) A 4-tube, 5-color flow cytometric assay designed to detect all hematopoietic neoplasms. In this assay, a PE-Texas Red conjugated CD45 antibody is included in each tube, to ensure comparability of cell identification (gating) across the tubes when used in conjunction with side-scatter and forward scatter. Tube 1 takes advantage of the mutually exclusive nature of immunoglobulin light chain (kappa/lambda) expression on B cells and CD4/CD8 expression on T cells, which allows this tube to contain fluorescein isothiocyanate (FITC)–conjugated kappa and CD8 antibodies and phycoerythrin (PE)-conjugated lambda and CD4 antibodies in the same tube. The CD3 and CD20 antibodies in this tube allow initial separation of T cells and B cells, respectively, among which kappa:lambda and CD4:CD8 ratios can be respectively determined. (*B*) Shows the proof of concept for BL diagnosis by the 4-tube, 5-color flow assay. The flow histograms (*dot plots*) in this figure show an experiment in which the Ramos BL cell line was added to benign pleural fluid at approximately 25% of the total cells. The flow assay easily identifies the tumor cells, which are colored black throughout the figure. As expected for BL, the tumor cells expressed the leukocyte-common antigen CD45, the pan–B-cell antigens CD19, CD20, and HLA-DR, and the germinal center B-cell antigens CD10 and CD38; the tumor cells lambda light chain-restriction, confirming monoclonality; and increased forward scatter (FS INT), indicating increased cell size.

pathogens makes BL the most common childhood cancer in Uganda and many other countries in SSA.

There are more than 70 pediatric cases of suspected BL seen each year at the UCI, where it was first described by Denis Burkitt[65] in 1958. These children are now followed through a clinical care project, which assures that all patients receive a tumor biopsy and pathology diagnosis. For many of these patients a diagnosis from 2 pathology laboratories is available, both of which rely on just H&E staining. A discordance rate between the 2 pathology laboratories as high as 40% (McGoldrick S, Kussick S, unpublished data) was noted.

To investigate inaccuracy in pediatric BL diagnosis at the UCI, the original FFPE blocks from the local pathology laboratories were obtained for approximately 60 purported BL cases after Institutional Review Board approval. These blocks were re-embedded and sectioned in the new, state-of-the-art histopathology laboratory built on the UCI campus through a UCI-FHCRC collaboration. As part of this collaboration, a Ugandan histotechnologist was trained by a highly skilled US histotechnologist. Because IHC is not yet online in this laboratory, the sections were sent to a commercial laboratory in the United States (PhenoPath Laboratories, Seattle, Washington), where the sections were immunostained and interpreted by a US-based pathologist, according to the LMIC-targeted algorithm in **Fig. 5**A. The algorithm was designed to minimize both the number of immunostains required for definitive diagnosis of each individual case and the total number of different immunostains required for the laboratory to effectively diagnose both hematopoietic and nonhematopoietic cancers. Underlying this emphasis on efficiency was the hope that the stains can be performed manually, without the need for expensive automated stainers or expensive proprietary reagents.

For the diagnosis of BL, the algorithm proved successful, in that the use of only 3 stains — an H&E plus CD20 and c-Myc IHC — enabled definitive recognition of all cases of BL (see **Fig. 5**B, C). Confirming the algorithm's utility for BL diagnosis were follow-up in situ hybridization studies showing the expected presence of EBV early RNA (EBER-1) in all IHC-identified BL cases. Terminal deoxynucleotidyl transferase (TdT) IHC was included as a third initial immunostain but did not provide significant information beyond the CD20 and c-Myc IHC, suggesting that TdT IHC can be omitted from the upfront diagnostic work-up of suspected BL.

Although the success of the algorithm was striking, it was disconcerting that approximately 20% of the 60 purported BL cases were misdiagnosed (unpublished data). Nevertheless, the algorithm did allow the large majority of non-BL cases to be classified, with the range of diagnoses including B-cell non-Hodgkin lymphoma of non-BL type, myeloid sarcoma, rhabdomyosarcoma, and neuroendocrine neoplasms of apparent epithelial or nonepithelial origin.

In parallel with the development of the IHC algorithm for FFPE, a 4-tube, 5-color MFC assay capable of identifying the full range of hematopoietic neoplasms from a fresh specimen (blood, bone marrow, tissue, and/or body fluid) was designed and validated. MFC is particularly appropriate for settings in which urgent diagnosis is required, for example, suspected acute leukemia or impending superior vena cava syndrome or spinal cord compression. The assay design appears in **Fig. 6**A and is based on new, dried-down antibody technology that obviates cold chain for antibody transport and is, therefore, ideal for LMICs in warm climates, such as SSA. Although this assay has not yet been used on African patient material, it has been validated in a US flow cytometry laboratory (PhenoPath, Seattle, Washington) on a large number of normal and abnormal specimens, with the abnormal specimens including a variety of different hematopoietic neoplasms. **Fig. 6**B shows the ability of this assay to identify Ramos BL cells (colored black) in a background of normal lymphocytes.

Impact on Clinical Care of Patients with Cancers in Low-income and Middle-income Countries

Diagnostic inaccuracies and uncertainties have a significant impact on the treatment of patients with cancers in LMICs. Physicians may not be able to rely solely on the histologic diagnosis and their clinical impressions become much more important, which is problematic because many cancers can mimic each other. Uncertainty surrounding the pathology diagnosis leads to questions as to whether a patient is receiving the most appropriate tumor-directed treatment, especially when patients do not respond to treatment. Misdiagnosis wastes valuable resources and can also financially strain families and fragile health care systems. Studies like these can help streamline diagnosis while delivering high-quality and accurate results.

Breast Cancer Treatment in Sub-Saharan Africa

Breast cancer, the most common cancer in SSA with approximately 100,000 persons diagnosed in 2012 (and likely underestimated), is characterized by poor survival with fewer than half of women diagnosed with the disease alive at 5 years in most countries and remains the second leading cause of cancer death in SSA.[8,66,67] There are a variety of factors responsible for the poor survival among women with breast cancer in SSA compared with resource-rich regions, including late stage at presentation and inadequate diagnostics.

Among patients with breast cancer, an accurate determination of the receptor status (ie, estrogen receptor, progesterone receptor, and expression of the human epidermal growth factor receptor 2) is essential to guide therapeutic decision making, yet this information is often unavailable in resource-limited regions. Even when available, data on receptor status often have been limited by poor specimen quality attributable to tissue degradation and improper storage and may yield falsely negative test results.[68–70] A recent systematic review that assessed 26 studies from SSA and incorporating approximately 5000 women found vast heterogeneity with a majority of estimates of estrogen receptor–positive disease, ranging from 20% to 70%.[71] Often, receptor targeted agents (eg, tamoxifen) are given empirically when available but not informed by pathologic characteristics. As such, the clinical efficacy of the medication may be limited and the potential for harm is greater.

There are plans to expand research at the UCI-FHCRC to

1. Characterize the molecular portrait and subtype prevalence of women presenting with breast cancer
2. Evaluate the potential to use widely available molecular technology to improve the diagnosis of breast cancer in resource-limited settings
3. Determine the feasibility of an oral chemotherapy regimen for the treatment of locally advanced breast cancer

SUMMARY

Although these 3 research efforts are diverse in subject and scope, they share commonalities. The first is that a great deal of knowledge can be gained by systematically studying patients and disease states in sufficient numbers to draw meaningful conclusions. In the case of the malaria studies in Malawi, valuable insight was gained concerning the pathogenesis of cerebral malaria, including information about the importance of increased brain volume and variability in the sequestration of parasitized red cells. In the case of the HIV studies in South Africa, the researchers have been able to gain insights into TB-associated mortality in HIV-infected individuals, the barriers to HIV transmission, and the composition and location of genital mucosal cells and antibodies. Pathology approaches are planned to inform the mucosal pharmacokinetics of HIV prevention strategies, such as the passive transfer of broadly neutralizing monoclonal antibodies. Finally, in the case of cancer diagnostic testing research in Uganda, the researchers were able to capitalize on a large patient population and existing tissue collection system to establish pared down but valuable diagnostic approaches for BL that make regional testing more feasible.

In every case, productive collaborations were established and sustained among multicountry investigators, physicians, health care providers, and technicians. In all the cases, African partners were necessary for funding, study design, ethical review, informed consent of patients, collecting samples, and processing material for long-term study. All these collaborations resulted in opportunities for partners to develop and hone new skills and to address research questions relevant to their LMIC needs.

The foreign investigators benefited greatly from research. In the case of HIV prevention research, mucosal characterization is more relevant in individuals at risk of HIV, because inflammation at the mucosal/genital compartments can be greater[37,38] and interventions less efficacious.[39–41] The malaria researchers in Malawi developed a more nuanced cultural perspective over the course of their study, which enhanced trust between all members of the research team, the patients, and their families. This sensitivity also ensured that vulnerable sectors of the community were protected from exploitation through thoughtful consenting so that factors, such as poverty, did not play a role in the decision to participate in studies.

Logistical challenges are more common in many countries in Africa. Depending on the location, the infrastructure may not include access to high-quality water, liquid nitrogen, or ice. The power supply can be variable, which has an impact on air conditioning and refrigeration. All these can damage instrumentation, impede specimen collection, or damage the integrity of tissue samples. Procuring the supplies and reagents required to perform assays or preserve tissue can be complicated. In many cases in SSA, there is little or no access to formalin, so tissue might be fixed in alcohol solutions or, worse, left unfixed for long periods of time. In addition, there is often a lack of high-quality ethanol and dehydrating solutions, which can effect downstream assays. These variables can greatly affect the outcome of many assays and limit the usefulness of the samples for diagnosis and research. And there may be insufficient human resources to perform assays or assemble the necessary teams for activities like rapid autopsy and so forth.

Investigators frequently find a dearth of individuals with technical knowledge in low-resource areas, often resulting from a lack of pathology training and a lack of or superficial training in histopathology. Advances like digital pathology and organizations working to improve access to collaborating pathologists from other regions are helping to address this need. Further attention, however, needs to be placed on more and better trained histology professionals. Basic skills from tissue fixation, adequate paraffin processing, correct frozen tissue preservation, sectioning, and H&E staining are paramount. South Africa has implemented training in basic histology and effort should then be placed on training technicians in other areas. Then there should be additional training in special stains and IHC followed by flow cytometry and molecular techniques. In addition, a culture of quality assurance and quality control needs to be instituted so that the value of samples collected and used is guaranteed and maintained. A great example of this is the newly implemented histopathology laboratory at the UCI-FHCRC clinic. An experienced histotechnican from the United States lived in Kampala for more than a year and trained 2 Ugandan technicians in basic histology. Because of the excellence of their work, the BL group was able to perform high-quality IHC on FFPE samples collected at the UCI. HIV prevention clinical studies in South Africa depend on locally trained technicians and pathologists, who could support training of other African nations with less capacity.

The outcome of sustained engagement in pathology research in Africa will continue to benefit scientists by producing meaningful and novel insight into the pathogenesis of disease while building relationships, capacity, and infrastructure in low-resource areas. Efforts directed toward building histology and pathology capacity should be complemented by efforts directed toward gaining a better understanding into cultural aspects of health care.

REFERENCES

1. UNAIDS. The gap report. Geneva (Switzerland): UNAIDS; 2014.
2. UNAIDS. Global AIDS update 2016. Geneva (Switzerland): UNAIDS; 2016.
3. World malaria report 2015. World Health Organization; 2015. Available at: http://apps.who.int/iris/bitstream/10665/200018/1/9789241565158_eng.pdf?ua=1. Accessed December 22, 2017.
4. Ferlay J, Shin HR, Bray F, et al. Estimates of worldwide burden of cancer in 2008: GLOBOCAN 2008. Int J Cancer 2010;127(12):2893–917.
5. Mathers CD, Loncar D. Projections of global mortality and burden of disease from 2002 to 2030. PLoS Med 2006;3(11):e442.
6. Torre LA, Bray F, Siegel RL, et al. Global cancer statistics, 2012. CA Cancer J Clin 2015;65(2):87–108.
7. Torre LA, Siegel RL, Ward EM, et al. Global cancer incidence and mortality rates and trends–An update. Cancer Epidemiol Biomarkers Prev 2016;25(1):16–27.
8. Bray F, Jemal A, Grey N, et al. Global cancer transitions according to the human development index (2008-2030): a population-based study. Lancet Oncol 2012; 13(8):790–801.
9. Taylor TE, Molyneux ME, Wirima JJ, et al. Blood glucose levels in Malawian children before and during the administration of intravenous quinine for severe falciparum malaria. N Engl J Med 1988;319:1040–7.
10. Ansari NA, Kombe AH, Kenyon TA, et al. Pathology and causes of death in a series of human immunodeficiency virus-positive and -negative pediatric referral hospital admissions in Botswana. Pediatr Infect Dis J 2003;22(1):43–7.
11. Oluwasola AO, Fawole OI, Otegbayo JA, et al. Trends in clinical autopsy rate in a Nigerian tertiary hospital. Afr J Med Med Sci 2007;36(3):267–72.
12. Molyneux ME, Taylor TE, Wirima JJ, et al. Clinical features and prognostic indicators in paediatric cerebral malaria: a study of 131 comatose Malawian children. Q J Med 1989;71(265):441–59.
13. Taylor TE. Caring for children with cerebral malaria: insights gleaned from 20 years on a research ward in Malawi. Trans R Soc Trop Med Hyg 2009; 103(Suppl):S6–10.
14. Lewallen S, Taylor TE, Molyneux ME, et al. Ocular fundus findings in Malawian children with cerebral malaria. Ophthalmology 1993;100(6):857–61.
15. Mfutso-Bengo JM, Taylor TE. Ethical jurisdictions in international biomedical research. Trends Parasitol 2002;18(5):231–4.
16. Milner DA, Dzamalala CP, Liomba NG, et al. Sampling of supraorbital brain tissue after death: improving on the clinical diagnosis of cerebral malaria. J Infect Dis 2005;191:805–8.
17. Moxon CA, Wassmer SC, Milner DA Jr, et al. Loss of endothelial protein C receptors links coagulation and inflammation to parasite sequestration in cerebral malaria in African children. Blood 2013;122(5):842–51.
18. Seydel KB, Kampondeni SD, Valim C, et al. Brain swelling and death in pediatric cerebral malaria. N Engl J Med 2015;72(12):1126–37.
19. Taylor TE, Fu W, Carr R, et al. Differentiating the pathologies of cerebral malaria by postmortem parasite counts. Nat Med 2004;10(2):143–5.
20. Milner DA Jr, Lee JJ, Frantzreb C, et al. Quantitative assessment of multiorgan sequestration of parasites in fatal pediatric cerebral malaria. J Infect Dis 2015; 212(8):1317–21.

21. Montgomery J, Milner DA, Tse MT, et al. Genetic analysis of circulating and sequestered populations of Plasmodium falciparum in fatal pediatric malaria. J Infect Dis 2006;194(1):115–22.

22. Wassmer SC, Taylor T, Maclennan CA, et al. Platelet-induced clumping of Plasmodium falciparum-infected erythrocytes from Malawian patients with cerebral malaria-possible modulation in vivo by thrombocytopenia. J Infect Dis 2008; 197(1):72–8.

23. Milner DA Jr, Whitten RO, Kamiza S, et al. The systemic pathology of cerebral malaria in African children. Front Cell Infect Microbiol 2014;4:104.

24. SANAC. South Africa global AIDS progress report. Pretoria (South Africa): S.A.N.A.C; 2015. p. 1–69. Available at: http://sanac.org.za/wp-content/uploads/2016/06/GARPR_report-high-res-for-print-June-15-2016.pdf. Accessed December 22, 2017.

25. Lan G, Blom A, Kamalski J, et al. A decade of development in Sub-Saharan African science, technology, engineering & mathematics research. Washington, DC: World Bank; 2014. Available at: https://openknowledge.worldbank.org/bitstream/handle/10986/23142/9781464807008.pdf?sequence=1. Accessed December 22, 2017.

26. Pouris A. Science in South Africa: the dawn of a renaissance? S Afr J Sci 2012; 108(7/8):1–6.

27. Shisana O, Rehle T, Simbayi LC, et al. South African national HIV prevalence, incidence and behaviour survey 2012. Cape Town (South Africa): HSRC Press; 2014.

28. Belyakov IM, Isakov D, Zhu Q, et al. A novel functional CTL avidity/activity compartmentalization to the site of mucosal immunization contributes to protection of macaques against simian/human immunodeficiency viral depletion of mucosal CD4+ T cells. J Immunol 2007;178(11):7211–21.

29. Perreau M, Welles HC, Harari A, et al. DNA/NYVAC vaccine regimen induces HIV-specific CD4 and CD8 T-cell responses in intestinal mucosa. J Virol 2011;85(19): 9854–62.

30. Ferre AL, Lemongello D, Hunt PW, et al. Immunodominant HIV-specific CD8+ T-cell responses are common to blood and gastrointestinal mucosa, and Gag-specific responses dominate in rectal mucosa of HIV controllers. J Virol 2010; 84(19):10354–65.

31. Yang OO, Ibarrondo FJ, Price C, et al. Differential blood and mucosal immune responses against an HIV-1 vaccine administered via inguinal or deltoid injection. PLoS One 2014;9(2):e88621.

32. Lemos MP, Karuna ST, Mize GJ, et al. In men at risk of HIV infection, IgM, IgG1, IgG3, and IgA reach the human foreskin epidermis. Mucosal Immunol 2016;9(3): 798–808.

33. Baden LR, Liu J, Li H, et al. Induction of HIV-1-specific mucosal immune responses following intramuscular recombinant adenovirus serotype 26 HIV-1 vaccination of humans. J Infect Dis 2015;211(4):518–28.

34. Haaland RE, Hawkins PA, Salazar-Gonzalez J, et al. Inflammatory genital infections mitigate a severe genetic bottleneck in heterosexual transmission of subtype A and C HIV-1. PLoS Pathog 2009;5(1):e1000274.

35. Lewis GK, DeVico AL, Gallo RC. Antibody persistence and T-cell balance: two key factors confronting HIV vaccine development. Proc Natl Acad Sci U S A 2014;111(44):15614–21.

36. Taha TE, Hoover DR, Dallabetta GA, et al. Bacterial vaginosis and disturbances of vaginal flora: association with increased acquisition of HIV. AIDS 1998;12(13): 1699–706.

37. Kaul R, Prodger J, Joag V, et al. Inflammation and HIV transmission in sub-Saharan Africa. Curr HIV/AIDS Rep 2015;12(2):216–22.
38. Naranbhai V, Abdool Karim SS, Altfeld M, et al. Innate immune activation enhances hiv acquisition in women, diminishing the effectiveness of tenofovir microbicide gel. J Infect Dis 2012;206(7):993–1001.
39. Moodie Z, Metch B, Bekker LG, et al. Continued follow-up of phambili phase 2b randomized HIV-1 vaccine trial participants supports increased HIV-1 acquisition among vaccinated men. PLoS One 2015;10(9):e0137666.
40. Benlahrech A, Harris J, Meiser A, et al. Adenovirus vector vaccination induces expansion of memory CD4 T cells with a mucosal homing phenotype that are readily susceptible to HIV-1. Proc Natl Acad Sci U S A 2009;106(47):19940–5.
41. Karat AS, Tlali M, Fielding KL, et al. Measuring mortality due to HIV-associated tuberculosis among adults in South Africa: comparing verbal autopsy, minimally-invasive autopsy, and research data. PLoS One 2017;12(3):e0174097.
42. Karat AS, Omar T, von Gottberg A, et al. Autopsy prevalence of tuberculosis and other potentially treatable infections among adults with advanced HIV enrolled in out-patient care in South Africa. PLoS One 2016;11(11):e0166158.
43. Auvert B, Taljaard D, Lagarde E, et al. Randomized, controlled intervention trial of male circumcision for reduction of HIV infection risk: the ANRS 1265 Trial. PLoS Med 2005;2(11):e298.
44. Bailey RC, Moses S, Parker CB, et al. Male circumcision for HIV prevention in young men in Kisumu, Kenya: a randomised controlled trial. Lancet 2007; 369(9562):643–56.
45. Gray RH, Kigozi G, Serwadda D, et al. Male circumcision for HIV prevention in men in Rakai, Uganda: a randomized trial. Lancet 2007;369(9562):657–66.
46. UNAIDS/WHO/SACEMA Expert Group on Modelling the Impact and Cost of Male Circumcision for HIV Prevention. Male circumcision for HIV prevention in high HIV prevalence settings: what can mathematical modelling contribute to informed decision making? PLoS Med 2009;6(9):e1000109.
47. Njeuhmeli E, Forsythe S, Reed J, et al. Voluntary medical male circumcision: modeling the impact and cost of expanding male circumcision for HIV prevention in eastern and southern Africa. PLoS Med 2011;8(11):e1001132.
48. Chigorimbo-Tsikiwa NG, Nyat Z, Bekker LG, et al. Protein correlates of HIV prevention in the male genital tract, in R4P research for prevention. Chicago: 2016.
49. Farmer P, Frenk J, Knaul FM, et al. Expansion of cancer care and control in countries of low and middle income: a call to action. Lancet 2010;376(9747):1186–93.
50. Kingham TP, Alatise OI, Vanderpuye V, et al. Treatment of cancer in sub-Saharan Africa. Lancet Oncol 2013;14(4):e158–67.
51. Cazap E, Magrath I, Kingham TP, et al. Structural barriers to diagnosis and treatment of cancer in low- and middle-income countries: the urgent need for scaling up. J Clin Oncol 2016;34(1):14–9.
52. Gupta S, Howard SC, Hunger SP, et al. Treating childhood cancer in low- and middle-income countries. In: Gelband H, JP, Sankaranarayanan R, et al, editors. Cancer: disease control priorities, vol. 3, 3rd edition. Washington, DC: The International Bank for Reconstruction and Development/The World Bank; 2015. Chapter 7.
53. Rodriguez-Galindo C, Friedrich P, Alcasabas P, et al. Toward the cure of all children with cancer through collaborative efforts: pediatric oncology as a global challenge. J Clin Oncol 2015;33(27):3065–73.
54. Hudson MM, Link MP, Simone JV. Milestones in the curability of pediatric cancers. J Clin Oncol 2014;32(23):2391–7.

55. Magrath I, Steliarova-Foucher E, Epelman S, et al. Paediatric cancer in low-income and middle-income countries. Lancet Oncol 2013;14(3):e104–16.

56. Steliarova-Foucher E, Colombet M, Ries LAG, et al, editors. International incidence of childhood cancer, vol. III. Lyon (France): International Agency for Research on Cancer; 2017. Electronic version.

57. Orem J, Mbidde EK, Lambert B, et al. Burkitt's lymphoma in Africa, a review of the epidemiology and etiology. Afr Health Sci 2007;7(3):166–75.

58. Tumwine LK, Orem J, Kerchan P, et al. EBV, HHV8 and HIV in B cell non Hodgkin lymphoma in Kampala, Uganda. Infect Agent Cancer 2010;5:12.

59. Adesina A, Chumba D, Nelson AM, et al. Improvement of pathology in sub-Saharan Africa. Lancet Oncol 2013;14(4):e152–7.

60. Barnabas M, Ngbea JA, Innocent E, et al. Role of pathology in improving health care in poor resource environments. Niger J Med 2014;23(3):263–6.

61. Naresh KN, Raphael M, Ayers L, et al. Lymphomas in sub-Saharan Africa–what can we learn and how can we help in improving diagnosis, managing patients and fostering translational research? Br J Haematol 2011;154(6):696–703.

62. Ogwang MD, Zhao W, Ayers LW, et al. Accuracy of Burkitt lymphoma diagnosis in constrained pathology settings: importance to epidemiology. Arch Pathol Lab Med 2011;135(4):445–50.

63. Orem J, Sandin S, Weibull CE, et al. Agreement between diagnoses of childhood lymphoma assigned in Uganda and by an international reference laboratory. Clin Epidemiol 2012;4:339–47.

64. Brady G, MacArthur GJ, Farrell PJ. Epstein–barr virus and Burkitt lymphoma. J Clin Pathol 2007;60(12):1397–402.

65. Burkitt D. A sarcoma involving the jaws in African children. British Journal of Surgery 1958;46:218–23.

66. Rambau PF. Pathology practice in a resource-poor setting: Mwanza, Tanzania. Arch Pathol Lab Med 2011;135(2):191–3.

67. Sankaranarayanan R, Swaminathan R, Brenner H, et al. Cancer survival in Africa, Asia, and Central America: a population-based study. Lancet Oncol 2010;11(2):165–73.

68. Bird PA, Hill AG, Houssami N. Poor hormone receptor expression in East African breast cancer: evidence of a biologically different disease? Ann Surg Oncol 2008;15(7):1983–8.

69. Kantelhardt EJ, Mathewos A, Aynalem A, et al. The prevalence of estrogen receptor-negative breast cancer in Ethiopia. BMC Cancer 2014;14:895.

70. Nalwoga H, Arnes JB, Wabinga H, et al. Frequency of the basal-like phenotype in African breast cancer. APMIS 2007;115(12):1391–9.

71. Eng A, McCormack V, dos-Santos-Silva I. Receptor-defined subtypes of breast cancer in indigenous populations in Africa: a systematic review and meta-analysis. PLoS Med 2014;11(9):e1001720.

Lymphoma and Pathology in Sub-Saharan Africa
Current Approaches and Future Directions

Tamiwe Tomoka, MD[a], Nathan D. Montgomery, MD, PhD[b],
Eric Powers, BA[b], Bal Mukunda Dhungel, MBBS, MD[c],
Elizabeth A. Morgan, MD[d], Maurice Mulenga, MBBS, MD[c],
Satish Gopal, MD, MPH[a,e], Yuri Fedoriw, MD[b,e,*]

KEYWORDS

- Lymphoma • Africa • Pathology • Laboratory
- Low-income and middle-income countries

KEY POINTS

- Clinical and pathologic studies of patients not infected with human immunodeficiency virus with hematolymphoid malignancies are severely lacking in sub-Saharan Africa (SSA), but are necessary to inform and support effective treatment strategies.
- Most chemotherapeutic agents used for lymphoma treatment are inexpensive and available. As such, access to these therapies depends on accurate diagnosis and not necessarily funding.
- Targeted therapies for some lymphomas require specific diagnostic tools beyond the standard histology that is implementable in SSA.

INTRODUCTION

Cancer is a major cause of morbidity and mortality in developing countries where health systems are poorly equipped to deal with this challenge.[1] In the sub-Saharan region of Africa, the incidence of hematolymphoid malignancies is escalating in large part because of the human immunodeficiency virus (HIV) epidemic as well as population growth and aging.[2] Despite the increasing burden, infrastructure for diagnosis and treatment of hematolymphoid malignancies remains inadequate in sub-Saharan Africa

Disclosures: The authors have no relevant conflicts of interest to disclose.
[a] UNC Project Malawi, Tidziwe Centre, Private Bag A-104, Lilongwe, Malawi; [b] Department of Pathology and Laboratory Medicine, The University of North Carolina School of Medicine, CB 7525, Chapel Hill, NC 27599-7525, USA; [c] Kamuzu Central Hospital, PO Box 149, Lilongwe, Malawi; [d] Brigham and Women's Hospital, 75 Francis Street, Amory Building, Boston, MA 02115, USA; [e] Lineberger Comprehensive Cancer Center, CB 7295, Chapel Hill, NC 27599-7295, USA
* Corresponding author. Department of Pathology and Laboratory Medicine, The University of North Carolina School of Medicine, CB 7525, Chapel Hill, NC 27599-7525.
E-mail address: Yuri.Fedoriw@unchealth.unc.edu

(SSA). In high-income countries (HICs), lymphoma diagnosis and classification rely heavily on expensive ancillary tools like flow cytometry, immunohistochemistry (IHC), and cytogenetics, which are, as yet, largely unavailable in SSA and other low-income to middle-income countries (LMICs). Likewise, intensive cytotoxic chemotherapy regimens are often not tolerable in settings with limited supportive care. Despite these limitations, strategies to improve care in SSA can be devised and successfully implemented. This article describes regional lymphoma epidemiology, current local approaches to laboratory and pathologic diagnosis, and ongoing research efforts in SSA.

REGIONAL LYMPHOMA EPIDEMIOLOGY

Although limited by data quality, GLOBOCAN 2012 estimates the age-standardized rate (ASR) of non-Hodgkin lymphoma (NHL) in SSA to be approximately 3.9 per 100,000 person years, with an age-standardized mortality of 3.2 per 100,000 person years.[3] Classic Hodgkin lymphoma (CHL) further contributes to lymphoma burden with an ASR of 0.9%.[3] Even when considering only expected growth and aging of the population without increasing incidence rates, the annual number of new lymphoma cases in SSA is expected to nearly double over the next 2 decades, from approximately 25,000 in 2012 to more than 48,000 by 2035.[3]

Lymphoma epidemiology in SSA is critically influenced by the important role of infectious disease in lymphomagenesis in this region. Oncogenic herpesviruses, HIV, and holoendemic malaria all contribute to a high burden of lymphoma and a disproportionate percentage of aggressive NHL.[1,4]

Among pediatric patients, endemic Burkitt lymphoma (eBL) predominates in much of SSA, representing more than 80% of all hematologic malignancies and more than 90% of NHLs in some published cohorts.[5] eBL is almost invariably associated with Epstein-Barr virus (EBV) and follows a distribution that mirrors the malaria belt through central Africa.[1,4] Although the precise mechanistic relationship between these pathogens remains incompletely understood, prevailing models suggest that malaria infection may either inhibit EBV-specific immune responses or promote EBV lytic reactivation, in either case ultimately leading to the development of eBL.[6] Other common pediatric lymphoid malignancies in SSA include CHL, which is also generally EBV associated in this setting, and acute lymphoblastic leukemia/lymphoma (ALL).[5,7,8] Although T-cell ALL (T-ALL) accounts for approximately 15% of pediatric ALL in Western cohorts, studies have shown an increased proportion of T-ALL compared with B-cell ALL in children and adolescents of African descent in the United States (25.8% vs 14%).[9,10] Review of 58 cases of pediatric (<18 years old) ALL from Rwanda similarly reflects a higher proportion of T-ALL cases (36%) among Rwandan patients (Elizabeth Morgan, personal communication, 2017).

Among adults, lymphoma epidemiology is largely driven by the ongoing HIV epidemic in SSA. Since the early 1990s, lymphoma incidence has steadily increased throughout the region. For instance, in Kampala, Uganda, NHL ASR increased 3.0-fold and 2.3-fold in women and men, respectively, between 1991 and 2010.[11] Although this trend is not entirely attributable to HIV, the epidemic is clearly the primary driver. HIV-associated lymphomas are disproportionately aggressive B-cell malignancies, such as diffuse large B-cell lymphoma (DLBCL), Burkitt lymphoma (BL), and plasmablastic lymphoma.[7] These lymphomas are associated with high mortality in African cohorts, in which access to modern chemotherapy and supportive care is limited.[12] Although improving access to antiretroviral therapy (ART) is likely to reduce the incidence of some HIV-associated malignancies, other lymphomas, including CHL and

BL, are equally common or even more common in patients on ART.[8] Hence, HIV is likely to be an important driver of lymphoma epidemiology in SSA for decades to come. Notably, in HICs with universal access to ART, lymphoma remains the primary cause of cancer-related death in individuals infected with HIV.[13]

Well-designed studies of lymphoma epidemiology in HIV-negative adults are generally lacking in SSA. Cancer registries tend to be limited by poor rates of histologic confirmation,[14] and series with pathology-confirmed disease are likely to have considerable sampling bias, missing both patients with indolent lymphoma who choose not to present to medical care and patients with aggressive lymphomas who die at home before they can seek medical attention. Despite these limitations, the available data (including our own experience in Malawi) support a wide spectrum of B-cell and T-cell NHL and CHL.[7] Indolent lymphomas and T-cell NHLs seem to represent a larger percentage of diagnoses in HIV-negative populations than in their HIV-positive counterparts.[7]

CURRENT THERAPIES AND INFRASTRUCTURE

Treatment of lymphoma at present in SSA is possible but also challenging.[1] It should be emphasized that standard chemotherapy backbones for lymphoma treatment even in HIC typically use old drugs with generic formulations and can thus often be applied at acceptable cost even in LMICs, especially for curative-intent treatment. However, high HIV prevalence, high endemic opportunistic infection burden, and poor supportive care limit the complexity and intensity of the chemotherapy that can be safely administered in most SSA environments.[1] Limited supportive care in particular includes supplies, personnel, and infrastructure for oncology nursing, infusional treatment, hematopoietic growth factor support, blood cultures, antimicrobial treatment, laboratory monitoring, and tumor lysis syndrome management (rasburicase, dialysis). Many groups are working to address these gaps and slowly build capacity, but there is clearly a cytotoxic ceiling for lymphoma treatment imposed by most SSA settings that is lower than for the same diseases in HIC. In addition, novel, targeted, noncytotoxic agents that have become accepted standards of care in HIC remain unavailable to most public sector patients in SSA, including rituximab, which received United States approval in 1991 and for which a less expensive, existing biosimilar is commercially available worldwide.[15]

As therapies become available and are shown to be effective and safe in SSA, patient selection through accurate diagnosis and classification is critical. For example, CD20 immunophenotyping is necessary for targeted therapy with rituximab, and expression by IHC is an inclusion criteria for safety and efficacy in an ongoing clinical trial in Malawi.[16] Some patients screened for this study thought likely to have DLBCL had CD20-negative tumors. Without histopathologic and immunophenotypic confirmation, patients would have been misenrolled and mistreated, compromising their care and study objectives. Access to routine immunophenotyping can also serve as a tool for discovery, which is a common practice in HIC. Recently, human herpes virus 8 (HHV-8) multicentric Castleman disease was definitively identified in SSA by latency-associated nuclear antigen expression, leading to improved diagnosis and treatment.[17,18]

Adopting and implementing other advanced ancillary diagnostic testing is also within reach for LMIC. EBV plasma viral load can serve as an additional diagnostic, prognostic, and predictive biomarker for BL and additional applications in LMIC are being investigated.[19] Thorough molecular classification and subcategorization of lymphoma cases from SSA have been completed in the United States.[20] With appropriate infrastructure, such on-site testing can enhance and guide effective therapy.

Although piecemeal efforts to improve the treatment landscape are underway, a comprehensive regional solution is likely to be elusive until there are international, multilateral, public-private commitments for cancer similar to those that eventually made HIV treatment possible in SSA.[21] Until then, many standard chemotherapy regimens from HIC likely can be safely and effectively applied in SSA at experienced centers with structured, resource-appropriate algorithms for monitoring and dose adjustment. These regimens include CHOP (cyclophosphamide, doxorubicin, vincristine, prednisone) for many aggressive NHL subtypes,[12,22,23] CVP (cyclophosphamide, vincristine, prednisone) for indolent NHL, and ABVD (doxorubicin, bleomycin, vinblastine, dacarbazine) for CHL.[24] For pediatric BL, regimens incorporating high-dose methotrexate, as implemented by the French-African Pediatric Oncology Group (GFAOP), have seemed more promising in SSA than anthracycline-based approaches,[25–28] although nursing and supportive care requirements for safe systemic methotrexate administration are not trivial and require careful attention if this approach is to be successful. Regional standards for salvage chemotherapy after first-line failure, or for very aggressive, less common NHL subtypes like extranodal natural killer/T-cell lymphoma, are less clear. In addition, for lymphoma subtypes that are frequently causally associated with EBV, like CHL or pediatric BL, peripheral blood EBV measurement may be an implementable tool in SSA to allow better prognostication and response assessment during treatment, potentially optimizing the therapeutic index and minimizing treatment-related morbidity, in light of the supportive care limitations highlighted earlier.[19,24]

INADEQUACY OF PATHOLOGY SERVICES

Tissue diagnosis is essential in the provision of clinical and public health services for cancer.[29] From screening for malignant disease; through diagnosis, staging, guiding, and monitoring treatment; to evaluating the complications of treatment, every step requires the support of pathology investigations.[30] In a review of a population-based cancer registry data in Malawi, just 18% of all cancer diagnoses had a pathologically confirmed diagnosis. The remaining cancers were diagnosed based on clinical suspicion alone or with the aid of radiology in some cases.[14] As therapies become more accessible, accurate tissue-based diagnosis will prevent overtreatment/undertreatment of potentially curable diseases.

Adequate pathology services are particularly important in the accurate diagnosis and classification of lymphomas, which may clinically mimic infectious diseases like tuberculosis. Striking differences still exist in the reliability of lymphoma diagnosis between HIC and LMIC. In 2011, the International Network of Cancer Treatment and Research (INCTR) conducted an evaluation of infrastructure for diagnosing lymphoma in 4 sub-Saharan countries: Kenya, Tanzania, Nigeria, and Uganda.[31] Key findings included wide use of fine-needle aspiration cytology as a diagnostic tool, lack of IHC or other immunophenotyping tools, variable equipment and personnel, and variable turnaround times. Many of the histologic and cytologic preparations were deemed suboptimal. However, as expected, metrics of quality were highly tied to available resources, and some centers collaborating with institutions in developed countries had well-established infrastructure and turnaround times of less than a week. Overall, pathologists were well trained but few in number, with inadequate numbers of trainees. Molecular and cytogenetic techniques, which are core elements of hematopathology, were not available in any of the centers.[31]

In light of the significant need, collaborative efforts to improve diagnostic pathology services in the region are ongoing at many levels. For instance, the National Cancer

Institute (NCI) is currently supporting the Sub-Saharan Africa Lymphoma Consortium, a grouping of 10 regional referral centers with an aim of characterizing lymphomas. In large part because of international investments such as this one, substantial progress has been made in recent years.

KAMUZU CENTRAL HOSPITAL, MALAWI

Although diagnostic pathology services remain insufficient in the region, they are not entirely absent.[32] General uniformity and structure between programs is lacking, and infrastructure, staffing, and financial support are highly variable. In some areas, support from government and/or partnering academic institutions is significant, and laboratory capacity matches that in HIC. In contrast, some laboratories depend heavily on volunteers and donations, which adds logistical complexity.

The hematopathology services at the Kamuzu Central Hospital (KCH) were developed more recently, through the close collaborative efforts of the Malawi Ministry of Health and the University of North Carolina (UNC). Located in the capital city of Lilongwe, KCH is one of 2 national teaching hospitals in Malawi and has a referral base of approximately 4 million to 5 million people. The laboratory was established in 2011 with financial backing from both institutional and governmental sources.

In 2016, the laboratory processed a total of 5611 histology and 1998 cytology cases. Most of these cases were interpreted by one of 2 local pathologists without international consultation or additional stains. However, difficult cases, as well as diagnostic specimens from all patients enrolled in the ongoing KCH Lymphoma Study, are additionally reviewed at a weekly telepathology conference attended by Malawian clinicians, Malawian pathologists, and their counterparts in the United States. The basic work flow for such cases is outlined in **Fig. 1**. Briefly, bone marrow and tissue biopsies or cytology specimens are processed and then initially reviewed by a local pathologist, who develops an impression, which is often shared with the treating clinician. In some cases, an initial panel of IHC stains may be ordered (**Box 1**). Relevant slides are scanned using an Aperio slide scanner and then uploaded to a secure online server. Cases are then reviewed in a weekly telepathology conference attended by Malawi-based clinicians and pathologists, as well as their colleagues in the United States. After discussion at this conference, and often after additional rounds of IHC stains, a consensus diagnosis is rendered by the local pathologist.

To ensure quality control and to facilitate research studies, tissue blocks and glass cytology slides are sent to collaborators in the United States quarterly. Histology cases are then further characterized by a broader panel of IHC and in situ hybridization stains. After glass slide review and expanded immunophenotyping, a final diagnosis is rendered. In a cohort of KCH patients with lymphoma and other lymphoproliferative disorders, concordance between initial diagnosis in Malawi and final diagnosis in the United States was very high.[8] Although expanded immunophenotyping permits more granular classification of some lymphomas, the initial diagnosis made in Malawi led to treatment appropriate to this setting in 95% of cases.

In addition to the immediate impacts on patient care, the robust pathology service at KCH has had several additional impacts. First, as described later, it has facilitated involvement in several regional and international clinical trials. Second, and equally important, the growth of services and infrastructure has attracted Malawian pathologists and technologists to a center that lacked any pathology services just 6 years ago.

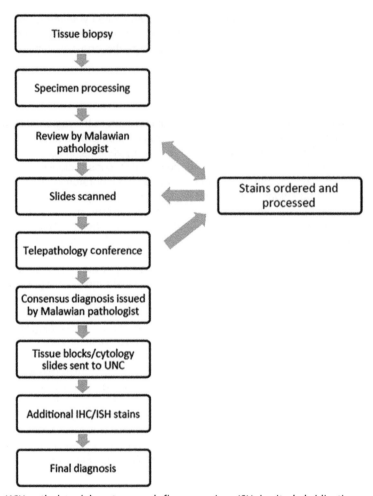

Fig. 1. KCH pathology laboratory work flow overview. ISH, in situ hybridization.

Box 1
Immunohistochemical stains available at the Kamuzu Central Hospital pathology laboratory

Available stains:
   CD45
   CD3
   CD20
   Ki67
   TdT
   BCL2
   CD30
   CD138
   HHV8 (latency-associated nuclear antigen)
   Synaptophysin
   AE1/AE3

ONGOING REGIONAL AND INTERNATIONAL CLINICAL TRIALS

In addition to important individual efforts, there are 2 cooperative groups sponsored by the NCI focused on lymphoma treatment in SSA. First, the AIDS Malignancy Consortium includes several SSA centers, and to date has implemented treatment studies for Kaposi sarcoma and cervical cancer. A clinical trial is also being implemented for HIV-associated DLBCL, with patients randomized to receive either CHOP or low-dose oral metronomic treatment, based on results from an earlier pilot study in Kenya and Uganda for this population before ART was widely available.[33,34] NCI is also working to convene a pediatric BL network spanning multiple SSA countries. Similar multicenter studies for pediatric BL specifically have been successfully completed by GFAOP and INCTR, as well as other groups.[25,35,36] All of these efforts convincingly suggest that harmonized studies across countries using a standardized protocol is achievable in SSA even for complex interventions like lymphoma treatment, and continued support for these efforts is vital to test innovative approaches and define optimal standards of care in LMIC.

FUTURE DIRECTIONS

Diagnostic pathology services are paramount for routine care and implementing impactful lymphoma trials. Although substantive progress has been made to document the extent to which pathology services are lacking, resources necessary to help guide the development and/or sustainability of anatomic pathology laboratories in the region are limited. Creation of universal best-practice guidelines, however, may be unrealistic because of intraregional variability in existing laboratory infrastructure, support, and staffing. Nonetheless, defining local needs, developing sustainable fiscal models to support pathology, and implementing quality-assurance standards are necessary for wider scale-up of lymphoma diagnostics in SSA.

Intensive laboratory accreditation processes necessary to maintain diagnostic consistency and accuracy in HICs. Although these standards are incrementally being addressed in the clinical pathology laboratories in SSA,[37–40] the anatomic pathology services required for lymphoma diagnosis lag behind. This difference likely reflects complexities of more manual (rather than automated) testing and paucity of infrastructure and expertise. However, as obstacles to lymphoma treatment in SSA are overcome, there is increasing need for ongoing, region-specific proficiency testing and laboratory accreditation processes. Comprehensive assessment of current pathology laboratory capacity is clearly necessary, as are creative approaches to testing and sustainability. Collaborative approaches and resource sharing may significantly improve diagnostic quality throughout the region.

SUMMARY

The care of patients with lymphoma relies heavily on accurate tissue diagnosis. However, in SSA, where lymphoma burden is increasing because of population growth, aging, and persistent epidemic levels of HIV infection, diagnostic pathology services are often inadequate to support resource-appropriate lymphoma care. Improvement of regional capacity to accurately classify tumors is paramount to understanding true disease epidemiology and to establish effective treatment strategies. Although regionally lacking, successful pathology laboratories capable of supporting strong lymphoma clinical and research efforts have been established. Continued development of sustainable diagnostic approaches and implementation of quality control initiatives are likely to have far-reaching effects on improving lymphoma patient outcomes in the region.

REFERENCES

1. Gopal S, Wood WA, Lee SJ, et al. Meeting the challenge of hematologic malignancies in sub-Saharan Africa. Blood 2012;119(22):5078–87.
2. Gopal S, Krysiak R, Liomba NG, et al. Early experience after developing a pathology laboratory in Malawi, with emphasis on cancer diagnoses. PLoS One 2013; 8(8):e70361.
3. Ferlay J, Soerjomataram I, Ervik M, et al. Cancer incidence and mortality worldwide: IARC CancerBase No. 11 [Internet]. Lyon, France: International Agency for Research on Cancer; 2013. Available at: http://globocan.iarc.fr. Accessed December 14, 2015.
4. Rogena EA, De Falco G, Schurfeld K, et al. A review of the trends of lymphomas in the equatorial belt of Africa. Hematol Oncol 2011;29(3):111–5.
5. Sinfield RL, Molyneux EM, Banda K, et al. Spectrum and presentation of pediatric malignancies in the HIV era: experience from Blantyre, Malawi, 1998-2003. Pediatr Blood Cancer 2007;48(5):515–20.
6. Moormann AM, Bailey JA. Malaria - how this parasitic infection aids and abets EBV-associated Burkitt lymphomagenesis. Curr Opin Virol 2016;20:78–84.
7. Montgomery ND, Liomba NG, Kampani C, et al. Accurate real-time diagnosis of lymphoproliferative disorders in Malawi through clinicopathologic teleconferences: a model for pathology services in sub-Saharan Africa. Am J Clin Pathol 2016;146(4):423–30.
8. Engels EA, Pfeiffer RM, Goedert JJ, et al. Trends in cancer risk among people with AIDS in the United States 1980-2002. AIDS 2006;20(12):1645–54.
9. Pui CH, Relling MV, Downing JR. Acute lymphoblastic leukemia. N Engl J Med 2004;350(15):1535–48.
10. Pui CH, Sandlund JT, Pei D, et al. Results of therapy for acute lymphoblastic leukemia in black and white children. JAMA 2003;290(15):2001–7.
11. Wabinga HR, Nambooze S, Amulen PM, et al. Trends in the incidence of cancer in Kampala, Uganda 1991-2010. Int J Cancer 2014;135(2):432–9.
12. Gopal S, Fedoriw Y, Kaimila B, et al. CHOP chemotherapy for aggressive non-Hodgkin lymphoma with and without HIV in the antiretroviral therapy era in Malawi. PLoS One 2016;11(3):e0150445.
13. Silverberg MJ, Lau B, Achenbach CJ, et al. Cumulative incidence of cancer among persons with HIV in North America: a cohort study. Ann Intern Med 2015;163(7):507–18.
14. Msyamboza KP, Dzamalala C, Mdokwe C, et al. Burden of cancer in Malawi; common types, incidence and trends: national population-based cancer registry. BMC Res Notes 2012;5:149.
15. Gota V, Karanam A, Rath S, et al. Population pharmacokinetics of Reditux, a biosimilar rituximab, in diffuse large B-cell lymphoma. Cancer Chemother Pharmacol 2016;78(2):353–9.
16. Rituximab plus CHOP chemotherapy for diffuse large B-cell lymphoma. Available at: https://clinicaltrials.gov/ct2/show/NCT02660710. Accessed August 22, 2017.
17. Gopal S, Liomba NG, Montgomery ND, et al. Characteristics and survival for HIV-associated multicentric Castleman disease in Malawi. J Int AIDS Soc 2015; 18:20122.
18. Gopal S, Fedoriw Y, Montgomery ND, et al. Multicentric Castleman's disease in Malawi. Lancet 2014;384(9948):1158.

19. Westmoreland KD, Montgomery ND, Stanley CC, et al. Plasma Epstein-Barr virus DNA for pediatric Burkitt lymphoma diagnosis, prognosis and response assessment in Malawi. Int J Cancer 2017;140(11):2509–16.
20. Morgan E, Sweeny MP, Tomoka T, et al. Targetable subsets of non-Hodgkin lymphoma in Malawi define therapeutic opportunities. Blood Adv 2016;1(1):84–92.
21. Gopal S. Moonshot to Malawi. N Engl J Med 2016;374(17):1604–5.
22. de Witt P, Maartens DJ, Uldrick TS, et al. Treatment outcomes in AIDS-related diffuse large B-cell lymphoma in the setting roll out of combination antiretroviral therapy in South Africa. J Acquir Immune Defic Syndr 2013;64(1):66–73.
23. Bateganya MH, Stanaway J, Brentlinger PE, et al. Predictors of survival after a diagnosis of non-Hodgkin lymphoma in a resource-limited setting: a retrospective study on the impact of HIV infection and its treatment. J Acquir Immune Defic Syndr 2011;56(4):312–9.
24. Westmoreland KD, Stanley CC, Montgomery ND, et al. Hodgkin lymphoma, HIV, and Epstein-Barr virus in Malawi: longitudinal results from the Kamuzu Central Hospital lymphoma study. Pediatr Blood Cancer 2017;64(5). https://doi.org/10.1002/pbc.26302.
25. Harif M, Barsaoui S, Benchekroun S, et al. Treatment of B-cell lymphoma with LMB modified protocols in Africa–report of the French-African Pediatric Oncology Group (GFAOP). Pediatr Blood Cancer 2008;50(6):1138–42.
26. Stanley CC, Westmoreland KD, Heimlich BJ, et al. Outcomes for paediatric Burkitt lymphoma treated with anthracycline-based therapy in Malawi. Br J Haematol 2016;173(5):705–12.
27. Molyneux E, Schwalbe E, Chagaluka G, et al. The use of anthracyclines in the treatment of endemic Burkitt lymphoma. Br J Haematol 2016. https://doi.org/10.1111/bjh.14440.
28. Buckle G, Maranda L, Skiles J, et al. Factors influencing survival among Kenyan children diagnosed with endemic Burkitt lymphoma between 2003 and 2011: a historical cohort study. Int J Cancer 2016;139(6):1231–40.
29. Adesina A, Chumba D, Nelson AM, et al. Improvement of pathology in sub-Saharan Africa. Lancet Oncol 2013;14(4):e152–7.
30. Stefan DC. Childhood cancer in Africa: an overview of resources. J Pediatr Hematol Oncol 2015;37(2):104–8.
31. Naresh KN, Raphael M, Ayers L, et al. Lymphomas in sub-Saharan Africa–what can we learn and how can we help in improving diagnosis, managing patients and fostering translational research? Br J Haematol 2011;154(6):696–703.
32. Mpunga T, Tapela N, Hedt-Gauthier BL, et al. Diagnosis of cancer in rural Rwanda: early outcomes of a phased approach to implement anatomic pathology services in resource-limited settings. Am J Clin Pathol 2014;142(4):541–5.
33. Mwanda WO, Orem J, Fu P, et al. Dose-modified oral chemotherapy in the treatment of AIDS-related non-Hodgkin's lymphoma in East Africa. J Clin Oncol 2009;27(21):3480–8.
34. Intravenous chemotherapy or oral chemotherapy in treating patients with previously untreated stage III-IV HIV-associated non-Hodgkin lymphoma. Available at: https://clinicaltrials.gov/ct2/show/NCT01775475. Accessed August 22, 2017.
35. Ngoma T, Adde M, Durosinmi M, et al. Treatment of Burkitt lymphoma in equatorial Africa using a simple three-drug combination followed by a salvage regimen for patients with persistent or recurrent disease. Br J Haematol 2012;158(6):749–62.
36. Hesseling PB, Molyneux E, Tchintseme F, et al. Treating Burkitt's lymphoma in Malawi, Cameroon, and Ghana. Lancet Oncol 2008;9(6):512–3.

37. Schroeder LF, Amukele T. Medical laboratories in sub-Saharan Africa that meet international quality standards. Am J Clin Pathol 2014;141(6):791–5.
38. Kibet E, Moloo Z, Ojwang PJ, et al. Measurement of improvement achieved by participation in international laboratory accreditation in sub-Saharan Africa: the Aga Khan University Hospital Nairobi experience. Am J Clin Pathol 2014; 141(2):188–95.
39. Amukele TK, Michael K, Hanes M, et al. External quality assurance performance of clinical research laboratories in sub-Saharan Africa. Am J Clin Pathol 2012; 138(5):720–3.
40. Gershy-Damet GM, Rotz P, Cross D, et al. The World Health Organization African region laboratory accreditation process: improving the quality of laboratory systems in the African region. Am J Clin Pathol 2010;134(3):393–400.

Building Laboratory Capacity to Strengthen Health Systems
The Partners In Health Experience

Juan Daniel Orozco, DPH[a],*, Lauren A. Greenberg, BA[a],
Ishaan K. Desai, BA[a,b], Fabienne Anglade, MD[a,c,d],
Deogratias Ruhangaza, MD[e], Mira Johnson, BA[f],
Louise C. Ivers, MD, MPH[a,b,g], Danny A. Milner Jr, MD, MSc(Epi)[f,h],
Paul E. Farmer, MD, PhD[a,b]

KEYWORDS

- Health systems strengthening • Partners In Health • Pathology • Cancer care
- Tuberculosis • Diagnostics • Haiti • Rwanda

KEY POINTS

- Moving beyond providing only "basic" services in health care to identifying and striving to meet essential patient needs allows for more effective and comprehensive responses to local burdens of disease.
- A well-functioning laboratory system constitutes the backbone of a public health system and is critical to the prevention, diagnosis, treatment, and ongoing surveillance of disease.
- Staff, stuff, space, and systems are central to the equitable delivery of quality diagnostic services and clinical care.
- Partners In Health has demonstrated successful laboratory systems strengthening in multiple settings of poverty with measurable impact.

Disclosure Statement: The authors declare that they have no conflicts of interest.
[a] Partners In Health, 800 Boylston Street, Suite 300, Boston, MA 02199, USA; [b] Department of Global Health and Social Medicine, Harvard Medical School, 641 Huntington Avenue, Boston, MA 02115, USA; [c] United States and Canadian Academy of Pathology, 404 Town Park Boulevard, Suite 201, Evans, GA 30809, USA; [d] University Hospital of Mirebalais, Route Départementale 11, Mirebalais Arrondissement, Centre Department, Haiti; [e] Ministry of Health, Butaro Hospital, Base Road, Butaro, Burera District, Rwanda; [f] American Society for Clinical Pathology, 33 West Monroe Street, Chicago, IL 60603, USA; [g] Center for Global Health, Massachusetts General Hospital, 125 Nashua Street, Suite 722, Boston, MA 02114, USA; [h] Department of Pathology, Brigham and Women's Hospital, 75 Francis Street, Boston, MA 02115, USA
* Corresponding author.
E-mail address: dorozco@pih.org

Clin Lab Med 38 (2018) 101–117
https://doi.org/10.1016/j.cll.2017.10.008
0272-2712/18/© 2017 Elsevier Inc. All rights reserved.
labmed.theclinics.com

BACKGROUND

Well-functioning laboratories constitute the backbone of effective clinical and public health systems and are critical to the prevention, diagnosis, treatment, and ongoing surveillance of disease. In places burdened by poverty and weak health systems, the absence of the staff, stuff, space, and systems needed to detect outbreaks of infectious disease, such as the recent Ebola epidemic in West Africa, and diagnose other medical conditions has underscored the need to not only set up diagnostic equipment in places where it is scarce but also invest resources into training laboratory personnel, introducing laboratory regulations, developing strategic plans that are aligned with national and international standards, and strengthening linkages between laboratories and the clinical facilities they are intended to support.

In recent decades, there have been new, if insufficient, efforts to improve diagnostic services in poor settings. Among the primary catalysts for this interest in laboratory strengthening has been the significant infusion of resources into the prevention, diagnosis, and treatment of HIV and tuberculosis (TB).[1–3] In certain instances, vertical funding to rein in these global pandemics has been leveraged to improve care delivery for a range of chronic conditions and, in the process, to strengthen laboratories, diagnostic services, and supply chains.[4] In many low-income countries, however, such investments have borne fruit only in national or reference laboratories, if at all; diagnostic capacity at lower and intermediate levels of care remains weak. In such settings, it is common practice to establish small laboratories or testing centers linked to rural health facilities, without proper assessment of local needs, context, or epidemiology.[5] These laboratories are often constrained by frequent stock-outs and unreliable supplies of reagents and commodities; obsolete equipment and technology, much of which is phased out from hospitals and larger health facilities; and insufficient staffing and training. Additionally, they lack systems and protocols—from essential diagnostics lists and safety standards to comprehensive guidelines and workflow practices—that can steer service delivery.[6] They are further bereft of adequate referral and transportation systems capable of connecting patients and health centers to national and regional laboratories for more advanced diagnostic procedures.[7]

As a result of such deficits, health systems in most low-income countries can deliver only the most rudimentary of diagnostic services, which often do not correspond to local burdens of disease. This *basic package* or *minimum standard* of services, as it is often termed in poor places, excludes several clinical, microbiological, and pathology diagnostics that are routinely provided by laboratories in high-income countries, rendering readily diagnosable and treatable conditions untreatable and, in many cases, disabling or fatal. Basic or minimum, in other words, is not equivalent to essential.

This article describes recent efforts of the medical nonprofit Partners In Health (PIH) to establish high-quality laboratory networks in some of the poorest parts of the world. With a focus on the expansion of pathology and TB diagnostics at PIH-supported sites in Haiti and Rwanda, it discusses the ways in which robust commitments to building laboratory capacity and to accompanying national health authorities can yield better and higher standards of care while strengthening the public health sector.

PARTNERS IN HEALTH IN HAITI: THE LABORATORY NETWORK

Haiti is the poorest country in the Western Hemisphere, with approximately 60% of the population living under the national poverty line.[8] In a list of 188 nations ranked by human development index—a composite measure of population health, education, and income—the United Nations' 2016 *Human Development Report* ranked Haiti at 163.[9] The country has some of the world's worst health indicators, including one of the highest burdens of HIV in the Caribbean region,[10] and the highest rate of TB in the Western Hemisphere (194 new TB cases per 100,000)[11] as well as rising rates of cancer and other noncommunicable diseases.[12]

But in Haiti, laboratories face enormous constraints and, when present, are largely inaccessible to the poor. The country has limited laboratory infrastructure, equipment, and supplies; a severe shortage of trained laboratory technicians and managers; and extremely limited quality-assurance and data-management systems required for public health surveillance.[13–15] This scarcity has tragic impacts on health and well-being in Haiti. Limited quality-assured diagnostics leave clinicians unable to provide patients with accurate and timely diagnosis, leading to severe consequences for those requiring urgent treatment and care for deadly and disabling diseases.[16,17]

For more than 30 years, PIH and its Haitian sister organization, Zanmi Lasante (ZL), have been working to improve access to high-quality health care for the poor and marginalized in rural central Haiti. With approximately 6000 staff, most of whom are Haitian nationals, PIH/ZL accompanies the country's public health sector and helps operate clinics, hospitals, and community-based health programs that serve a region of 4.5 million people. Among these health facilities is University Hospital of Mirebalais (Hôpital Universitaire de Mirebalais), the flagship, 300-bed public teaching hospital supported by PIH/ZL. The largest solar-powered hospital in the developing world, University Hospital provides a level of tertiary health care and clinical education never before available in the Haitian public sector.[18]

In earlier years, as it sought to expand access to primary care and treatment of TB, HIV, and other common afflictions, PIH/ZL rapidly recognized the need for comprehensive and integrated diagnostic capacity to more completely respond to the true burden of disease.[1] Through decades of investment and partnership with Haiti's Ministry of Health (Ministère de la Santé Publique et de la Population) and its National Public Health Laboratory (Laboratoire National de Santé Publique), PIH/ZL now supports laboratories that provide basic, intermediate, and referral diagnostic services for a network of 12 public health care facilities across the Central Plateau and the lower Artibonite, 2 of the country's poorest regions.

Mirebalais Regional Reference Laboratory

In early 2015, PIH/ZL began construction of a modern, 15,800–sq ft regional reference laboratory in Mirebalais, Haiti, that, when fully functional, will provide an unprecedented standard for advanced diagnostics and innovation in Haiti and dramatically improve clinical case management. Situated on the grounds of University Hospital, Mirebalais Regional Reference Laboratory serves as the premier reference laboratory for the hospital as well as the network of other PIH/ZL-supported health centers and hospitals in the region (**Fig. 1**). In September 2016, after construction was completed, PIH/ZL`implemented the first phase of diagnostic services—an anatomic pathology laboratory to support cancer care in rural Haiti—despite the logistical and financial challenges of such an endeavor. Moreover, in spring 2017, PIH/ZL received and commissioned equipment from the US Centers for Disease Control and Prevention office in Haiti for the forthcoming biosafety level (BSL)-3 section of the laboratory, which will assure safe operations related to airborne infectious disease and enhance the detection of TB and multidrug-resistant TB (MDRTB).

Over the next year, Mirebalais Regional Reference Laboratory will be fully capacitated to provide clinical and anatomic pathology testing as well as more advanced

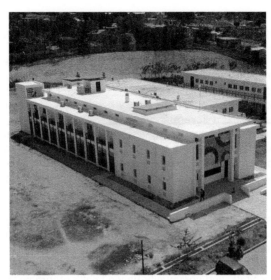

Fig. 1. Mirebalais Regional Reference Laboratory, located on the campus of University Hospital of Mirebalais, in rural central Haiti. Architect: Shepley Bulfinch. (*Courtesy of* Andrew Jones, Build Health International.)

testing in the new BSL-2 and BSL-3 facilities. These diagnostic services will cover high-priority clinical areas, including microbiology, TB, and MDRTB, as well as routine monitoring for patients receiving cancer treatment and antiretroviral therapy. The laboratory is designed to not only expand access to quality-assured diagnostic services but also serve as a hub to cultivate holistic, systems-level improvements in laboratory management in the public health sector.

Over the next 5 years, the new reference laboratory will work with local and international partners to seek accreditation and adopt various protocols and procedures to meet national and international laboratory standards, such as uniform documentation, data management, biosafety, quality assurance, training, and an uninterrupted supply chain. Furthermore, because infectious pathogens contribute to a substantial portion of the disease burden in Haiti, the laboratory will facilitate the regional and national surveillance of various infectious diseases, such as HIV, hepatitis, meningitis, cholera, Zika, and chikungunya. Consistent with PIH's goal of linking care delivery with efforts to generate new knowledge and to train staff, the laboratory will ultimately support multiple research projects and provide training and continuing education to clinicians, pathology residents, technicians, and laboratory specialists.

As the largest and most advanced in the existing PIH/ZL laboratory network, Mirebalais Regional Reference Laboratory will also seek to provide ongoing inpatient and outpatient testing support—including advanced chemistry, immunology, and hematology technologies—for those treated at other PIH/ZL-supported health facilities. To improve transportation between health facilities and communities, PIH/ZL is working with partners to launch a pilot project that uses drones to speed up specimen transport and referral from peripheral centers to the reference laboratory. This project aims to reduce turnaround time for diagnosis and thereby accelerate the initiation of effective therapy for various conditions.[19,20] Ultimately, the new reference laboratory seeks to cooperate with Haiti's National Public Health Laboratory to provide diagnostic referral support across the entire country.[21–23]

Strengthening Clinical Laboratory Systems

To make optimal use of its clinical laboratories and diagnostic equipment, PIH/ZL prioritizes the development of a skilled cadre of local laboratory professionals. Given the shortage of health workers and training facilities in Haiti,[14] PIH/ZL adheres to an accompaniment-based educational model, whereby local training opportunities are coupled with supervision provided by expatriate and in-country clinicians and laboratory experts. PIH/ZL has hired and trained several Haitian laboratory technicians and managers, including a medical pathologist, a quality management systems officer, a consultant on MDRTB diagnostics, 3 histotechnicians, a facilities manager, and a laboratory store manager. To support these professionals' career development, PIH/ZL works with various funders and implementing partners to organize capacity-building and mentorship initiatives (**Fig. 2**). Advanced training was recently offered in Mirebalais, Haiti, for employees working in the newly opened pathology section of Mirebalais Regional Reference Laboratory; specialists from Boston's Brigham and Women's Hospital and the Dana-Farber Cancer Institute conducted the training, offering on-site mentorship to laboratory personnel on the processing of specimens for cancer diagnosis.

In March 2017, PIH/ZL staff attended a cross-site laboratory training in Toulouse, France, which brought together professionals from PIH's Boston headquarters and from 8 countries in which PIH works for a weeklong workshop designed to improve laboratory skills, share expertise and best practices in global laboratory medicine, and strengthen collaborations among laboratory professionals working in places with weak health systems. The attendees also discussed methods to standardize laboratory policies, procedures, and strategies across sites and mapped essential diagnostic tests that should be available at each level of a health care delivery system, from communities to referral hospitals. Additional training was then provided on the operation and maintenance of diagnostic tools, such as the GeneXpert molecular technology—developed by Cepheid, which is based in Toulouse, France—for rapid diagnosis and monitoring of TB, including drug-resistant strains; HIV infection, including viral load and testing for early infant diagnosis; and markers of certain cancers.[24]

Other recent capacity-building initiatives hosted by PIH/ZL included a training on diagnosis of sickle cell disease, conducted by a specialist from Boston Children's Hospital; specimen collection and storage for Zika diagnosis; an annual workshop for more than 30 laboratory managers and technicians from PIH-supported health

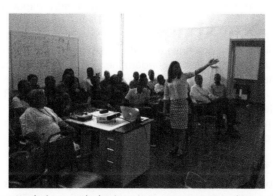

Fig. 2. Dr Fabienne Anglade, a pathologist, gives a presentation during a PIH workshop in March 2017 on laboratory systems in Haiti. (*Courtesy of* Daniel Orozco/Partners In Health.)

facilities; and a training for biomedical technicians on the maintenance of microscopes. In the coming years, as PIH/ZL expands its diagnostic services in microbiology, TB/MDRTB, and anatomic pathology, it will offer advanced training on these topics, on site and abroad.

In addition to developing highly skilled laboratory professionals and equipping them with the tools of their trade, PIH/ZL establishes rigorous protocols to ensure efficient, consistent, and high-quality diagnostic operations, while cultivating systems that can help achieve optimal clinical outcomes. These efforts have been facilitated by the implementation of a comprehensive data management tool in collaboration with the National Public Health Laboratory. PIH/ZL has established a laboratory management structure led by a Lab Coordination Team, which guides implementation and outlines strategy. PIH/ZL is also currently reviewing and updating a laboratory formulary to ensure that essential supplies are always available and accessible at PIH/ZL-supported facilities and that maintenance plans are in place for laboratory equipment. The organization continues to refine standard operating procedures and is currently pursuing accreditation for Mirebalais Regional Reference Laboratory. It has conducted a baseline assessment using World Health Organization guidelines and is developing a 5-year implementation plan to ultimately achieve accreditation based on International Organization for Standardization standards.

Improving care delivery in rural Haiti through the strengthening of diagnostic networks has demanded substantial financial and infrastructural resources. PIH/ZL has leveraged catalytic investments and donations to finance its laboratory operations—including the founding of Mirebalais Regional Reference Laboratory—and has established diverse partnerships spanning the public, private, and philanthropic sectors. These partnerships have involved Haitian public health institutions, academic medical centers, international health agencies, donors, philanthropic foundations, and various nongovernmental organizations. With the help of future fundraising and communications efforts, PIH/ZL's laboratory division is seeking to build new collaborations with research groups and advance surveillance of Haiti's burden of disease.

PATHOLOGY AS A PRIORITY: FROM HAITI TO RWANDA

According to a 2011 World Health Organization report, by 2030, cancer incidence will increase by 65% and cancer deaths by 71%, with more than 70% of the total burden occurring in the developing world.[25] Despite the massive burden of cancer in such settings, both oncology and pathology services are often absent or of poor quality in many low-income countries. Without adequate laboratory capacity, cancer cases go undiagnosed and untreated, often leading to death.

As discussed by Binagwaho and colleagues,[26] the provision of cancer care in low-income and middle-income countries has often been depicted as too complex and too costly; such dismissive attitudes have undermined efforts to introduce and link clinical oncology services and pathology laboratory services in poor places.[26] The costs of inaction prove to be much higher, however.[27] In both Haiti and Rwanda, PIH has debunked such faulty assumptions by effectively delivering cancer care in rural settings and achieving improved clinical outcomes.[28] These efforts have benefitted thousands of cancer patients.

Pathology in Rural Haiti

Prior to the establishment of PIH/ZL's cancer care program, cancer patients in Haiti would often wait months for a diagnosis or never receive one. These delays were in part due to the lack of accessible laboratories capable of providing pathology services and a paucity of pathologists in the country. Even today, there is, by some accounts, only 1 pathologist in Haiti working outside of the capital city, Port-au-Prince.

In 2011, PIH/ZL formalized an ongoing partnership, which began informally in 2003, with 2 academic medical centers in Boston, Massachusetts—the Dana-Farber Cancer Institute and Brigham and Women's Hospital—to offer free pathology services to patients at PIH/ZL-supported facilities in central Haiti.[29] Before the pathology section of Mirebalais Regional Reference Laboratory was opened in 2016, PIH/ZL sent patient samples from Haiti to Brigham and Women's Hospital for processing and diagnosis, while Dana-Farber Cancer Institute provided financial and clinical support for patient care and treatment. During this period, diagnosis still took months to accomplish, and patients, already presenting with late-stage disease, would become more ill and treatments more complex. Although challenging, however, pathologic diagnoses remain absolutely essential to cancer care. PIH/ZL's partnership with the Dana-Farber Cancer Institute and Brigham and Women's Hospital created a system in which clinical suspicion of cancer could be linked to biopsy, technical support from Boston-based oncologists, and treatment, if needed. A woman in rural Haiti with breast cancer, for example, can present at a PIH/ZL-supported health facility, obtain a diagnosis (with hormone receptor status), and subsequently receive appropriate hormone therapy or chemotherapy.[30]

Even as this system was refined over several years to expand the volume of pathologic diagnoses and accelerate the speed at which they were made, PIH/ZL deemed a high-quality, *local* pathology laboratory a critical priority for its network of health facilities. In October 2016, as an initial step toward this vision, PIH/ZL established and began operations of the pathology section of Mirebalais Regional Reference Laboratory (**Fig. 3**). That month, pathology specialists from Boston trained a team of 4 Haitian staff—3 technicians and 1 pathologist—and provided on-site training and mentorship. Clinical laboratory technicians were taught histopathology techniques, such as grossing and processing tissue collected by surgeons and oncologists at University Hospital. As a result, pathology samples are now grossed and processed into blocks on site, in rural Haiti itself, whereas in the past, such tasks were conducted by staff at the partnering Boston institutions (**Fig. 4**).

Since October 2016, the new laboratory has processed approximately 800 oncology-related biopsies taken at University Hospital and has created more than

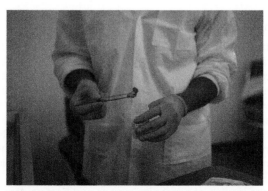

Fig. 3. Mirebalais, Haiti—November 17, 2016: Prophete Lagrénade, from Mirebalais Regional Reference Laboratory, holds a sample. Despite construction, technicians work at the new pathology laboratory at University Hospital of Mirebalais. (*Courtesy of* Cecille Joan Avila/Partners In Health.)

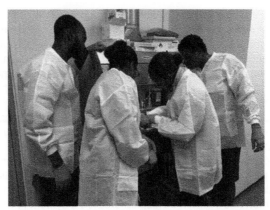

Fig. 4. Mirebalais, Haiti—October 19, 2016: Dr. Fabienne Anglade (*third from left*), a Partners In Health pathologist, trains laboratory histotechnicians (*from left*) Prophete Lagrénade, Bellevue Chantal, and Myrlene Mompremier in the newly opened pathology section of Mirebalais Regional Reference Laboratory. (*Courtesy of* Lauren Greenberg/Partners In Health.)

2000 paraffin blocks to be conveyed to Boston for further processing and reading. During this first phase of implementation, PIH/ZL is beginning to see a reduction in turnaround time between sample collection and results. Lower turnaround times ensure that patients receive the timely diagnoses needed to provide prompt access to care. In just a few months, the pathology section of Mirebalais Regional Reference Laboratory has directly elevated PIH/ZL's capacity to save lives and provide the highest quality care for the patients it serves.[31]

Currently, PIH/ZL and partners are in the process of installing new laboratory equipment, such as microtomes and embedding centers, and conducting further training. PIH/ZL anticipates further reductions in turnaround time and dramatic increases in on-site diagnostic capacity as Mirebalais Regional Reference Laboratory is expanded, which includes the addition of telepathology through collaboration with the American Society for Clinical Pathology. With investments in pathology diagnostics, training, and service delivery, the same Haitian woman with breast cancer will be able to receive a diagnosis in just days, as opposed to months.

Pathology in Rural Rwanda

Since 2005, PIH has partnered with the government of Rwanda to help build health systems in 3 rural districts of the country. Known locally as Inshuti Mu Buzima (IMB), PIH has accompanied the national health authorities in achieving some of the largest improvements in health outcomes and reductions in premature mortality ever seen in the world.[32] During this time, as it has combatted the heavy burden of chronic infectious diseases, including HIV and TB, and improved maternal and child health, Rwanda's Ministry of Health has also invested resources into the prevention and treatment of noncommunicable diseases and cancers. The country, with a population of approximately 12 million people, had just 1 oncologist, posing challenges to the treatment of cancer patients, especially in rural regions.

In response to the burden of cancer in Rwanda and Eastern Africa, as well as the gap in services to treat it, PIH/IMB worked with the Ministry of Health to establish in 2012 the first cancer center in rural Rwanda, the Butaro Cancer Center of Excellence, located in the northern Burera district. The Butaro Cancer Center serves as a national referral center and has seen thousands of patients in just a few years.[33] In partnership with the Dana-Farber/Brigham and Women's Cancer Center, PIH/IMB has pioneered a unique cancer care delivery model, whereby generalist physicians, internists, and nurses can provide oncology services.[34] Moreover, PIH/IMB has also developed nationally endorsed treatment protocols to apply and disseminate models pioneered at the Butaro Cancer Center.

When the Butaro Cancer Center was launched, PIH/IMB and the Rwandan government also created a pathology laboratory to strengthen the center's ability to provide accurate diagnosis and to link patients into timely oncology care.[35] Technicians were selected by the Ministry of Health to travel to the United States and receive intensive pathology training at Brigham and Women's Hospital. On their return to Rwanda, supplies and equipment were procured and pathology services implemented. Because no on-site pathologists were available at the time, technicians would initially create only paraffin blocks, which were subsequently sent to Brigham and Women's Hospital for cutting, staining, and diagnosis. As capacity was built, cutting, hematoxylin-eosin staining, and, eventually, immunohistochemistry techniques were conducted locally at the Butaro Cancer Center's pathology laboratory (**Fig. 5**). Now, approximately 90% of histology diagnoses are made locally. The Center's histopathology unit also serves patients from neighboring countries, such Burundi, Democratic Republic of the Congo, and Uganda. Laboratories send fresh formalin-fixed samples or tissue blocks for immunohistochemistry and consultation.

Telepathology was also initiated to bridge the human resource gap. Through an online telemedicine platform known as iPath, static images were uploaded by technicians in Rwanda and reviewed by pathologists in the United States and Europe, who commented and rendered diagnoses for patients seen at the Butaro Cancer Center. One recent study of this telepathology triage system showed 93% to 97% concordance between static image and standard glass-slide diagnosis (**Fig. 6**).[36] In 2016, a full-time pathologist was hired at the Butaro Cancer Center. Samples can now be read on site in less than 1 week, and cancer patients can initiate treatment soon

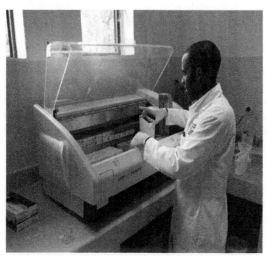

Fig. 5. Gaspard Muvugabigwi, histotechnician, prepares the automated staining machine at the pathology laboratory of the Butaro Cancer Center of Excellence in Rwanda in 2013. (*Courtesy of* David Shulman, Partners In Health.)

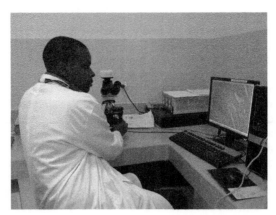

Fig. 6. Irenee Nshimiyimana, histotechnician, takes static images of a patient sample in the pathology laboratory of the Butaro Cancer Center of Excellence in 2015. (*Courtesy of* David Shulman/Partners In Health.)

thereafter. As a result of this phased approach, PIH/IMB's pathology services—once limited in scope and delivery—are now comprehensive and accessible, with services provided both on site and (with the help of the telepathology system) by more than 15 pathologists based outside of Rwanda.

In 2016, the Butaro Cancer Center developed a novel partnership with the American Society for Clinical Pathology, which, in collaboration with the Ministry of Health, has installed automated high-throughput histology equipment and a whole-slide imaging telepathology system. This leapfrog technology will aid the cancer center in becoming a pathology center of excellence for the entire country of Rwanda. Samples can be sent to Butaro, and complex oncology cases will be referred to this northern rural cancer center. As a result of this partnership and of several years of investments in capacity building, the Butaro Cancer Center of Excellence has become a beacon rural health facility and has shown that with prompt diagnosis and treatment, cancer need not be a death sentence in the poorest parts of the world.

CHALLENGES TO BUILDING LABORATORY CAPACITY

As PIH has learned, building laboratory capacity in places of privation brings with it several challenges. Identifying primary obstacles to successful clinical laboratories is the first step in overcoming them. In PIH's experience, these obstacles generally fall into 4 categories: laboratory workforce (staff), equipment and supplies (stuff), physical infrastructure (space), and the necessary systems to produce desired health outcomes (systems).

Staff

As with other components of a health system, laboratories across the globe suffer shortages of qualified staff. Remuneration for technicians and other cadres of laboratory workers is low. Moreover, formal training opportunities are limited and generally available only for basic laboratory techniques, limiting staff's potential for career development and clinical impact. The more specialized techniques discussed in this article, such as pathology diagnostics for cancer care and microbiology services for infectious diseases, are often available only at national reference laboratories or in the private sector, where the price of services prevents the poor from accessing them. Many laboratory personnel are appointed without having the academic credentials and technical expertise needed to carry out their responsibilities. Collectively, these circumstances lead to low staff retention, burnout, and chronically understaffed laboratories.[37,38]

Stuff

Even when laboratory workers are present, they often lack access to the tools of their trade, which include well-equipped laboratories, essential diagnostic tests that correspond to the burden of disease, and laboratory supplies and reagents.[39] As a result, laboratory personnel struggle to accept the low quality of care afforded to patients living in poverty but lack the means to improve it. Many under-resourced laboratories make use of obsolete technologies and rely excessively, for certain conditions, on rapid diagnostic tests, which are often used outside of laboratory settings without sufficient quality assurance.[40,41] The lack of equipment maintenance, servicing plans, and warranties further exacerbates the scarcity of diagnostic resources. Additionally, as laid bare by epidemics of infectious disease, like the recent Ebola epidemic in West Africa, the lack of personal protective equipment can compromise staff safety and lead to hazardous work conditions.[42]

Space

In many poor and remote parts of the world, laboratories are located in small spaces, often in the corners of clinics and hospitals. Services and operations, from specimen collection to testing, washing, recording, and reporting, are often conducted in a single room. Many clinical laboratories do not have consistent water supply or electricity, jeopardizing the safety, reliability, and timeliness of diagnostic testing.[43]

Systems

Without the staff, stuff, and space needed to deliver even the most basic diagnostic services, few laboratories are capable of considering the importance of developing systems, strategic plans, and protocols to incrementally improve their operations and strengthen patient care. Quality, biosafety, standardization, maintenance, and accurate recording and reporting are critical to well-functioning laboratories[44,45] but are often overlooked or deemed insignificant in the face of resource constraints. Laboratory guidelines and policies published by health ministries are often outdated, fail to adhere to international standards, and are frequently not even communicated to public laboratory staff around the country.

LESSONS LEARNED AND THE WAY FORWARD

Although challenging, PIH's work to create and expand laboratory capacity has been transformative for the patients it serves. PIH strives to provide a preferential option for the poor in health care by delivering the fruits of modern medicine and public health, with quality, to patients living in poverty, while accompanying governments in their efforts to build strong national health systems. As described in this article, after years of investments in Haiti and Rwanda, PIH now supports 2 reference laboratories—linked to 2 tertiary referral hospitals—in rural parts of both countries, an accomplishment few considered possible in settings that are often termed resource-poor.

Given the challenges that have been outlined previously, it is worth interrogating current trends in global laboratory medicine. One trend includes burgeoning efforts to decentralize laboratory capacity and incorporate rapid testing services at smaller, peripheral health centers without sufficiently introducing the staff, stuff, space, and systems needed to diagnose disease. Without consideration of such resource constraints, these efforts have largely failed to close the diagnostic gap in rural settings. Testing at such peripheral laboratories is done precariously, without proper materials, supervision, quality control, supply chains, and monitoring practices. Evidence shows that quality assurance is a concept widely understood by technicians and managers but rarely implemented in rural and peripheral health facilities. When done, laboratory staff often deem it an additional burden in the face of already large workloads and insufficient pay.[46,47] Because laboratories are made up of not only equipment and supplies but also people and systems, governments and their partners must invest more in training opportunities and operational planning to achieve clinical impact and population-level health gains. PIH's work in Haiti and Rwanda, although incomplete and having substantial room for improvement, provides 2 examples of how equitable diagnostic service delivery can be achieved.

PIH's laboratory experience supports alternative approaches to the tendency to decentralize without quality. Building proper transportation and referral networks—and better connecting peripheral laboratories to reference ones—can be an important provisional step as diagnostic capacity is decentralized. In conceptualizing Mirebalais Regional Reference Laboratory and laboratories in Rwanda, including that of the Butaro Cancer Center, PIH has found several benefits to strengthening reference laboratories. Regional reference centers can offer a more comprehensive menu of testing and diagnostics, of which pathology services are 1 example. They can also serve as sites for training and career development and help generate systems, protocols, training materials, and guidelines that can then be adapted and used at peripheral sites. Furthermore, the throughput of reference laboratories allows for greater automation and volume of services as well as lower overall costs for maintenance and servicing; they can, therefore, make better use of existing human, infrastructural, and financial resources and overcome the logistical constraints of replicating diagnostic operations across numerous sites. Because space is often limited in peripheral settings, central laboratories connected to smaller health centers can improve the storage and distribution of supplies, especially those requiring cold chains and consistent power when stored.

Of course, PIH's experience, which has largely been in rural and remote parts of Haiti and sub-Saharan Africa, does not support the termination of diagnostic services in peripheral health centers. Instead, in the same way that improving tertiary and district hospitals can strengthen care delivery at every level of a health system, investing in regional reference laboratories can have broad spillover effects. Several technologies available today—such as drone delivery and telemedicine, both of which PIH and its partners are piloting or currently employing—allow for easier transportation, shorter turnaround time, and improved connectivity between a reference laboratory and its corresponding network of health and testing centers. The reference laboratory plays a fundamental role in ensuring that operations in peripheral centers are streamlined and well supervised, and it fills critical gaps in services not routinely available.

Ultimately, future laboratory efforts should be patient-centered and build systems capable of supporting and integrating the chain of services needed to advance health equity. The 2013 to 2016 epidemic of Ebola virus disease in West Africa, for example, laid bare the hazards of inadequate diagnostic laboratory systems in settings of poverty and offers relevant lessons for the future of global laboratory medicine. In the years after the region's civil wars, plans to rebuild health systems and strengthen laboratory capacity were not executed and remained underfinanced, yielding limited capacity to diagnose hemorrhagic fevers and other diseases.[48] As a result, public health authorities failed to identify Ebola virus infections until March 2014—months after the start of the outbreak—and would continue to miss future cases within and across the porous borders of Guinea, Liberia, and Sierra Leone; initially, chains of illness and death were mistakenly attributed to other infectious afflictions causing similar symptoms.[49,50] Later in the epidemic, even as access to nucleic acid tests was expanded to boost laboratory confirmation of Ebola virus infection, most health facilities and Ebola treatment units lacked basic biochemical and hematologic diagnostics to monitor volume status, electrolyte abnormalities, and blood counts, impeding the delivery of effective supportive care and contributing to high case-fatality rates—by some estimates, more than 70%—during the epidemic.[51,52] By contrast, in settings in which clinical laboratory systems were strong and supportive and critical care could be delivered, local transmission was limited and clinical outcomes markedly better: of the 27 Ebola patients treated in the United States and Europe in 2014 and 2015, more than 80% survived.[53] Thus, in West Africa, weak laboratory systems undermined both surveillance of new cases and quality of patient care, compromising the integration of preventive and therapeutic interventions needed to halt epidemics of Ebola and other infectious pathogens.[54]

The case of Ebola in West Africa further buttresses another lesson that PIH has learned over several decades of building health systems in impoverished places: the importance of linking laboratory services with patient care. Diagnostic networks alone—that is, laboratories that are detached from clinical settings and unresponsive to local burdens of disease—are unable to facilitate care delivery and may therefore fail to affect health outcomes. At one hospital in eastern Sierra Leone, for example, investments by academic consortia and US government institutions had resulted in substantial improvements in laboratory infrastructure and research capacity prior to the outbreak. In the face of funding restrictions and in the absence of commensurate commitments to patient care, however, few improvements were made to the clinical facilities to which the hospital's laboratory was linked.[48] It was not surprising then that this part of Sierra Leone, even with its superior diagnostic capabilities, became an epicenter of the outbreak, suffering high rates of Ebola-associated mortality and health care worker infections.[55,56] In the outbreak's aftermath, with the departure of humanitarian groups and withdrawal of funding earmarked for disease containment, the region's health systems, including its laboratories and laboratory workforce, remain depleted of the staff, stuff, space, and systems needed to detect and treat disease.

The PIH experience, as summarized in this article, offers an alternative to such anemic, short-term approaches to cycles of poverty and disease. It challenges recent trends in global laboratory medicine to roll out basic or minimum packages of diagnostic services across health centers in low-income countries. Although such policy initiatives often have good intentions, they can neglect key health problems and fail to adequately capture local burdens of disease. Many tests are considered too expensive or not cost effective. The costs of not diagnosing (and, subsequently, not treating) certain conditions, however, often outweigh those of doing so. Moreover, surveillance of certain conditions and accurate understandings of disease burden remain limited without more comprehensive diagnostic capacity. PIH's delivery of pathology services in rural Haiti and Rwanda, for example, uncovered large numbers of previously undiagnosed cases of cancer and led to their treatment—in many instances, for the first time in the catchment areas served. This experience shows how national and international health authorities, along with their implementing partners, can reframe their approaches to laboratory medicine. Shifting from packages of basic diagnostic services based on tenuous notions of cost and feasibility to essential services based on disease burden and gaps in delivery can produce health systems that are both more effective and more equitable.[57]

ACKNOWLEDGMENTS

The authors express deep gratitude to the many partners—including the Haitian health authorities and various academic institutions, donors, funders, and local and international organizations—whose contributions have supported PIH's efforts to build quality clinical laboratory systems in service to the destitute sick. The authors also thank Cecille Joan Avila and the PIH Communications team for their assistance with figures and for their commitments to vividly illustrating the work of PIH.

REFERENCES

1. Walton DA, Farmer PE, Lambert W, et al. Integrated HIV prevention and care strengthens primary health care: lessons from rural Haiti. J Public Health Policy 2004;25(2):137–58.
2. Parsons LM, Somoskövi Á, Gutierrez C, et al. Laboratory diagnosis of tuberculosis in resource-poor countries: challenges and opportunities. Clin Microbiol Rev 2011;24(2):314–50.
3. Ridderhof JC, van Deun A, Kam KM, et al. Roles of laboratories and laboratory systems in effective tuberculosis programmes. Bull World Health Organ 2007; 85(5):354–9.
4. Farmer PE. Chronic infectious disease and the future of health care delivery. N Engl J Med 2013;369:2424–36.
5. Dominique JK, Ortiz-Osorno AA, Fitzgibbon J, et al. Implementation of HIV and tuberculosis diagnostics: the importance of context. Clin Infect Dis 2015; 61(S3):S119–25.
6. Petti CA, Polage CR, Quinn TC, et al. Laboratory medicine in Africa: a barrier to effective health care. Clin Infect Dis 2006;42(3):377–82.
7. Kebede Y, Fonjungo PN, Tibesso G, et al. Improved specimen-referral system and increased access to quality laboratory services in Ethiopia: the role of the public-private partnership. J Infect Dis 2016;213(Suppl 2):S59–64.
8. The World Bank. The World Bank in Haiti. 2015. Available at: http://www.worldbank.org/en/country/haiti/overview. Accessed July 29, 2017.
9. UNDP. Human Development Report 2016. United Nations Development Programme 1 UN Plaza, New York, NY 10017 USA. 2017. Available at: http://hdr.undp.org/sites/default/files/2016_human_development_report.pdf. Accessed July 29, 2017.
10. UNAIDS. HIV and AIDS estimates (2015). 2016. Available at: http://www.unaids.org/en/regionscountries/countries/haiti. Accessed July 29, 2017.
11. WHO. Tuberculosis Country Profiles – Haiti. 2016. Available at: http://www.who.int/tb/country/data/profiles/en/. Accessed July 29, 2017.
12. PIH. Cervical Cancer Program Expands in Haiti. 2016. Available at: https://www.pih.org/article/cervical-cancer-program-expands-in-haiti. Accessed July 29, 2017.
13. Louis FJ, Osborne AJ, Elias VJ, et al. Specimen referral network to rapidly scale-up CD4 testing: the hub and spoke model for Haiti. J AIDS Clin Res 2015;6(8): 1000488.
14. USAID. Health Infrastructure Fact Sheets – Haiti. 2017. Available at: https://www.usaid.gov/sites/default/files/documents/1862/FINAL_HealthInfrastructure_March_2017_0.pdf. Accessed July 29, 2017.
15. PEPFAR. The PEPFAR perspective on laboratory infrastructure. 2013. Available at: http://www.poweringhealth.org/index.php/community/stories/item/337-the-pepfar-perspective-on-laboratory-infrastructure. Accessed July 29, 2017.

16. RAND Corporation. Estimating the global health impact of improved diagnostic tools for the developing world. Research highlights. 2007. Available at: http://www.rand.org/content/dam/rand/pubs/research_briefs/2007/RAND_RB9293.pdf. Accessed July 29, 2017.
17. Drain PK, Hyle EP, Noubary F, et al. Evaluating diagnostic point-of-care tests in resource-limited settings. Lancet Infect Dis 2014;14(3):239–49.
18. PIH. Haiti. 2017. Available at: https://www.pih.org/country/haiti. Accessed July 29, 2017.
19. Amukele TK, Street J, Carroll K, et al. Drone transport of microbes in blood and sputum laboratory specimens. J Clin Microbiol 2016;54:2622–5.
20. Amukele TK, Sokoll LJ, Pepper D, et al. Can unmanned aerial systems (Drones) be used for the routine transport of chemistry, hematology, and coagulation laboratory specimens? PLoS One 2015;10(7):e0134020. Available at: https://doi.org/10.1371/journal.pone.0134020.
21. PIH. New Reference Laboratory to open in Haiti. 2016. Available at: https://www.pih.org/article/new-reference-laboratory-to-open-in-haiti. Accessed July 30, 2017.
22. PIH. Haiti's new Pathology lab accelerates cancer diagnosis. 2016. Available at: https://www.pih.org/article/haitis-new-pathology-lab-accelerates-cancer-diagnosis. Accessed July 30, 2017.
23. The Haitian Times. Hopital Universitaire De Mirebalais' New Lab Will Help Save Lives. 2016. Available at: http://haitiantimes.com/2016/07/11/hopital-universitaire-de-mirebalais-new-lab-will-help-save-lives/. Accessed July 30, 2017.
24. PIH. PIH Hosts First Cross-Site Lab Training. 2017. Available at: https://www.pih.org/article/pih-hosts-first-cross-site-lab-training. Accessed July 30, 2017.
25. WHO: International Agency for Research on Cancer. International cancer community welcomes global initiative for cancer registry development in low- and middle-income countries. 2011. Available at: http://www.iarc.fr/en/media-centre/iarcnews/pdf/GICR.pdf. Accessed July 30, 2017.
26. Binagwaho A, Wagner CM, Farmer PE. A vision for global cancer medicine: pursuing the equity of chance. J Clin Oncol 2015;34(1):3–5.
27. John R, Ross H. The global economic cost of cancer. Atlanta (GA): American Cancer Society and Livestrong; 2010.
28. Neal C, Rusangwa C, Borg R, et al. Cost of providing quality cancer care at the Butaro Cancer Center of Excellence in Rwanda. J Glob Oncol 2017. [Epub ahead of print].
29. Carlson JW, Lyon E, Walton D, et al. Partners in pathology: a collaborative model to bring pathology to resource-poor settings. Am J Surg Pathol 2010;34:118–23.
30. Sharma K, Costas A, Damuse R, et al. The Haiti breast cancer initiative: initial findings and analysis of barriers-to-care delaying patient presentation. J Oncol 2013;2013:206367.
31. Available at: https://www.pih.org/article/haitis-new-pathology-lab-accelerates-cancer-diagnosis. Accessed July 30, 2017.
32. Farmer PE, Nutt CT, Wagner CM, et al. Reduced premature mortality in Rwanda: lessons from success. BMJ 2013;346:f65.
33. Tapela NM, Mpunga T, Hedt-Gauthier B, et al. Pursing equity in cancer care:implementation, challenges and preliminary findings of a public cancer referral center in rural Rwanda. BMC Cancer 2016;16:237–48.
34. Rubagumya F, Greenberg L, Manirakiza A, et al. Increasing global access to cancer care: models of care with non-oncologists as primary providers. Lancet Oncol 2017;18(8):1000–2.

35. Mpunga T, Tapela N, Hedt-Gauthier BL, et al. Diagnosis of cancer in rural Rwanda: early outcomes of a phased approach to implement anatomic pathology services in resource-limited settings. Am J Clin Pathol 2014;142: 541–5.

36. Mpunga T, Hedt-Gauthier BL, Tapela N, et al. Implementation and validation of telepathology triage at cancer referral center in rural Rwanda. J Glob Oncol 2016;2(2):76–82.

37. Scott K. The Laboratory Workforce Shortage Demands New Solutions. 2015. Clinical Laboratory News.

38. Carden R, Allsbrook K, Thomas R. An examination of the supply and demand for clinical laboratory professionals in the United States. Transfusion 2009;49(11pt2): 2520–3.

39. Olmsted SS, Moore M, Meili RC, et al. Strengthening laboratory systems in resource-limited settings. Am J Clin Pathol 2010;134(3):374–80.

40. Mukadi P, Gillet P, Lukuka A, et al. External quality assessment of reading and interpretation of malaria rapid diagnostic tests among 1849 end-users in the democratic republic of the Congo through short message service (SMS). PLoS One 2013;8:e71442.

41. Seidahmed OME, Mohamedein MMN, Elsir AA, et al. End-user errors in applying two malaria rapid diagnostic tests in a remote area of Sudan. Trop Med Int Health 2008;13:406–9.

42. Hinshaw D. Ebola virus: for want of gloves, doctors die. Wall Str J 2014. Available at: https://www.wsj.com/articles/ebola-doctors-with-no-rubber-gloves-1408142137. Accessed July 29, 2017.

43. Abimiku AG, Institute of Human Virology, University of Maryland School of Medicine PEPFAR Program (AIDS Care Treatment in Nigeria [ACTION]). Building laboratory infrastructure to support scale-up of HIV/AIDS treatment, care, and prevention: in-country experience. Am J Clin Pathol 2009;131(6): 875–86.

44. Nkengasong JN, Nsubuga P, Nwanyanwu O, et al. Laboratory systems and services are critical in global health: time to end the neglect? Am J Clin Pathol 2010; 134(3):368–73.

45. Carter JY. External quality assessment in resource–limited countries. Biochem Med (Zagreb) 2017;27(1):97–109.

46. Klarkowski DB, Orozco JD. Microscopy quality control in Médecins Sans Frontières programs in resource-limited settings. PLoS Med 2010;7(1):e1000206.

47. Soares BEC. Quality of medical laboratory services in resource-limited settings. Afr J Infect Dis 2012;6(1):10–1.

48. Bausch DG. The year that Ebola virus took over West Africa: missed opportunities for prevention. Am J Trop Med Hyg 2015;92(2):229–32.

49. Baize S, Pannetier D, Oestereich L, et al. Emergence of Zaire Ebola virus disease in Guinea. N Engl J Med 2014;371(15):1418–25.

50. Sack K, Fink S, Belluck P, et al. How Ebola roared back. New York Times 2014.

51. Lamontagne F, Clément C, Fletcher T, et al. Doing today's work superbly well — treating Ebola with current tools. N Engl J Med 2014;371(17):1565–6.

52. WHO Ebola Response Team. West African Ebola epidemic after one year—slowing but not yet under control. N Engl J Med 2015;372(6):584–7.

53. Uyeki TM, Mehta AK, Davey RTJ, et al. Clinical management of Ebola virus disease in the United States and Europe. N Engl J Med 2016;374(7):636–46.

54. Farmer P. Diary. London Review of Books 2014;36(20):38–9.

55. Goba A, Khan SH, Fonnie M, et al. An outbreak of Ebola virus disease in the Lassa fever zone. J Infect Dis 2016;214(suppl 3):S110–21.
56. Schieffelin JS, Shaffer JG, Goba A, et al. Clinical illness and outcomes in patients with Ebola in Sierra Leone. N Engl J Med 2014;371(22):2092–100.
57. Schroeder LF, Guarner J, Elbireer A, et al. Time for a model list of essential diagnostics. N Engl J Med 2016;374(26):2511–4.

Building Cross-Country Networks for Laboratory Capacity and Improvement

Miriam Schneidman, MA, MPH[a],*, Martin Matu, PhD, MSc, MBA[b],
John Nkengasong, PhD, MSc[c], Willie Githui, PhD[d],
Simeon Kalyesubula-Kibuuka, MD, MPH[e],
Kelly Araujo Silva, MBA, MPH[f]

KEYWORDS

- Laboratory networks • Epidemiologic surveillance • Disease outbreak response
- Global health security

KEY POINTS

- Cross-country networks require well-defined governance structures, clear mandates, and concrete deliverables.
- Cross-country networks are effective in supporting peer-to-peer learning, and have the potential to generate efficiencies in responding to disease outbreaks and in conducting joint research and training.
- Networks have the potential to strengthen regional cooperation and foster mutual accountability.
- Drawing lessons from subregional networks can potentially be useful in informing the design of broader continent-wide disease control and surveillance initiatives.
- Consolidating and sustaining achievements of cross-country networks remains a key challenge going forward.

Disclosure Statement: The investigators report no conflict of interests.
[a] World Bank, Health, World Bank, 1818 H Street, NW, Washington, DC 20433, USA; [b] East, Central and Southern Africa Health Community, Plot 157, Olorien, Njiro Road, PO Box 1009, Arusha, Tanzania; [c] Africa Centers for Disease Control and Prevention, African Union Headquarters, PO Box 3243, Roosvelt Street (Old Airport Area), W21K19, Addis Ababa, Ethiopia; [d] Mycobacteriology Research Laboratory, Centre for Respiratory Diseases Research, Kenya Medical Research Institute, Kenyatta National Hospital Grounds, PO Box 47855, Nairobi 00200, Kenya; [e] Uganda National Health Laboratory Services, Plot 1062-106 Butabika Road Luzira, Kampala, Uganda; [f] Lacliv – Laboratorio de Analises Clinicas de Valenca, Travessa Silva Jardim, Centro 13 Valenca, Bahia, Brazil
* Corresponding author.
E-mail address: mschneidman@worldbank.org

Clin Lab Med 38 (2018) 119–130
https://doi.org/10.1016/j.cll.2017.10.009
0272-2712/18/© 2017 Elsevier Inc. All rights reserved.

BACKGROUND

Cross-country laboratory networks have historically played a critical role in supporting epidemiologic surveillance, accelerating disease outbreak response, and tracking drug resistance. Laboratory networks and enhanced diagnostic capacity are essential components of national and regional efforts to comply with the International Health Regulations and to build strong International Disease Surveillance and Response (IDSR) systems.[1] In the modern interconnected world with the increased risk of the spread of infectious diseases, having strong capacity to rapidly identify emerging pathogens, to contain the spread of diseases, and to notify others of outbreaks of international public health importance has taken on a new importance.[2]

In low-income and middle-income countries in sub-Sahara Africa, several cross-country networks have been established to facilitate timely sharing of epidemiologic information, build capacity, and introduce quality assurance systems to improve standards across participating sites.[3] Many of the networks have built on a historical record of collaboration among different stakeholders, with well-defined governance structures, common goals, and external support. The increase in funding for global health over the past decade[4,5] from the US President's Emergency Plan for AIDS Relief, President Obama's Global Health Initiative, and other bilateral donors offered an important opportunity to end the historical neglect of laboratory systems and services.

Laboratory networks are vital to well-functioning public health systems and to the global health security agenda, with innovative proposals to promote better integration of laboratory networks, surveillance systems, and public health institutes.[6] The recently launched Africa Centres for Disease Control and Prevention is expected to play a key role in this regard by strengthening disease intelligence and improving outbreak response and prevention capacity through surveillance and laboratory networks. Africa Centres for Disease Control and Prevention established 5 regional integrated surveillance and laboratory networks (RISLNET) that will offer a platform to better coordinate public health responses around the rescue coordinating centers (RCCs) in Egypt, Nigeria, Gabon, Zambia, and Kenya. RISLNET and the RCCs will provide opportunities for early detection and response to outbreaks, enhance disease intelligence, and combat antimicrobial resistance. The Africa RISLNET will ensure that public health assets in each geographic region are better leveraged to contribute to the broader agenda of disease management on the continent. Drawing lessons from subregional networks can potentially be useful in informing the design of broader continent-wide initiatives. One of the nascent laboratory networks, led by policy makers in East Africa, and supported by the World Bank, is the East Africa Public Health Laboratory Network.

INTRODUCTION

In 2010, policy makers in East Africa came together to establish a network of high-quality, accessible public health laboratories to combat the spread of communicable diseases in cross-border areas. All countries faced similar challenges, including emergence of multidrug-resistant tuberculosis (MDR-TB), frequent disease outbreaks, and limited laboratory confirmation of causative agents. Less than 1% of public sector laboratories on the continent were accredited, reflecting the poor state of facilities, lack of trained personnel, and weak quality management systems. Peripheral facilities had limited capacity to diagnose suspected MDR-TB cases, and needed to send sputum samples to the national reference laboratories for culture, which resulted in lengthy delays and risk of patient default. The continent had only 1 tuberculosis (TB) supranational reference laboratory (SRL), which could not respond to the growing demand from countries for technical support. Officials recognized that lack of access to quality laboratory services contributed to misdiagnosis, compromised patient care, and inability to detect public health threats efficiently.

Building on a long-standing record of cooperation, East African officials established a network that promoted mutual accountability and fostered solidarity. The network operates on the principle of not leaving anyone behind, recognizing that one country's inability to control the spread of infectious diseases can have negative spillover effects for neighboring countries.[7] The laboratory network supports the introduction of regional quality standards; facilitates the rollout and evaluation of new diagnostic tools; and serves as a platform for training, research, and knowledge sharing. Each country leads in a technical area, piloting innovations, disseminating good practices, and supporting neighboring countries (**Fig. 1**). The East, Central, and Southern Africa Health Community (ECSA-HC), an intergovernmental body that facilitates collaboration in the health sector, provides regional oversight and supports knowledge sharing. The network works through communities of practitioners that comprise experts in specialized areas such as laboratory accreditation, disease surveillance, and operational research. The governance structures are spelled out in legal agreements with clearly delineated roles and responsibilities for each party within the network. At the end of the first phase in early 2016 the network supported 32 laboratories that serve as centers of excellence in the 5 countries in East Africa (Burundi, Kenya, Rwanda, Tanzania, and Uganda). These laboratories have benefitted from state-of-the art investments, capacity building, and mentorship with more than 10,000 experts trained since 2010.[8] Building on the initial achievements, the financing was extended to 2020 with a total of US$128.5 million provided by the World Bank since 2010.

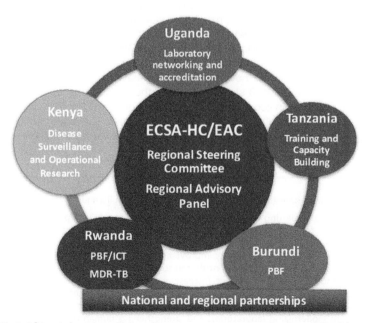

Fig. 1. East Africa Laboratory Network governance structure and model with countries' technical leadership and regional coordination. EAC, East Africa Community; ECSA-HC, East Central and Southern Africa Health Community; ICT, information communication technology; PBF, performance-based financing.

KEY RESULTS
Quality Assurance and Accreditation

Recognizing that high standards of laboratory practice are required to ensure reliable, timely, and reproducible results for clinical care and disease outbreak response, the network gave priority to introducing quality management systems toward accreditation.[9] Laboratory accreditation was widely viewed as an important aspirational goal of the networked facilities, given its role in benchmarking performance, instilling a culture of continuous quality improvements, and bolstering confidence of clinicians in laboratory results.[10,11] All facilities enrolled in the World Health Organization (WHO) Regional Office for Africa (AFRO) Stepwise Laboratory Improvement Process Towards Accreditation (SLIPTA) scheme and the related gold standard training program (Strengthening Laboratory Management Towards Accreditation [SLMTA]). A unique regional peer audit mechanism was introduced, whereby certified assessors trained by the African Society for Laboratory Medicine (ASLM) conduct annual peer assessments of laboratories in neighboring countries, promoting knowledge sharing, ensuring objectivity and transparency, and generating cost efficiencies.

Participation in the laboratory network has provided a structured and supportive process for piloting innovations. The network has promoted strong collaboration among practitioners, engendered healthy competition, and fostered mutual accountability. Participating facilities have shared good practices and received recognition awards for their achievements. Although non–project-supported laboratories in these countries also participate in the SLIPTA/SLMTA programs, the main advantages of being part of the network are the supportive environment for innovations and the efficiency gains from joint training, research, and knowledge sharing activities. Countries that have used multiple strategies, including intensive mentorship, facility improvement grants, and performance-based financing linking incentive payments to progress on the SLIPTA scores, have done well (**Box 1**).

Progress on quality management systems has been steady but occasional slippages have occurred. As of March 2017, more than 96% of project-supported facilities attained at least 2 stars, which was the original target, compared with 20% at baseline (2011). Most of the networked facilities have surpassed the initial target (**Fig. 2**) and a new target of 3 stars was set for the second phase. There has been considerable variability in scores within and across countries over time, with some facilities experiencing difficulties sustaining their star levels. The most frequent factors explaining slippages are staff turnover, equipment maintenance problems (contracts

---

Box 1
Performance-based financing for public health laboratories in Rwanda

An evaluation of the piloting of performance-based financing (PBF) for public health laboratories in Rwanda found improved laboratory performance at all project-supported sites as measured by the SLIPTA scores.[12] For the first time, laboratories were bringing in PBF revenues, instilling a culture of continuous quality improvements, and focusing management attention on accreditation. PBF seems to have contributed to an accelerated change, with PBF laboratories experiencing an overall greater increase in SLIPTA scores compared with project-supported laboratories in other countries. Although it was difficult to differentiate the effects of different interventions, the evaluation found a system-strengthening value to combining investments in modernizing laboratories, and strengthening human resources through PBF. Relationships between laboratory staff and clinicians improved, with laboratory managers having a greater voice in hospital management and laboratory staff increasingly valued and respected.

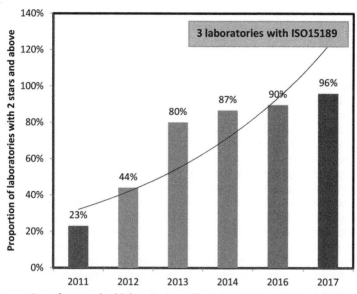

Fig. 2. Proportion of networked laboratories with at least 2 stars, 2011 to 2017.

and calibration), external quality assurance (EQA; comprehensive panel coverage), and reagent stock-outs. Three laboratories in the network have reached ISO (International Organization for Standardization) 15189 accreditation, including the Uganda Supranational TB Regional Laboratory (SRL), which now serves as part of the prestigious WHO SRL network. ECSA-HC mobilized a US$6.1 million regional grant from the Global Fund to operationalize the Uganda SRL, which is now providing specialized services and technical assistance to more than 20 National TB Reference Laboratories (NTRLs) on the continent, highlighting the importance of building African institutions and the power of networking.[13]

New Diagnostic Technologies

The laboratory network has supported the rollout and testing of new TB diagnostics, such as the GeneXpert, to improve access to more accurate testing for underserved populations in cross-border areas. The GeneXpert machine, approved by the WHO in 2010, was expected to revolutionize TB care, which continued to rely on sputum smear microscopy dating back to 1882 when Robert Koch showed the bacilli under a microscope.[14] "The launching of GeneXpert is a major milestone in diagnosis of TB. This is particularly important for us in Wajir, where patients travel hundreds of miles to get services," said one medical officer in Kenya. Since project inception, 35 units were deployed to the project-supported satellite laboratories in the 5 countries for use in rapid diagnosis of TB and detection of resistance to rifampicin, the first-line drug for treatment of TB and to provide an indication of possible MDR-TB.[15] A cross-sectional descriptive study was conducted to assess the contribution of the networked facilities to the national effort and to determine the number of potential cases of MDR-TB detected at these sites.[16] With the GeneXpert machines, facilities were able to conduct roughly 104,500 tests, accurately diagnosing MDR-TB (rifampicin resistance) within several hours, rather than waiting months for culture results, implying that drugs could be prescribed with greater accuracy, potentially saving time and money. Overall, out of 3847 MDR-TB cases detected at the networked facilities since the installation of the GeneXpert machines, 956 MDR-TB cases were confirmed at the networked laboratories. The distribution of MDR-TB cases detected from the networked laboratories and their relative share out of the national total was as follows: Tanzania (386; 35.1%), Kenya (147; 7.9%), Rwanda (35; 25%), Uganda (245; 41.1%), and Burundi (143; 98.6%).

Although these findings are encouraging in terms of improving access to rapid, accurate diagnosis and picking up missing cases, implementation challenges need to be addressed continuously. These challenges can prevent the scale-up of this novel technology with access remaining a major challenge for patients in low-income and middle-income countries.[17] An analysis conducted in Uganda found that, compared with using microscopy, some laboratory staff reported that this automated technology relieved workloads, served as a good proxy for MDR-TB detection, and reduced turnaround time to a few hours. At the same time, laboratory personnel encountered several operational challenges, such as limited operational funds, inadequate demand, equipment downtime, and poor specimen transport. Adequate financial resources for procuring warranty extensions, spare parts, and power backup systems was an impediment during the initial phase. Advocacy from different stakeholders resulted in the government including GeneXpert supplies in the national credit line system, so that the National Medical Stores can take over the procurement and distribution of these supplies. User acceptance was also a significant problem at project inception and required continuous sensitization (ie, clinicians' handbook, circulars, policy statements) of both clinicians and laboratory personnel with an increased uptake over time. Equipment downtime is not as frequent as it was at the initial stage, with the Uganda NTRL now supporting EQA and equipment maintenance nationwide. The manufacturer also recruited a representative to deal with technical repairs and maintenance, reducing the module annual breakdown rate to about 10%. As in other countries, the quality of the sputum sample and its efficient transport from other facilities influenced the accuracy of the results. Uganda incorporated TB samples into its HUB system to facilitate the collection, packaging, and shipment of samples (**Fig. 3**).[18] The TB Specimen and Results Transport System reduced turnaround time for receiving TB specimens from an average of 17 days in 2008 to 3 days by 2011, with the rate of sample rejection because of packaging-related issues decreasing to less than 10%. In light of the high rate of laboratory staff turnover, continual staff training is critical to maintaining high standards. Another challenge experienced in Uganda was related to the need to adopt clear guidelines. At inception, it was at the discretion of laboratory staff to subject only those sputum samples that were smear negative on microscopy to the GeneXpert. With the latest changes in algorithm for confirming TB, all presumptive individuals with TB receive GeneXpert screening without passing through microscopy.[19]

Operational Research

The network adopted an evidence-based approach with a strong emphasis on generating knowledge to inform public policy. In total, 3 multicountry, multisite studies were conducted through premiere national research institutes in the 5 countries. Likewise, staff from the networked laboratories were trained to perform more than 20 offshoot studies, in the spirit of empowering front-line workers. Under the leadership of the Operational Research Secretariat at the Kenya Medical Research Institute (KEMRI), a common methodological framework was developed for the 3 main multicountry studies that dealt broadly with reemerging diseases, including MDR-TB, *Escherichia coli* pathotypes, and malaria drug–resistant *Plasmodium* strains. The countries were

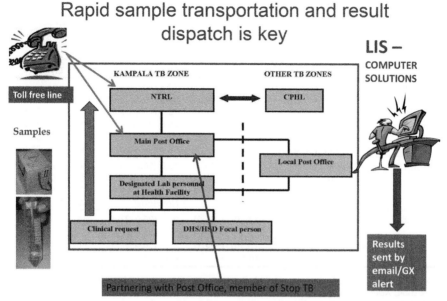

Fig. 3. TB and results transport system in Uganda, NTRL, MoH, 2016. DHS/HSD, District Health Services/Health sub-District; LIS, Laboratory Information System; MoH, Ministry of Health; NTRL, National TB Reference Laboratory; SMS, short message servive.

concerned with reemerging infectious diseases that are occurring with greater frequency in the subregion.[20] The offshoot studies dealt with a wide range of critical issues, such as identifying causes of loss to follow-up of patients with TB diagnosed and referred for specialized care (Tanzania). Eight articles were published in a supplement of the *African Journal of Health Sciences* (December 2014) and several newsletters of the KEMRI Secretariat (April 2016, June 2016, and October 2016). Participants from the national and regional study sites have shared results from the various studies at several seminars, workshops, and conferences. A comprehensive review of the study results is underway with a view to identifying potential policy implications.

The GeneXpert was found to have incremental value in detecting TB in smear-negative culture-positive, as well as human immunodeficiency virus (HIV)–positive, populations. As shown in **Table 1**, GeneXpert was able to detect TB in a higher proportion of HIV positive cases compared with fluorescence microscopy in Kenya (92%, 66%), Tanzania (96%, 80%), and Rwanda (72%, 57%). In addition, analysis using combined HIV-positive and HIV-negative samples indicated that sensitivity of the GeneXpert was higher than that of fluorescent microscopy in Kenya (86%, 74%) and Tanzania (93%,74%). The Kenya results were comparable with previously published data.[21] Specificity of GeneXpert was more than 90% in Kenya, Tanzania, and Rwanda. GeneXpert MTB/RIF showed excellent reproducibility of results and comparable performance of diagnostic tools, regardless of geographic setting in Kenya.[22]

The enteric study documented high and increasing resistance to commonly used antimicrobials for management of pathogenic *E coli* and *Shigella*, as seen in **Table 2**. There was variation in the rate of detection of enteric pathogens in different countries but at least 1 circulating enteric pathogen was detected in 4% of patients. Among the pathogens identified, *E coli* strains were found in up to 18% of patients in Kenya and considerably less in other countries. In Kenya, high resistance levels

Table 1
Sensitivity and specificity of different tuberculosis diagnostic tools among populations positive and negative for human immunodeficiency virus

Performance Assessment	Diagnostic Tool	Kenya % (95% CI)	Tanzania % (95% CI)	Rwanda % (95% CI)
Sensitivity stratified by HIV status	HIV positive: ZN	60.6 (48.8–72.4)	72.6 (68.9–76.2)	Not done
	HIV negative: ZN	75.1 (69.0–81.3)	75.8 (73.2–78.5)	Not done
	HIV positive: FM	65.6 (53.7–77.5)	79.8 (76.8–82.8)	57.1 (37.1–75.5)
	HIV negative: FM	77.6 (71.4–83.8)	75.8 (73.2–78.5)	51.1 (34.2–71.2)
	HIV positive: Xpert	92.3 (77.8–100)	96.3 (94.4–98.2)	71.4 (51.3–86.7)
	HIV negative: Xpert	83.3 (70.0–96–7)	96.4 (94.6–98.1)	50.0 (37.0–63.0)
Sensitivity	ZN microscopy	71.4 (65.8–76.9)	70.8 (66.2–75.4)	Not done
	FM microscopy	74.5 (68.9–80.9)	74.4 (70.1–78.7)	[a]49.8 (39.0–60.8)
	Genexpert	86.0 (75.7–96.4)	92.6 (90.3–94.9)	[a]67.1 (56.3–76.7)
	MGIT	Not done	Not done	94.0 (87.2–98.0)
Specificity	ZN microscopy	93.6 (92.2–95.0)	96.7 (96.0–97.4)	Not done
	FM microscopy	94.1 (92.6–95.5)	96.8 (96.1–9v 7.5)	96.0 (92.1–97.4)
	Genexpert	91.1 (87.1–95.1)	96.7 (96.0–97.4)	94.2 (65.1–95.9)
	MGIT	Not done	Not done	99.2 (98.2–99.7)

Abbreviations: CI, confidence interval; FM, fluorescence microscopy; MGIT, mycobacteria growth index tube; Xpert, GeneXpert; ZN, Ziehl-Neelsen.
[a] Significantly lower sensitivity values.

were observed, especially for sulfamethoxazole (93%), ampicillin (88%), and tetracycline (73%) among the *E coli* isolates. Among *Shigella* isolates, resistance was observed for sulfamethoxazole (89%) and ampicillin (88%). Emerging resistance to quinolones (ciprofloxacin and nalidixic acid) and gentamycin was observed for *E coli* (up to 18%), and *Shigella* (up to 39%) isolates.[23] In Rwanda, high resistance levels of *Shigella* isolates were found, especially to tetracycline (76%), ampicillin (67%), and sulfamethoxazole (61%).

The malaria study found an efficacy level of antimalarial drugs that was lower than the expected WHO threshold in Kenya, Tanzania, and Rwanda. The study used a single-blinded randomized, 2 arm, noninferiority clinical trial to assess the efficacy of dihydroartemisinin-piperaquine (DP) with artemether-lumefantrine (AL) as the comparative drug. The primary outcome was adequate clinical and parasitologic response (ACPR) at days 28 and 42. Overall, at day 42, findings showed the efficacy (ACPR) of 67.5% in patients on DP (arm A) and 79.7% in patients on AL (arm B) (**Table 3**). In Uganda, ACPR was 66% for the DP arm and results from the Al arm are pending. These efficacy levels in the two countries were less than the WHO standard, which states that an effective antimalarial drug is expected to give an ACPR of more than 90% (Kimani F, Omar S, Githui W. Evaluation of the efficacy of artemisinin combination therapy in children aged between 6 months and 12 years from EAPHLNP study sites in East Africa, unpublished data, 2017).

Disease Surveillance and Outbreak Preparedness

The networked laboratories played a key role in supporting disease surveillance and outbreak preparedness. Given frequent disease outbreaks in the region, policymakers aimed to bolster capacity to diagnose pathogens accurately, and to share information in real time. The 5 East African countries experienced outbreaks of various diseases, including Rift Valley fever, cholera, pandemic influenza, Ebola, and other viral hemorrhagic fevers. Most facilities had limited capacity to conduct outbreak investigations.

Table 2
Resistance profiles of enteric pathogenic *Escherichia coli* and *Shigella* to commonly prescribed antibiotics at the network facilities

	Amp % (95% CI)	Chl % (95% CI)	Cip % (95% CI)	Tc % (95% CI)	Nal % (95% CI)	Fur % (95% CI)	Gen % (95% CI)	Ery % (95% CI)	Ctx % (95% CI)	Stx % (95% CI)
E coli										
Kenya (n = 232)	88 (83–92)	25 (19–31)	15 (10–19)	73 (67–79)	29 (23–35)	14 (9–18)	14 (9–18)	86 (81–90)	19 (18–24)	93 (90–96)
Shigella										
Kenya (n = 99)	88 (81–94)	42 (33–52)	26 (18–35)	77 (68–85)	55 (45–64)	23 (15–32)	30 (21–39)	88 (81–94)	21 (13–29)	89 (83–95)
Rwanda (n = 82)	67 (57–77)	—	—	76 (67–85)	4 (0–8)	—	—	—	—	61 (50–72)

Abbreviations: Amp, ampicillin; Chl, chloramphenicol; Cip, ciprofloxacin; Ctx, cefotaxime; Ery, erythromycin; Fur, furazolidone; Gen, gentamicin; Nal, nalidixic acid; Stx, sulfamethoxazole; Tc, tetracycline.

Table 3
Adequate clinical and parasitologic response to dihydroartemisinin-piperaquine and artemether-lumefantrine at day 42

Country (ITT Population)	Arm A % (95% CI)	Arm B % (95% CI)	Expected (%)
Kenya	77 (72.2–81.3)	68 (62.0–72.5)	>90
Rwanda	83 (77.8–87.2)	78 (72.4–82.7)	>90
Tanzania	79.1 (73.5–83.9)	56.3 (49.9–62.4)	>90
Overall	79.7 (76.9–82.4)	67.5 (55.7–79.4)	>90

Abbreviation: ITT, intent to treat population.

Laboratory personnel were often not properly trained, or were involved in outbreak investigations. Health and animal health specialists worked in an uncoordinated manner. Critical information about events of public health importance experienced lengthy delays before reaching neighboring countries.

With the upgraded facilities, including new infrastructure, novel technologies, staff training, and modern information and communication systems, the countries are better equipped to cope with outbreaks. A cross-border surveillance and response framework was developed, and was endorsed by the East African Community ministers of health. The framework provided a new governance structure to facilitate intercountry collaboration on outbreak management. A greater number of outbreaks in cross-border areas were investigated jointly (eg, 2012 Marburg and Ebola outbreaks in Uganda; 2012 cholera outbreaks between Kenya and Uganda in the Mbale region; and a 2015 cholera outbreak at the border of Burundi and Tanzania). Cross-border multidisciplinary committees were established in 8 hot-spot disease transmission areas. These committees brought together disease surveillance coordinators, laboratory experts, veterinary officers, and immigration officials to develop joint plans. A regional, Web-based, electronic reporting system (electronic IDSR) was designed to capture critical data on 6 priority diseases (ie, measles, cholera, meningitis, malaria, MDR-TB, bloody diarrhea). Although this system represents an important step forward in terms of timely sharing of information, it involves challenges, because some countries are reluctant to share the type of information that may deter tourists and investors, and there are lingering concerns with quality and reliability. In addition, laboratory confirmation of outbreaks has greatly improved, with more than 88% of networked facilities reporting etiologic confirmation by 2016 compared with less than 20% at baseline (2011).

The network supported capacity building to enhance disease outbreak preparedness. Various tabletop simulation exercises in cross-border areas were conducted to strengthen capacity to deal effectively with epidemics. Training on novel approaches for managing outbreaks was performed in cross-border areas (eg, avian influenza in Busia, 2014; Ebola virus disease in Mbarara, 2014; viral hemorrhagic fever/yellow fever, Muyinga, 2012; Ebola virus disease in Namanga, 2016). All project-supported countries enrolled participants in the gold standard Field Epidemiology and Laboratory Training Program (FELTP), with more than 25 residents trained in this 2-year course. The FELTP residents were used strategically to support countries to investigate and respond to outbreaks, including the Marburg outbreak in Uganda (2012) and several cholera outbreaks that occurred in the region.

SUMMARY

- Cross-country networks need to adopt clear governance structures, agree on common goals, and leverage national structures. The roles and responsibilities of each party need to be clearly articulated and mechanisms and modalities for collaboration identified. Country capacity needs to be leveraged to contribute to regional goals. Adequate financial resources are critical to sustain network activities.

- Cross-country networks are effective for supporting peer-to-peer learning, and have the potential to generate efficiencies in responding to disease outbreaks and in conducting joint research and training. A notable example is the regional peer audit mechanism, which has proved to be an effective tool for facilitating cross-country learning and tracking performance. This model is not only novel and innovative but is also easily scalable to other countries and regions.
- Substantial improvements in quality management systems can be attained in a short time with countries learning from each other. Although progress is not always linear and slippages occur, remedial actions need to be taken to address common bottlenecks, such as staff turnover, equipment maintenance, and irregular supplies and reagents. Quality improvement indicators, as reflected by the SLIPTA scores, are important but not sufficient for assessing performance. Additional metrics (ie, test volumes, accuracy of test results, and turnaround time) will be useful to measure performance of networked facilities.
- Consolidating and sustaining achievements of the cross-country network will remain one of the key challenges going forward. Given that the network activities are donor funded, creative ways to mainstream innovations and sustain key interventions need to be identified. Some countries (Kenya, Rwanda) have absorbed personnel recruited under the project. Video conferencing capacity established at participating sites is facilitating ongoing communications and serves as a platform for continual knowledge sharing. Strong ownership of key stakeholders augurs well for institutional sustainability.

REFERENCES

1. Masanza MM, Nqobile N, Mukanga D, et al. Laboratory capacity building for the International Health Regulations (IHR[2005]) in resource-poor countries: the experience of the African Field Epidemiology Network (AFENET). BMC Public Health 2010;10(Suppl 1):S8.
2. Knobler S, Mahmoud A, Lemon S, et al. The impact of globalization on infectious disease emergence and control: exploring the consequences and opportunities: workshop summary. Washington, DC: National Academies Press (US); 2006. Summary and Assessment. Available at: https://www.ncbi.nlm.nih.gov/books/NBK56579/. Accessed April 11, 2017.
3. RESAOLAB– Fondation Mérieux. Available at: http://www.fondation-merieux.org/reinforcing-access-and-quality-of-biological-diagnosis-in-west-africa-resaolab. Accessed on April 2, 2017.
4. McCoy D, Chand S, Sridhar D. Global health funding: how much, where it comes from and where it goes. Health Policy 2009;24:407–17.
5. Ravishankar N, Gubbins P, Cooley RJ, et al. Financing of global health: tracking development assistance for health from 1990 to 2007. Lancet 2009;373:2113–24.
6. Onyebujoh P, Thirumala A, Ndihokubwayo J. Integrating laboratory networks, surveillance systems and public health institutes in Africa. Afr J Lab Med 2016;5(3): 431. Available at: http://www.ajlmonline.org/index.php/ajlm/article/view/431/718. Accessed April 19, 2017.
7. World Bank. Tackling communicable diseases in East Africa: power of laboratory networking. Available at: http://www.worldbank.org/en/news/video/2016/06/07/

east-africa-public-health-laboratory-power-of-networking. Accessed October 19, 2017.

8. World Bank. Rwanda works with a regional lab network to prevent epidemics. Available at: http://www.worldbank.org/en/news/video/2014/08/19/rwanda-works-with-a-regional-lab-network-to-prevent-epidemics. Accessed October 19, 2017.

9. World Bank. How can better diagnostics improve health in East Africa? Available at: http://www.worldbank.org/en/news/video/2013/03/22/how-can-better-diagnostics-improve-health-in-east-africa. Accessed October 19, 2017.

10. Opio A, Wafula W, Amone J, et al. Country leadership and policy are critical factors for implementing laboratory accreditation in developing countries. Am J Clin Pathol 2010;134(3):381–7.

11. The advantages of being an accredited laboratory. Available at: http://www.cala.ca/ilac_the_advantages_of_being.pdf. Accessed March 10, 2017.

12. Kumar M, Lehmann J, Rucogoza A, et al. East Africa public health laboratory networking project: evaluation of performance-based financing for public health laboratories in Rwanda. Health, nutrition and population discussion paper. World Bank; 2016. Available at: https://openknowledge.worldbank.org/handle/10986/24400. Accessed November 18, 2017.

13. ECSA-HC. Global Fund Laboratory Strengthening Project. Available at: http://www.ecsahc.org/wp-content/uploads/2016/08/The-Global-Fund-Project-Newsletter.pdf. Accessed April 19, 2017.

14. WHO. Xpert MTB/RIF implementation manual. Technical and operational 'how-to': practical considerations; 2014. Available at: http://www.who.int/tb/publications/xpert_implem_manual/en/. Accessed September 5, 2016.

15. World Bank. Saving lives with science: East Africa laboratory networks expand access to diagnostic services. Available at: http://www.worldbank.org/en/news/video/2016/06/08/saving-lives-with-science-east-africas-laboratory-networks-expand-access-to-diagnostic-services. Accessed October 19, 2017.

16. Mushi B, Matu M, Schneidman M, et al. Improved diagnosis of TB, including MDR-TB, using new TB diagnostic technology through the East Africa Public Health Laboratory Networking Project, ASLM, Cape Town (South Africa), December 6, 2016.

17. Pai M, Furin J. Tuberculosis innovations mean little if they cannot save lives. eLife 2017;6 [pii:e25956].

18. Schematic of National TB Specimen and Results Transport Network, Ministry of Health, Republic of Uganda, January 2012.

19. National TB Control Programme annual report 2015/16, Ministry of Health, Republic of Uganda, January 2017.

20. Mackey T, Liang B. Threats from emerging and re-emerging neglected tropical diseases (NTDs). Infect Ecol Epidemiol 2012;2(1):75–88.

21. Githui WA, Mwangi M, Orina F, et al. Performance of Ziehl-Neelsen microscopy, light emitting diode –FM and Xpert MTB/RIF in the diagnosis of tuberculosis in people with presumptive TB from EAPHLNP study sites in Kenya. Afr J Health Sci 2014;27(4):432–45.

22. Githui W, Mwangi M, Wanzala P, et al. Reproducibility of laboratory results and performance of TB diagnostic tools in different geographical settings in the Kenya World Bank – EAPHLN Project. Data presented at the 6th East African Health and Scientific Conference, Bujumbura (Burundi), March 29–31, 2017.

23. Sang W, Too R, Githii S, et al. Emerging antimicrobial resistance patterns of enteric pathogens isolated from children under 5 years of age in five EAPHLNP satellite sites in Kenya. Afr J Health Sci 2014;27(4 (issue No. 50)).

Strengthening Laboratory Management Toward Accreditation, A Model Program for Pathology Laboratory Improvement

Linda R. Andiric, MT(ASCP), MSc, EdD, Lawrence A. Chavez, PhD,
Mira Johnson, BA, Kenneth Landgraf, MSc,
Danny A. Milner Jr, MD, MSc(Epi)*

KEYWORDS

- SLMTA • SLIPTA • Laboratory • Training • Stepwise • Quality • Improvement
- History

KEY POINTS

- Strengthening Laboratory Management Toward Accreditation (SLMTA) and Stepwise Laboratory Quality Improvement Process Toward Accreditation (SLIPTA) have proved to be effective tools to empower laboratorians and improve laboratory quality in developing settings.
- Participants progressed more quickly when the laboratory leaders attended training and involved the entire laboratory staff in the improvements and changes needed.
- Access to mentors as well as supervisory visits were key to success.
- SLMTA/SLIPTA can serve as a useful model for improving laboratory quality across pathology disciplines.

BACKGROUND

Only 10 years ago, access to reliable diagnostic testing in sub-Saharan Africa was critically limited and misdiagnosis a common occurrence. Although reliable laboratory results can support clinical decision making and improve patient outcomes, unreliable

Financial Support: The American Society for Clinical Pathology (ASCP) is funded through the Centers for Disease Control and Prevention (CDC-RFA-GH13-1096) and the PEPFAR program (NU2GGH001096-04-01). The views and opinions expressed in this article are those of the ASCP staff and do not necessarily represent the views, opinions, or policies of the CDC or the President's Emergency Plan for AIDS Relief (PEPFAR) program.
Center for Global Health, American Society for Clinical Pathology, Chicago, IL 60603-5671, USA
* Corresponding author. American Society for Clinical Pathology, 33 West Monroe, Suite 1600, Chicago, IL 60603.
E-mail address: Dan.Milner@ascp.org

Clin Lab Med 38 (2018) 131–140
https://doi.org/10.1016/j.cll.2017.10.010
0272-2712/18/© 2017 Elsevier Inc. All rights reserved.

laboratory results prolonged illness or resulted in unnecessary or ineffective treatment regimens. With the wrong treatment, time and financial resources were wasted.[1] If and when diagnostic testing was available, the results were suspect. It was common for clinicians to ignore test results and proceed with patient care using only the patient's symptoms and the physician's clinical impression. Reyburn and colleagues[2] found that, among 4670 patients admitted to hospitals in Tanzania and treated for malaria, less than 50% had malaria confirmed by a blood smear. In the absence of high-quality laboratory testing, disease surveillance and epidemiology programs also lag behind.

Shortly after the millennium, in response to the growing human immunodeficiency virus (HIV)/acquired immunodeficiency syndrome (AIDS) epidemic, support for health systems strengthening in developing countries became a priority for many donors, including the World Bank; the United States (through the Global AIDS Program); and the Global Fund to Fight AIDS, Tuberculosis, and Malaria. Initially, funding was limited so efforts primarily focused on targeted technical assistance projects. With the introduction of the US President's Emergency Plan for AIDS Relief (PEPFAR) in 2003, spending scaled up rapidly and monies were directed to procure medications and direct patient care supplies. In order to deliver care to the number of individuals supported by these programs, it was quickly realized that efficient and reliable health systems, including quality laboratory services, needed to be supported. Laboratory infrastructure and personnel in Africa were insufficient to fill their role in the accurate diagnosis and treatment of infectious and chronic diseases.[3]

The best way for laboratories to ensure the quality of their testing results is to implement a robust quality management system (QMS). The International Standards Organization (ISO) has adopted ISO 15189 as the standard for laboratory quality and competence and this is designed to provide laboratories and laboratory auditors with a common set of standards for assessing a laboratory QMS. At the outset of PEPFAR, however, achieving international accreditation seemed like a daunting task for many laboratories in developing settings. In response, the World Health Organization (WHO) Regional Office in Africa (WHO-AFRO) began developing a stepwise program toward accreditation that provided a framework for auditing and monitoring laboratory quality and that rewarded incremental progress. On completion of the WHO-AFRO process, laboratories were ready to go forward to potentially achieve accreditation through ISO 15189. This approach was ratified and gained consensus during 7 meetings that took place through 2008 to 2011.[3]

1. The Maputo Declaration (2008) included 33 countries with the WHO; the World Bank; and the Global Fund to Fight AIDS, Tuberculosis, and Malaria. A declaration to strengthen laboratory systems was passed.
2. A meeting in Lyon, France, with WHO and the US Centers for Disease Control and Prevention (CDC) called for countries with limited resources to improve their quality systems by using a stepwise approach. It further recommended minimum standards be established.
3. At Yaoundé, Cameroon, in the 58th session of the Regional Committee (2008), a resolution was adopted emphasizing the urgency to strengthen laboratories with a request that WHO African Region support this effort to achieve improvement.
4. In Dakar, Senegal, at the fifth meeting of the Regional HIV/AIDS Network of Public Health Laboratories (2008), agreement was reached to support improvement for all laboratories without limitation to any specific disease.

5. In Kigali, Rwanda, in the presence of government health officials, WHO-AFRO in collaboration with CDC, The Clinton Health Access Initiative (CHAI), ASCP, and other partners launched the stepwise laboratory accreditation process (2009).
6. Later (2009) in Kigali, Rwanda, at the 59th session of the Regional Committee, among other infectious disease resolutions, a call for strengthening of public health laboratories was adopted.
7. In Nairobi in 2011, consensus of a key stakeholders meeting was achieved on the Stepwise Laboratory Quality Improvement Process Toward Accreditation (SLIPTA) Policy Guidance and Checklist.

The WHO-AFRO SLIPTA checklist, derived from ISO 15189, not only became the tool to assess a laboratory's stepwise progress in improvement but it also provided guidelines as to quality expectations for implementation. It gave credit for partial achievement rather than the pass-fail nature of ISO 15189 accreditation assessment.[3]

DEVELOPMENT OF STEPWISE LABORATORY QUALITY IMPROVEMENT PROCESS TOWARD ACCREDITATION: STRENGTHENING LABORATORY MANAGEMENT TOWARD ACCREDITATION

In addition to adopting the stepwise accreditation process for the 13 African countries during the first meeting in Kigali, Rwanda, a laboratory management improvement training called Strengthening Laboratory Management Toward Accreditation (SLMTA) was launched.[4] This program used 3 pillars, each essential in providing the necessary information for improvement in laboratory quality management.

Framework

The framework defined laboratory-specific management tasks that must be performed to accomplish quality outcomes in laboratory services. This list of tasks was created by ASCP, Clinton Health Access Initiative (CHAI), the Association of Public Health Laboratories (APHL), the American Society for Microbiology (ASM), the Clinical and Laboratory Standards Institutes (CLSI), and Becton Dickinson. The components of this framework were used to develop both the WHO-AFRO Laboratory Accreditation Checklist and the SLMTA training curriculum.

The framework organized laboratory quality management tasks into 4 levels (I–IV), which correlated to a typical tiered laboratory network. Level I tasks are those management tasks specific to national laboratories; level II for regional laboratories; level III for district laboratories; and level IV for community laboratories. Development partners decided to focus laboratory improvement at the regional and district levels, so the level II management tasks were used to guide the development of the SLMTA curriculum. Using the job task list as a guide, training was developed to detail: what to do, when to do it, and how to do it. An assessment checklist would then be used to observe the results.[5]

Strengthening Laboratory Management Toward Accreditation Curriculum

Based on the management tasks derived from the framework, training modules were developed to instruct laboratory managers (including managers of the laboratory, and quality and section heads) how to fulfill their duties in carrying out these tasks as expected. Rather than being descriptive or theoretic, SLMTA training was uniquely developed to be prescriptive and practical. Participants receive instructions for what to do and then perform the prescribed method either in the classroom or in their home laboratories. This hands-on approach provided assurance for both trainers and participants that the processes were understood and could be performed as intended.

Within the curriculum, there are 10 key areas of work tasks fundamental to level II to IV laboratories, as described in the framework. These key areas are:

1. Productivity management
2. Work area management
3. Inventory management
4. Procurement management
5. Preventive maintenance and equipment
6. Quality assurance
7. Specimen collection and processing
8. Laboratory testing
9. Test result reporting
10. Documents and records management

Training for these key areas consists not only of the expectations for accreditation but also how to accomplish and perform the tasks. Learning with hands-on activities as well as job aids provides practical use for participants' home laboratories.[5]

World Health Organization Regional Office in Africa Stepwise Laboratory Quality Improvement Process Toward Accreditation Checklist

The official accreditation tool to assess progress in laboratory improvement, the WHO-AFRO checklist, also functioned as a guide and an educational tool to instruct the exact expectations for quality and accreditation. The 12 sections of the WHO-AFRO checklist are based on the 12 CLSI quality system essentials (**Table 1**). By consensus of the 13 African countries, recognition for improvement in laboratory quality was to be awarded by a stepwise scheme of 1 to 5 stars, depending on the points accrued during a laboratory assessment using the WHO-AFRO checklist.

The checklist standards each have an assigned weighted value based on their complexity and/or importance. If fulfillment of a standard is incomplete but an

Table 1
Comparison of Clinical and Laboratory Standards Institutes 12 quality system essentials and Stepwise Laboratory Quality Improvement Process Toward Accreditation checklist sections

WHO-AFRO SLIPTA checklist version 2:2015	CLSI 12 quality system essentials
Documents and records	Documents and records
Management reviews	Personnel
Organization and personnel	Organization
Client management and customer service	Customer service
Equipment	Equipment
Evaluation and audits	Assessment
Purchasing and inventory	Purchasing and inventory
Process control	Process control
Information management	Information management
Identification of nonconformities, corrective and preventive actions	Process improvement
Occurrence management and process improvement	Occurrence management
Facilities	Facilities and safety

effort toward compliance is recognized, partial credit of 1 point is given. Laboratories are required to achieve at least 55% on the assessment to be awarded a 1-star recognition. When 95% or more is achieved, a laboratory is awarded a 5-star recognition and is deemed ready to apply for and receive ISO 15189 accreditation (**Fig. 1**).[3,6]

STRENGTHENING LABORATORY MANAGEMENT TOWARD ACCREDITATION MODEL

SLMTA is a hands-on, activity-based curriculum developed to provide and empower laboratory personnel with the skills and tools needed to implement laboratory improvement toward best laboratory practices as defined by the 12 CLSI quality system essentials and the standards of ISO 15189. The implementation of SLMTA consists of an initial baseline evaluation using the WHO checklist performed by an experienced assessor. Following the assessment, 3 week-long training sessions are conducted by individuals specifically qualified for teaching the SLMTA methodology. Each key area of laboratory management is guided by both the tasks needed for successful implementation of best practices within that key area (derived from the laboratory management framework) and the WHO checklist items that are related to it and must be accomplished before recognition is granted. At the end of each workshop the participants have either practiced the skill or task within the classroom setting or have in their possession the information they need to implement the learned improvements when they return to their home laboratories. Supervisory visits to home laboratories ensure that the skills are implemented as intended.

Between each training workshop, participants are expected to use the skills and tools provided in the workshop by implementing improvement projects in their laboratories. These projects are assigned at the end of each workshop according to the material covered most recently in the workshop and the specific gaps found during the laboratory's baseline evaluation. Trained mentors are often assigned to focus on specific laboratories to act as an immediate resource and to coach the laboratory staff in carrying out the assigned improvements. Mentors also assist with staff behavior change during this period of intense hands-on practice. Several supportive site visits by an overseer supervisory team of laboratory experts ensures that improvement projects are understood and are on track.

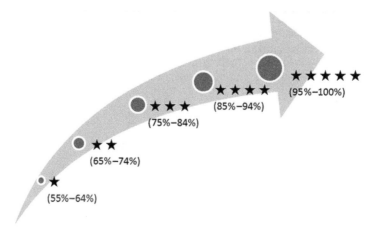

★ (55%–64%)
★★ (65%–74%)
★★★ (75%–84%)
★★★★ (85%–94%)
★★★★★ (95%–100%)

Fig. 1. SLIPTA tiers of recognition.

At the conclusion of 3 training sessions and 3 interim periods for implementation of improvements (typically 1 year), a second assessment of the laboratory using the WHO checklist is performed. From the second assessment, improvement is measured (**Fig. 2**).[5,6]

STRENGTHENING LABORATORY MANAGEMENT TOWARD ACCREDITATION TRAINING OF TRAINERS

After an initial pilot introduction of the SLMTA curriculum taught by SLMTA-trained instructors, most countries train a team of in-country trainers. Participants chosen for this training may be stakeholders, mentors, and other laboratory experts, and often are SLMTA participants from the pilot program who have excelled in making improvements using the SLMTA methods they learned. By training in-country trainers, countries take ownership of the SLMTA program in order to perpetuate the improvements throughout their countries.

The Training of Trainers (TOT) is a 2-week session conducted by SLMTA master trainers. The curriculum follows the same SLMTA modules, albeit not necessarily in the same order. During the first week, master trainers reteach the more complex offerings with special attention given to methodology, how to prepare visual aids, and how to encourage participant input. In addition to the SLMTA material, subject matter relating to methods on how adults learn best is given.

The second week is performed, for the most part, by the participants who have been assigned several SLMTA topics they and their small group will teach back to the master trainers, as if the master trainers were SLMTA participants. After each group teaching, the master trainer gives immediate feedback to the aspiring trainers that focuses on the positive aspects of the instruction as well as where improvement could be made. Statements such as: "I liked the way you..." or "I wish you would have..." are meant to be instructive rather than critical. Clarification of any misunderstanding of subject matter is also addressed at this time. At the conclusion of the second week of training, SLMTA master trainers typically recommend trainers who are ready to teach.

ESTABLISHMENT OF AFRICAN SOCIETY FOR LABORATORY MEDICINE AND ADOPTION OF THE WORLD HEALTH ORGANIZATION STEPWISE LABORATORY QUALITY IMPROVEMENT PROCESS TOWARD ACCREDITATION CHECKLIST

The African Society for Laboratory Medicine (ASLM) is a professional organization, partnered with the CDC, advocating for the important role and needs of laboratory medicine throughout Africa. The ASLM was established as a response to WHO Resolution AFR/RC58/R2 for strengthening public health laboratories and the Maputo Declaration on strengthening laboratory systems by working collaboratively with

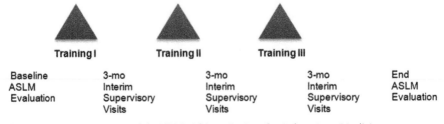

Fig. 2. SLMTA program model. ASLM, African Society for Laboratory Medicine.

governments, local and international organizations, implementing partners, and private sectors to achieve the following goals by 2020:

- Strengthening laboratory workforces by training and certifying laboratory professionals and clinicians through standardized frameworks
- Transforming laboratory testing quality by enrolling laboratories in quality improvement programs to achieve accreditation by international standards
- Developing strong, harmonized regulatory systems for diagnostic products as defined by the Global Harmonization Taskforce
- Building a network of national public health reference laboratories to improve early disease detection and collaborative research

In 2011, the ASLM began its role in certifying laboratories with the use of the WHO-AFRO checklist derived from ISO 15189 standards and the CLSI 12 quality system essentials. This checklist was implemented by ASLM and, along with the assessment process, became known as SLIPTA.

During a standardized process of application and assessment, SLIPTA measures and evaluates the progress that laboratories make toward international accreditation (ISO 15189). SLIPTA enables laboratories to develop their QMSs to improve and produce timely and accurate laboratory results in a stepwise manner. A certificate of recognition is awarded (0–5 star ratings) for the progress made at the time of the assessment. When 5-star recognition is awarded, laboratories are considered ready for international ISO 15189 accreditation.[7]

PARTICIPATING COUNTRIES AND PROGRESS

As of December 2016, 1103 laboratories in 47 countries have implemented the SLMTA program. In total, 63 master trainers have been trained, capable of rolling out SLMTA TOT workshops and supporting the dissemination of the curriculum.[8] Of participating laboratories, 38 (3.4%) have gone on to achieve ISO 15189 accreditation.[9]

Over the past 4 years, the ASLM has established its role as the lead auditor for the SLIPTA program. By the end of 2016, 242 laboratories in 19 countries had been audited by ASLM teams. ASLM has identified several common weaknesses across countries, regions, and laboratory tiers.[10] Of all laboratories audited by ASLM, 11.7% received 0 stars, 23.5% received 1 star, 33.2% received 2 stars, 23.5% received 3 stars, 7% received 4 stars, and 1% received 5 stars.[11] The topics of management reviews, internal audits, and corrective action are consistently identified as areas of weakness in the assessed laboratories. The ASLM has set ambitious goals for 2020: enrolling 2500 laboratories and supporting the accreditation of 250 laboratories to international standards. To accomplish this, they propose to scale-up training programs and further expand their team of qualified laboratory quality auditors.[10]

THE CONTRIBUTION OF THE AMERICAN SOCIETY FOR CLINICAL PATHOLOGY AND ITS MEMBERS TO THE STRENGTHENING LABORATORY MANAGEMENT TOWARD ACCREDITATION MOVEMENT

The American Society for Clinical Pathology (ASCP) has supported the SLMTA program since its inception in 2009. To date, ASCP has directly supported the training of 829 SLMTA participants in 22 training cohorts. In order to institutionalize SLMTA and build local capacity, the ASCP also provide SLMTA TOT workshops for 344 participants, and targeted mentorship training for 214. Building on these efforts, the ASCP initiated a program to institutionalize the SLMTA curriculum at the preservice level by providing SLMTA training to medical educators in 2 countries: Vietnam and

Lesotho. To address gaps in the original SLMTA training program, the ASCP has offered numerous specialized workshops in quality control, document management, biosafety, external quality assurance, and internal audits. Likewise, 42 participants from Mozambique and Ethiopia have completed the follow-up SLMTA 2 curriculum (described later). In total, SLMTA programs in 13 countries have received direct support through ASCP's PEPFAR program.

LESSONS LEARNED

Laboratories participating in SLMTA progressed more quickly when the laboratory manager and quality officer who were chosen to attend the SLMTA trainings returned to their laboratories and included the entire laboratory staff in the improvements and changes needed. When only the attendees to the training tried to implement the newly learned skills, there was often resistance to the changes by staff members who were accustomed to established routines. When mentors were assigned to sites and worked directly with staff in the implementation of modifications, they had the time to explain and convince staff members why the changes were necessary. At subsequent training sessions, laboratories shared their successes and how they overcame obstacles encountered during implementation.

Mentors as well as supervisory visits were key to success. On the occasions when a laboratory was remotely located and mentors were not accessible or available in the area and/or supervisory visits were difficult, a noticeable lag in improvement was noted. Time would be lost as laboratories that worked alone and isolated lost their training inspiration and even forgot or misunderstood what they had learned. It was important to keep up the momentum for improvement to have resources available for both clarification and encouragement.

The most successful laboratories during the initial phase of improvement were those facilities whose chief officers/administrator stakeholders were committed to the project. When this happened and the laboratory staff were encouraged and commended on progress by the chief operating officer, success continued to occur.

SLMTA teaches the development of many logs and checklists to document maintenance and all aspects of quality management with the warning that tasks not documented are not considered completed. After setting up procedures to accomplish these tasks, laboratories often failed to continue the record keeping. This failure was especially noted when a laboratory's WHO assessment was due and they had to wait a long time or if it was postponed. This long wait did not necessarily occur after the training sessions were complete, but sometimes occurred while awaiting an official assessment by the ASLM, which was initially backlogged with assessment requests.

It is noteworthy that SLMTA training, when completed successfully, provides laboratories the ability to implement changes necessary to obtain a 3-star recognition. The framework of tasks and the WHO SLIPTA checklist further guide the requirements necessary for 5-star recognition and for the requirements that need to be performed by countrywide policy changes, such health/safety and supply and capital equipment procurement. In addition, there are subject matters introduced in SLMTA training but not presented in depth:

- Quality control
- Writing SOPs (standard operating procedures)
- Management of documents and records

A supplemental SLMTA workshop focused on quality control was piloted in 2013 to partially address this gap. However, to address additional weaknesses identified in

SLMTA participants' SLIPTA postassessments, the SLMTA 2 program was launched in 2016. SLMTA 2 does not modify or replace the existing SLMTA curriculum but builds on it to provide the extra push laboratories need to achieve 5 stars. SLMTA 2 covers quality control, method validation, measurement analysis and improvement, internal audit, occurrence management, root cause analysis, and corrective action.

The SLMTA program, in combination with the SLIPTA checklist and process, has proved to be an effective tool to empower laboratorians and improve laboratory quality in developing settings. The SLIPTA checklist can provide useful program feedback to national and international partners, enabling them to create tailored education programs to address specific gaps. SLMTA, by providing practical tools and methods, has enabled thousands of laboratorians to implement quality system improvements in their laboratories, thus resulting in improved patient care. As shown by postassessment SLIPTA score, however, additional interventions after SLMTA are required for laboratories to reach the level of international accreditation. International partners should focus their efforts to address the specific needs of national laboratory quality programs and continue to support the adoption of quality standards and the establishment of national accreditation programs. Although the HIV/AIDS epidemic was the primary motivation for SLMTA and SLIPTA, the tools have been implemented in a wide variety of laboratories and disease programs. They can serve as a useful model for improving laboratory quality across pathology disciplines, and their content and training methodology can contribute to preservice laboratory training programs as well.

ACKNOWLEDGMENTS

The authors would like to acknowledge the long-standing contributions of Katy Yao (CDC) to the success of the SLMTA program as well as the World Health Organization for moving the program to the forefront of laboratory improvement. ASCP would like to especially thank Anna Murphy and Mary Kathryn Linde for their contributions to training in Africa through ASCP's PEPFAR-funded SLMTA activities.

REFERENCES

1. Petti CA, Polage CR, Quinn TC, et al. Laboratory medicine in Africa: a barrier to effective health care. Clin Infect Dis 2006;42:377–82.
2. Reyburn H, Mbatia R, Drakeley C, et al. Overdiagnosis of malaria in patients with severe febrile illness in Tanzania: a prospective study. BMJ 2004;329:1212–7.
3. Gershy-Damet G, Rotz P, Cross D, et al. The World Health Organization African region laboratory accreditation process. Am J Clin Pathol 2010;134:393–400.
4. Nkengasong JN. A shifting paradigm in strengthening laboratory health systems for global health. Am J Clin Pathol 2010;134:359–60.
5. Yao K, McKinney B, Murphy A, et al. An innovative training approach to accelerate laboratory accreditation. Am J Clin Pathol 2010;134:401–9.
6. Andiric LR, Masambu CG. Laboratory quality improvement in Tanzania. Am J Clin Pathol 2015;143:1–7.
7. ASLM.org.
8. Yao, K. SLMTA updates. SLIPTA/SLMTA symposium 2016. December 2016, Cape Town, South Africa. [Online]. Available at: https://slmta.org/uploads/category_file/28/1.3%20-%20SLMTA%20Updates.pdf. Accessed July 18, 2017.
9. SLMTA laboratories that have achieved accreditation. [Online]. Available at: https://slmta.org/accredited-labs/. Accessed August 11, 2017.

10. WHO/AFRO SLITPA update. SLIPTA/SLMTA symposium 2016. December 2016, Cape Town, South Africa. [Online]. Available at: https://slmta.org/uploads/category_file/29/1.4%20-%20SLIPTA%20Updates.pdf. Accessed July 18, 2017.

11. SLIPTA database analysis. [Online Query]. Available at: http://www.aslm.org/resource-centre/slipta-map/slipta-database-analysis/. Accessed August 11, 2017.

Practical Successes in Telepathology Experiences in Africa

Nathan D. Montgomery, MD, PhD[a], Tamiwe Tomoka, MD[b],
Robert Krysiak, MS[b], Eric Powers, BA[a], Maurice Mulenga, MBBS, MD[c],
Coxcilly Kampani, BS[b], Fred Chimzimu, BS[b],
Michael K. Owino, MPH[b], Bal Mukunda Dhungel, MBBS, MD[c],
Satish Gopal, MD, MPH[b,d], Yuri Fedoriw, MD[a,d,*]

KEYWORDS

- Telepathology • Digital pathology • Africa • Resource-limited setting
- Whole-slide imaging

KEY POINTS

- Anatomic pathology services are lacking in much of Africa.
- Telepathology infrastructure can help support local pathology services, clinical care, and research in this setting.
- The most important features of a successful program include consistent participation of team members and reliable Internet service.

INTRODUCTION

Across much of Africa, there is a critical shortage of pathology services. A survey from 2016 estimated that there are more than 500,000 people per pathologist in much of the

Disclosures: The authors have no relevant conflicts of interest to disclose.
Funding/Acknowledgments: The Kamuzu Central Hospital Pathology Laboratory is supported by grants from the National Institutes of Health (K01TW009488, R21CA180815, U54CA190152, P20CA210285), the Medical Education Partnership Initiative (U2GPS001965), the Lineberger Comprehensive Cancer Center (P30CA016086), and the UNC Center for AIDS Research (P30AI50410).
[a] Department of Pathology and Laboratory Medicine, The University of North Carolina School of Medicine, CB 7525, Chapel Hill, NC 27599-7525, USA; [b] UNC Project Malawi, Tidziwe Centre, Private Bag A-104, Lilongwe, Malawi; [c] Kamuzu Central Hospital, Tidziwe Centre, PO Box 149, Lilongwe, Malawi; [d] Lineberger Comprehensive Cancer Center, CB 7295, Chapel Hill, NC 27599-7295, USA
* Corresponding author. Department of Pathology and Laboratory Medicine, The University of North Carolina School of Medicine, CB 7525, Chapel Hill, NC 27599-7525.
E-mail address: Yuri.Fedoriw@unchealth.unc.edu

Clin Lab Med 38 (2018) 141–150
https://doi.org/10.1016/j.cll.2017.10.011
0272-2712/18/© 2017 Elsevier Inc. All rights reserved.

continent, with this ratio exceeding 5 million to 1 in some countries.[1] In large part, lack of diagnostic pathology mirrors access to other medical services. However, even in settings where specialty-level clinical care, such as medical oncology, is available, access to anatomic pathology services has often lagged behind.[1–3]

Cancer registries from the region reflect this problem. For instance, fewer than 20% of cancer cases were pathologically confirmed in the most recent registry from Malawi.[4] This discrepancy creates an untenable scenario where treating clinicians and their patients are often forced to make medical decisions without the benefit of a tissue diagnosis.[2] Even where pathologists are available, they often work in relative isolation with large case volumes and difficult case material. In our experience, cytology, dermatopathology, hematopathology, and pediatric pathology, all of which may require subspecialty training beyond residency in the United States, often represent a disproportionate percentage of cases.

Digital telepathology has been touted as a tool to help overcome the pathologist shortage in Africa, and some successful examples have been reported in the literature.[5–10] Such programs are generally supported by international collaborations between hospitals or medical schools in Africa and institutions in the United States or Europe.

In broad terms, there are four basic platforms for telepathology: (1) static images, (2) whole-slide scanning, (3) dynamic nonrobotic telemicroscopy, and (4) dynamic robotic telemicroscopy.[11] These approaches vary dramatically in terms of instrumentation cost, information technology (IT) support, and need for local pathology expertise (**Table 1**). For instance, static images have the benefit of requiring limited technical infrastructure (only a microscope, digital camera, and Internet connection) but depend on appropriate selection of diagnostic fields. With appropriate training of technologists, this approach has proven effective in some centers. A particularly successful example of this approach has been reported from the Butaro Cancer Center of Excellence in Rwanda, where a static-image telepathology system was established in collaboration with Partners in Health and the Dana-Farber Brigham and Women's Cancer Center.[12] After an intensive training period, static-image telepathology diagnoses were 97% concordant with subsequent glass slide review. These results highlight the potential for remarkable accuracy when applying this approach to appropriately selected cases. In the published Butaro experience, hematoxylin-eosin stained slides were available for all cases, and carcinomas represented nearly 90% of all malignant diagnoses. Field selection may be more challenging when applied to cytologic preparations and hematologic malignancies.

By comparison, whole-slide imaging systems allow the consulting pathologist to see the entire specimen at a range of magnifications. However, these advantages come at considerable cost, including purchase of slide scanning equipment, increased IT support, and server space to allow data storage. Both dynamic nonrobotic and robotic telemicroscopy systems allow consulting pathologists to review slides in real-time from a remote microscope. Dynamic nonrobotic telemicroscopy is technically much simpler and involves transmission of video images across any of several Internet-based teleconference systems, such as Skype or Zoom Video Communications.[13] Similarly to static-imaging systems, dynamic nonrobotic telemicroscopy works best when a skilled local pathologist is available to "drive" the microscope. Although dependent on image resolution/camera quality and Internet speed, this system provides the benefit of whole-slide review at much lower cost than whole-slide imaging systems. Finally, robotic telemicroscopy, a system that allows the consulting pathologist to control the stage and objectives of a microscope remotely, has been less frequently used in low-income countries because of cost and technical challenges. However, all of these approaches have been implemented with reported success in Africa.[5–10]

Table 1
Telepathology platform overview

Method	Relative Cost	Local Support	Published Examples

Static images	Low
	Specimen processing
	Microscope
	Digital camera
	Internet connection
	Minimal IT support
		Local technical expertise:
		  Essential: Necessary for specimen processing
		Local pathology expertise:
		  Essential: Local pathologic expertise necessary for selection of diagnostic fields
			Gimbel et al,[9] 2012

Whole-slide imaging	High
	Specimen processing
	Slide scanning equipment
	Internet connection
	Server space
	Substantial IT support
		Local technical expertise:
		  Essential: Necessary for specimen processing
		Local pathology expertise:
		  Not essential: Local pathology less critical given whole slide scanning
			Pagni et al,[6] 2011; Montgomery et al,[10] 2016

Dynamic nonrobotic telemicroscopy	Low
	Specimen processing
	Microscope
	Digital camera
	Internet connection
	Moderate IT support
		Local technical expertise:
		  Essential: Necessary for specimen processing
		Local pathology expertise:
		  Essential: Local pathologic expertise necessary for selection of diagnostic fields
			UNC Project Malawi (unpublished work, Robert Krysiak, MS, 2017)

Dynamic robotic telemicroscopy	High
	Specimen processing
	Microscope
	Digital camera
	Internet connection
	Robotic microscopy unit
	Substantial IT support
		Local technical expertise:
		  Essential: Necessary for specimen processing
		Local pathology expertise:
		  Not essential: Local pathologic less critical as microscope controlled remotely
			Wamala et al,[7] 2011

Abbreviation: IT, information technology.

Herein, we describe successful implementation of telepathology services to support local pathologists and clinical care, with an emphasis on our experience at Kamuzu Central Hospital (KCH) in Lilongwe, Malawi.

ROLE OF TELEPATHOLOGY IN OUR CLINICAL PRACTICE

The KCH Pathology Laboratory opened in 2011 as a collaborative effort between KCH, the Malawi Ministry of Health, and the University of North Carolina at Chapel Hill (UNC).[2,3] Two years later, we initiated a telepathology program using whole-slide imaging on the Aperio Digital Pathology System (Leica Biosystems, Buffalo Grove, IL) to support local pathologists, clinical care, and research efforts. Technical details of this system are outlined in the next section.

At KCH, biopsies and cytology specimens are submitted to the pathology laboratory, which is directed by a Malawian pathologist and provides basic cytology and histology processing, and a limited panel of manual immunohistochemical (IHC) stains.[3,10] Cases are initially reviewed by local pathologists, who generally communicate an initial impression to clinicians, often after ordering supporting IHC stains.

In difficult cases, and before enrollment in UNC-affiliated research studies, slides are then scanned and loaded to a secure server, which collaborating US pathologists access via a virtual private network connection. Once each week, Malawi-based clinicians and pathologists present these patients at a telepathology conference, which is attended by local providers and their counterparts in the United States (**Fig. 1**). After discussion and frequently after additional rounds of IHC stains, a consensus diagnosis is rendered by the pathologist in Malawi. This framework has provided critical support to the ongoing Kamuzu Central Hospital Lymphoma study. As part of that study, biopsies from all enrolled patients are shipped to the United States for final pathology review, typically after a much larger panel of IHC stains is performed. Even after incorporating additional immunophenotypic data, we have demonstrated that diagnoses rendered at the weekly telepathology conference are highly accurate (only ~5% major discordance) for guiding clinical care under local conditions.[10]

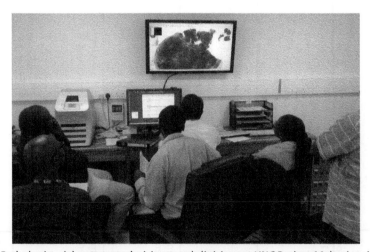

Fig. 1. Pathologists, laboratory technicians, and clinicians at UNC Project-Malawi review digital slides with their US collaborators in a telepathology conference using the Aperio system. Approximately 10 to 15 cases are reviewed at these weekly conferences.

From inception, incorporation of telepathology into the clinical workflow at KCH has been modeled after internal multidisciplinary tumor boards, with an emphasis on consensus diagnoses reached after conversations between local clinicians, local pathologists, and US pathologists. To this end, US-based participants are viewed as collaborators, not consultants. This model is intentionally in contrast to consultative pathology services popular in the United States, where diagnoses are rendered at a remote site by an expert pathologist often without direct communication with the submitting provider.

In light of this ethos, more recently, our group has begun to experiment with alternative teleconferencing solutions, primarily using the online Zoom Video Conferencing system (Zoom Video Communications, San Jose, CA). When coupled to a microscope-mounted digital camera, this system allows dynamic telemicroscopy driven not by the US-based collaborating pathologist (as would be the case in robotic telemicroscopy) but by local pathologists in Malawi. Although of this system is in its infancy in our program, potential advantages include a primary role for local pathologists in the conference, and lower up-front capital costs (mostly limited to the cost of a digital camera).

TECHNICAL INFRASTRUCTURE

The success of the UNC Project Malawi weekly telepathology conferences largely relies on a thoughtfully developed technical infrastructure and a dependable Internet connection. The KCH Pathology Laboratory houses the complete Aperio Digital Pathology System on site, which includes a ScanScope CS slide scanner, workstation CPU, and image server. The images of the scanned slides are stored on the image server, accessible for pathologists anywhere internationally once granted access through a username and password-protected virtual private network within our own server network.

Approximately 10 to 15 cases with 5 to 10 distinct slides are reviewed weekly. For histologic sections and immunohistochemical stains, the slides are scanned at ×20 magnification, whereas selected areas of cytology preparations and peripheral blood smears are scanned at ×40. The 0.75-TB server can store approximately 2000 images in a .sis file format, which can be deleted as necessary to preserve storage space for conference. Unless specifically requested to remain accessible on the server, the 600 oldest slides are deleted from the server whenever space becomes limited. Requested images can also be stored on an external hard drive, but all slides are archived and can be rescanned at any time.

Proprietary software (Spectrum Plus, Buffalo Grove, IL) installed on the image server is used to organize cases and slide information, and viewing software (Imagescope, Buffalo Grove, IL) is freely available and necessary to open stored images. The Imagescope viewing software also allows access to a Digital Slide Conferencing feature and provides a mechanism to control and annotate the image in real time. This allows either US or Malawian pathologists to identify relevant cells or fields for discussion and control the conference as need be.

The UNC Project–Malawi employs a four-person IT team on site, with a single IT member assigned to all pathology-related work. This pathology-dedicated IT specialist typically serves as the point of contact. IT support is provided either via email to a support email address or by calling the IT support office extension. The Project uses last mile fiber for its Internet connectivity. All internal connections within the building are either through a CAT 5e or 6 ethernet cable capable of a 100 Mps–1 Gbps connection. We are currently receiving 8 MB on a ratio of 1:1. In addition, we use networking tools that allow control of bandwidth usage, primarily a Barracuda Web

Filter 410 (Campbell, CA) that allows the IT team to prioritize bandwidth based on work-related Internet traffic. This Internet connection is sufficient to support clear voice calls through online messaging applications and the remote conferencing system described previously (Zoom Video Communications).

EXAMPLES OF OTHER PROGRAMS

Established telepathology systems between resource-limited settings and resource-rich academic centers have been described.[5–7,9,14–25] Although workflow design and specifics of implementation vary, these collaborations seem consistently effective. Representative examples of such programs are described next.

Wamala and colleagues[7] describe their experience with a telepathology platform between a hospital in Uganda and academic hospital in Germany. The collaborators used an Internet browser–based dynamic imaging system that provided clinical information, gross pathologic description, and a digitized microscopy platform. The remote pathologist had control of the microscope focus, brightness, magnification, and field selection. The authors report progress from the first year of their efforts, which included the random prospective selection of 96 surgical pathology cases for review by the remote pathologist following diagnosis by the local institution. Concordant diagnosis was made for 92 of the 96 cases (97%). The average time for transmission of the images and review by remote pathologist was 10 minutes per case, and the robotic microscope controls were easy to learn by the consultants, making this platform a feasible tool for remote consultation on challenging cases.

A static-image teledermatopathology system between four hospitals in Kenya and Tanzania and Massachusetts General Hospital is reported by Gimbel and colleagues.[9] The local pathologists would make an initial diagnosis based on hematoxylin-eosin-stained slides alone, with the option of referring difficult cases for second-opinion review at Massachusetts General Hospital. Representative images were taken by the referring pathologists and uploaded to an online World Wide Web platform. The authors report the first 29 cases referred for telepathologic consultation. A diagnosis was made by evaluation of the static images in 22 of 29 cases (76%), with the remaining seven cases partially or nondiagnostic because of lack of IHC staining or clinical information, and inadequate image quality. Glass slides from the 22 evaluable cases were then sent to the United States to blindly assess diagnoses made by static-image examination compared with the gold standard of traditional microscopy. A comparable diagnosis was made in 91% of these cases. Their experience demonstrates that a telepathology service for providing second opinions on challenging dermatologic cases is effective using a less-expensive telepathology imaging modality.

In settings with even less capacity, telepathology may provide the only access to pathology services. Pagni and colleagues[6] reported on a telepathology collaboration between their institution in Italy and a hospital in Zambia that previously did not have a pathology service. This system used whole-slide imaging to allow the Italian pathologists to make remote histologic and cytologic diagnoses on a variety of anatomic pathology specimens. Following 7 months of operation, the original glass slides were shipped to Italy to establish a true diagnosis, and these results were compared with those made via telepathology. Similar to our experience in Malawi, more than 85% of final diagnoses were either unchanged or had only minor differences on final review, and in only 3% of cases did a change in diagnosis occur that would have resulted in different treatment in Zambia. Agreement was even higher for cytology cases in this series, with no treatment-relevant differences between telepathology and final diagnoses.

Although programs like this one can overcome some resource limitations, infrastructure investments are still necessary, and local technical expertise remains essential even to process specimens before scanning. To this end, the Italian program supported the training of two Zambian technologists and provided the satellite server needed for transmission of the images. This study emphasizes the potential of telepathology to provide a much-needed service to health care centers without pathology capabilities, provided that resources exist to train personnel and establish and maintain equipment and servers.

Lastly, the American Society for Clinical Pathology (ASCP) has created an initiative, Partners for Cancer Diagnosis and Treatment in Africa, bringing together a large number of partners from academia, industry, governments, and NGOs to provide telepathology solutions that can meet the pathologist shortage in Africa today while training for future pathologists is ongoing.[26] The program began in 2015 with Butaro District Hospital receiving the first installation. With the advent of Food and Drug Administration approval of the first system in the United States for primary diagnosis of histology by telepathology, the role of telepathology in settings with few or no pathologists is likely to increase sharply and programs like the ASCP initiative, our Malawi program, and the previous described examples should flourish and expand to fill this major diagnostic need.

COMMON THEMES OF SUCCESSFUL PROGRAMS

In our experience, the main common ingredients of successful programs are strong commitments by participating pathologists, clinicians, and IT collaborators.[2,3,10] Rendering accurate diagnoses for complex diseases in real-time across continents and time zones will inevitably encounter logistical challenges. However, these are usually surmountable, provided that participating members value the activity sufficiently to find work-around solutions. Commitments to regular real-time conferences also serve to improve communication and build rapport between team members, thereby adding incremental value to the conferences over time as they become an integral and important vehicle for improving patient care and the overall academic environment. This is not dissimilar to ubiquitous tumor boards that take place in cancer centers worldwide in higher resource settings. Other key components for successful programs include minimum computing and image capture technologies, although these can be modest and low-tech while still serving as valuable and effective conference platforms. A reasonably stable source of funding is also important to maintain and replace equipment over time as required. Finally, for our group telepathology has become vitally important as an instrument for collaboration and mentorship even beyond service provision alone. Our program's success reflects significant engagement by team members in the activity as a key local resource for bilateral scientific engagement, capacity building, and career development for junior Malawian and US pathologists.

CHALLENGES AND OBSTACLES

Although the current system has met the need to support clinical trials at KCH, including studies sponsored by National Cancer Institute cooperative groups, there are notable challenges and limitations. Importantly, development and continued operation of the laboratory at KCH have been and remain heavily dependent on research grants. Initial renovation and equipment costs for the laboratory totaled approximately $200,000 USD, most of which was provided through funding from the US National Institutes of Health Medical Education Partnership Initiative, AIDS Malignancy

Consortium, and Division of AIDS. This initial investment included the $85,000 USD purchase of the Aperio ScanScope system.

Annual operating costs for the KCH laboratory total approximately $170,000 USD. Much of the laboratory's budget is devoted to salary support for employees. Equipment maintenance fees are approximately $16,000 USD per year, including a $4500 USD service contract for the Aperio system. Although KCH provides some support for consumable supplies in the laboratory, all other expenses are covered by external grant sources, which are often used to cover costs of routine pathology services in the Malawi public sector even outside research studies. To ensure sustainability of our program, we are actively diversifying funding sources beyond faculty research grants, to include revenue generated by the laboratory using locally appropriate fee schedules, philanthropic and foundation sources, and development partners. Other potential funding models include the ASCP Partners for Cancer Diagnosis and Treatment in Africa, which aims to increase access to telepathology resources.[26]

Beyond funding concerns, technologic limitations also create obstacles for our program. Despite efforts to manage traffic, bandwidth is occasionally insufficient for smooth communication and timely loading of scanned slides. Internet service provider outages are unpredictable in the region, leading to conference rescheduling approximately every other month. Conference interruptions and inconsistencies can result in delayed patient care and treatment.

Sufficient space is available for temporary image storage, but regular purging of stored images is nonetheless necessary because of the large size of whole-slide imaging files. This can be overcome with additional hardware upgrades and purchases but financial resources are not available at this time. This limitation does lead to the unfortunate loss of a potentially valuable educational resource for local trainees and pathologists. Smaller image files, such as static photographs of representative diagnostic fields, might be more easily adapted for generation of such educational resources.

The current cost of Internet service is $3300 USD/month for 8 MB contention at 1:1 ratio. Additional costs include the router license, the switch, and the wireless access point hardware used in the pathology building to provide access.

The Project faces extensive delays when sourcing materials is required to address repairs to the Aperio server. As with other technical skills, there are few personnel with the adequate skill set who are able to make repairs and adjustments to equipment and hardware. These challenges result in prolonged delays when maintenance is required.

We find that the magnification and image quality is sufficient to effectively and consistently evaluate histologic sections and immunohistochemical stains. However, cytologic evaluation of peripheral blood, bone marrow, and fine-needle aspirate smears can be limited with a maximum effective objective magnification of ×40. Moreover, identifying a plane of focus is challenging for the slide-scanning instrument, particularly for bone marrow aspirate preparations.

Finally, when working in a setting with substantial technologic limitations, we find that it is imperative to take full advantage of those resources that do exist, most importantly, local clinical expertise. In our experience, the thoughtful impressions of a skilled clinician can help to overcome many resource limitations. Such observations emphasize the need for clinical context in telepathology programs and remind us to be cautious when making interpretations that counter clinical impression.

SUMMARY

Despite limitations and challenges, the telepathology conferences have had a dramatic impact on diagnostic accuracy for direct patient care and have supported successful implementation of clinical trials.[10] These systems provide referral and educational opportunities for pathologists worldwide, and additionally can support quality control and improvement initiatives previously impossible in some regions of Africa. Furthermore, telepathology can make possible collaborative relationships and significant scientific opportunities for hospitals and academic institutions in sub-Saharan Africa. Groups interested in developing related processes in resource-limited settings have many options with respect to whole-slide imaging systems, digital microscopy, and conference format. However, we have found that the flexibility to deal with technical challenges and inclusion of clinicians and pathologists in weekly conferences is absolutely critical to program success.

REFERENCES

1. Adesina A, Chumba D, Nelson AM, et al. Improvement of pathology in sub-Saharan Africa. Lancet Oncol 2013;14(4):e152–7.
2. Gopal S, Krysiak R, Liomba G. Building a pathology laboratory in Malawi. Lancet Oncol 2013;14(4):291–2.
3. Gopal S, Krysiak R, Liomba NG, et al. Early experience after developing a pathology laboratory in Malawi, with emphasis on cancer diagnoses. PLoS One 2013; 8(8):e70361.
4. Msyamboza KP, Dzamalala C, Mdokwe C, et al. Burden of cancer in Malawi; common types, incidence and trends: national population-based cancer registry. BMC Res Notes 2012;5:149.
5. Fischer MK, Kayembe MK, Scheer AJ, et al. Establishing telepathology in Africa: lessons from Botswana. J Am Acad Dermatol 2011;64(5):986–7.
6. Pagni F, Bono F, Di Bella C, et al. Virtual surgical pathology in underdeveloped countries: the Zambia project. Arch Pathol Lab Med 2011;135(2):215–9.
7. Wamala D, Katamba A, Dworak O. Feasibility and diagnostic accuracy of Internet-based dynamic telepathology between Uganda and Germany. J Telemed Telecare 2011;17(5):222–5.
8. Sohani AR, Sohani MA. Static digital telepathology: a model for diagnostic and educational support to pathologists in the developing world. Anal Cell Pathol 2012;35(1):25–30.
9. Gimbel DC, Sohani AR, Prasad Busarla SV, et al. A static-image telepathology system for dermatopathology consultation in East Africa: the Massachusetts General Hospital experience. J Am Acad Dermatol 2012;67(5):997–1007.
10. Montgomery ND, Liomba NG, Kampani C, et al. Accurate real-time diagnosis of lymphoproliferative disorders in Malawi through Clinicopathologic Teleconferences: a model for pathology services in Sub-Saharan Africa. Am J Clin Pathol 2016;146(4):423–30.
11. Pantanowitz L. Digital images and the future of digital pathology. J Pathol Inform 2010;1. https://doi.org/10.4103/2153-3539.68332.
12. Mpunga T, Hedt-Gauthier BL, Tapela N, et al. Implementation and validation of telepathology triage at Cancer Referral Center in rural Rwanda. J Glob Oncol 2016;2(2):76–82.
13. Sirintrapun SJ, Cimic A. Dynamic nonrobotic telemicroscopy via skype: a cost effective solution to teleconsultation. J Pathol Inform 2012;3:28.
14. Halliday BE, Bhattacharyya AK, Graham AR, et al. Diagnostic accuracy of an international static-imaging telepathology consultation service. Hum Pathol 1997; 28(1):17–21.

15. Zhao C, Wu T, Ding X, et al. International telepathology consultation: three years of experience between the University of Pittsburgh Medical Center and KingMed diagnostics in China. J Pathol Inform 2015;6:63.
16. Rotimi O, Orah N, Shaaban A, et al. Remote teaching of histopathology using scanned slides via Skype between the United Kingdom and Nigeria. Arch Pathol Lab Med 2017;141(2):298–300.
17. Prieto-Egido I, Gonzalez-Escalada A, Garcia-Giganto V, et al. Design of new procedures for diagnosing prevalent diseases using a low-cost telemicroscopy system. Telemed J E Health 2016;22(11):952–9.
18. Streicher JL, Kini SP, Stoff BK. Innovative dermatopathology teaching in a resource-limited environment. J Am Acad Dermatol 2016;74(5):1024–5.
19. Farahani N, Riben M, Evans AJ, et al. International telepathology: promises and pitfalls. Pathobiology 2016;83(2–3):121–6.
20. Kumar N, Busarla SV, Sayed S, et al. Telecytology in East Africa: a feasibility study of forty cases using a static imaging system. J Telemed Telecare 2012;18(1): 7–12.
21. Micheletti RG, Steele KT, Kovarik CL. Robotic teledermatopathology from an African dermatology clinic. J Am Acad Dermatol 2014;70(5):952–4.
22. Santiago TC, Jenkins JJ, Pedrosa F, et al. Improving the histopathologic diagnosis of pediatric malignancies in a low-resource setting by combining focused training and telepathology strategies. Pediatr Blood Cancer 2012;59(2):221–5.
23. Kldiashvili E, Schrader T. Reproducibility of telecytology diagnosis of cervical smears in a quality assurance program: the Georgian experience. Telemed J E Health 2011;17(7):565–8.
24. Brauchli K, Jagilly R, Oberli H, et al. Telepathology on the Solomon Islands: two years' experience with a hybrid Web- and email-based telepathology system. J Telemed Telecare 2004;10(Suppl 1):14–7.
25. Mireskandari M, Kayser G, Hufnagl P, et al. Teleconsultation in diagnostic pathology: experience from Iran and Germany with the use of two European telepathology servers. J Telemed Telecare 2004;10(2):99–103.
26. White house announces global initiative to accelerate fight against cancer in Africa. Available at: http://www.ascp.org/Newsroom/White-House-Announces-Global-Initiative-to-Accelerate-Fight-Against-Cancer-in-Africa.html - NewsroomGrid. Accessed November 27, 2015.

World Health Organization List of Priority Medical Devices for Cancer Management to Promote Universal Coverage

CrossMark

André M. Ilbawi, MD[a],*, Adriana Velazquez-Berumen, MSc[b]

KEYWORDS

- Universal coverage • Laboratory medicine • Anatomic pathology
- Health system capacity • Medical devices • Cancer control

KEY POINTS

- In order to achieve sustainable development goals and universal coverage, current gaps in laboratory medicine pertaining to financing models, population coverage, and service availability must be identified and addressed. Defining core package of services to be financed by current pooled funds can improve access to laboratory services.
- The WHO list of priority medical devices for cancer management offers a framework for defining and expanding core cancer services. Priority medical devices, key competencies, and necessary infrastructure are delineated and prioritized.
- Laboratory medicine, including pathology, is dependent on a robust health system. A situational analysis should be used to inform national laboratory policies that are then linked to sustainable financing mechanisms and robust implementation strategies to ensure quality.

INTRODUCTION

The landscape of global health evolved radically in 2015 as governments around the world declared their commitment to the 2030 Agenda for Sustainable Development. As it pertains to health, Sustainable Development Goal (SDG) 3 is founded on the realization of health for all and builds on the right to health that has been recognized as a

Disclosure Statement: A.M. Ilbawi and A. Velazquez-Berumen are staff member of the World Health Organization (WHO). The authors alone are responsible for the views expressed in this article, and they do not necessarily represent the decisions, policy, or views of WHO. The authors have no commercial or financial conflicts of interest and have no funding sources.
[a] Management of Noncommunicable Disease Unit, Department for Management of Noncommunicable Diseases, Disability, Violence and Injury Prevention, World Health Organization, 20 Avenue Appia, Geneva 27 1211 Switzerland; [b] Innovation, Access and Use Unit, Essential Medicines and Health Products Department, World Health Organization, 20 Avenue Appia, Geneva 27 1211 Switzerland
* Corresponding author.
E-mail address: ilbawia@who.int

Clin Lab Med 38 (2018) 151–160
https://doi.org/10.1016/j.cll.2017.10.012
0272-2712/18/© 2017 Elsevier Inc. All rights reserved.

labmed.theclinics.com

basic human right since ratification of the WHO Constitution in 1946 then reaffirmed in the Declaration of Alma-Ata on Primary Health Care in 1978.

For decades, programs in health have been viewed predominantly through a disease-oriented lens, particularly shaped by the burden and consequences of communicable diseases. Yet, to achieve the SDGs, core health services cannot be fragmented or disregarded, and management strategies are needed for diseases that have received lower priority to date, such as noncommunicable disease (NCDs). Laboratory services, including pathology, are essential to achieving the SDGs and advancing health, ranging from diagnosing NCDs to surveillance of health risks and epidemics.[1] Accordingly, laboratory medicine should be viewed as a critical cross-cutting investment, affording it appropriate prioritization and commensurate funding.

Comprehensive laboratory services are essential to improve health outcomes in an efficient and equitable manner, consistent with SDG 3 and foundational to a strong health system. All the building blocks of the health system – technologies, well-trained health workforce, robust health information system with reporting of results, financing mechanisms, governance and regulatory structures, and quality and timely service delivery – pertain to laboratory services and should be considered when evaluating or implementing programs.

The global burden of NCDs is rising in low- and middle-income countries, and the threats of communicable diseases persist, placing increasing strain on laboratory services and health systems. In order to achieve universal health coverage articulated in the SDGs, as well as commitments made in Maputo Declaration (2008)[2] and resolutions such as the Political Declaration on NCDs adopted in 2011, accelerated action is needed (eg, World Health Assembly [WHA] resolutions 62.15, 63.12, 64.15, 64.17, 66.10, 66.24, 67.25, 70.12). By strengthening laboratory and pathology services, significant progress can be made toward global targets.

Within the broad range of interventions encompassed in laboratory medicine, particular emphasis in this article will be made on anatomic pathology and cancer. Anatomic pathology generally requires more advanced health system capacity and has critical importance in the management of NCDs. Approximately 66% of deaths in low- and middle-income countries are from NCDs, and the burden is rising rapidly in these settings.[3] Cancer, one of the four NCDs, requires high-quality pathology services as the foundation of diagnosis, effective treatment, and surveillance for tumor recurrence. With the recent WHA resolution on cancer prevention and control as well as the United Nations (UN) high-level meeting on NCDs in 2018, augmenting anatomic pathology services has particular prominence and urgency.

UNIVERSAL COVERAGE

Laboratory services are of central importance, used in 70% to 80% of all health care decisions affecting diagnosis or treatment, and these should be viewed through the lens of universal coverage.[4] When considering core health services, such as laboratory medicines and pathology, there must an acknowledgment that context-specific variations are needed, adapted by national authorities. Laboratory science is rapidly evolving, which complicates rationale purchasing of technologies and national strategic planning.

Nevertheless, mechanisms of developing national laboratory policies and adopting context-appropriate technologies are important for any health system to provide and finance universal coverage.[5] The 3 dimensions of universal coverage are: service coverage (ie, selection of interventions to be covered); population coverage (ie, communities and individuals who receive a service); and cost coverage (ie, proportion of costs covered by public contributions)[6] (**Fig. 1**).

WORLD HEALTH ORGANIZATION LIST OF PRIORITY MEDICAL DEVICES FOR CANCER MANAGEMENT

In response, WHO has highlighted improving access to medical products as central to the achievement of universal health coverage and is one of six WHO leadership priorities to attain equity in public health.[7] In May 2017, WHO published WHO List of Priority Medical Devices for Cancer Management to assist health planners provide universal coverage for cancer services by defining key interventions, identifying essential medical products, promoting population coverage, and facilitating efficient resource allocation.[8] This guidance document uses the cancer control continuum, organizing each chapter along that continuum with a summary of the basic devices, health workforce, and infrastructure required for key interventions (**Fig. 2**). The interventions selected can be considered a package of cancer services and were identified through comprehensive review of best practices and expert opinion.[8]

Once essential interventions have been defined, guidance is provided on how to design laboratory infrastructure, including robust procurement and supply chain management, to maximize population coverage and service coverage in accordance with national priorities. The section on clinical laboratory and pathology delineates the 63 capital equipment and more than 100 accessories/consumables required for basic service provision. The majority of clinical interventions related to pathology should be considered at all resource level (ie, they are the core package of services for universal coverage, Annex 1, WHO List of Priority Medical Devices for Cancer Management).

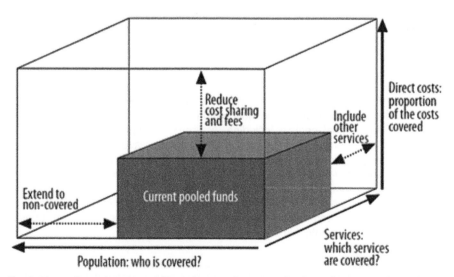

Fig. 1. Three dimensions to consider when moving toward universal coverage. (*From* World Health Organization. Health systems financing: the path to universal coverage. The World Health Report 2010. Geneva (Switzerland): World Health Organization; 2010. Available at: http://apps.who.int/iris/bitstream/10665/44371/1/9789241564021_eng.pdf. Accessed June 5, 2017.)

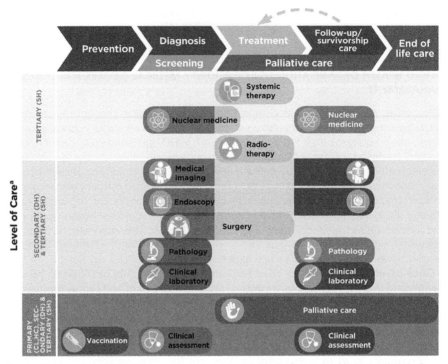

Fig. 2. Core services along the cancer continuum with level of care. [a] Appropriate level of care will depend on the particular intervention, setting, and available infrastructure and human resources. CL, community level health post; DH, district hospital, HC, health center, SH, specialized hospital. (*From* World Health Organization. WHO list of priority medical devices for cancer management. Geneva (Switzerland): World Health Organization; 2017. Available at: http://www.who.int/medical_devices/publications/priority_med_dev_cancer_management/en/. Accessed June 5, 2017.)

Other pillars of the health system required to deliver essential interventions are delineated in this document including trained health workforce and infrastructure requirements (**Fig. 3**). The core competencies for laboratory and pathology medicine are defined, recognizing that different occupations may perform the essential roles according to the national context including workforce availability and models.[8] For example, the development of standard operating procedures (SOPs) is a critical function in pathology services and can be performed by different cadre depending on the setting and regulatory environment; a particular competency should be performed by cadre officially recognized as per its scope of practice.[8]

Using the lens of universal coverage, the WHO List of Priority Medical Devices for Cancer Management can help policymakers optimize the impact of current pooled funds to achieve the greatest impact on outcomes.

Service Coverage

As the menu of diagnostic tests and therapeutic options expand, the sophistication and costs of laboratory services have increased exponentially. Policymakers at all income levels are encountering the challenge of identifying interventions that are resource-appropriate, affordable, cost-effective, and commensurate with health system capacity. In the diagnosis and management of cancer, the need to match

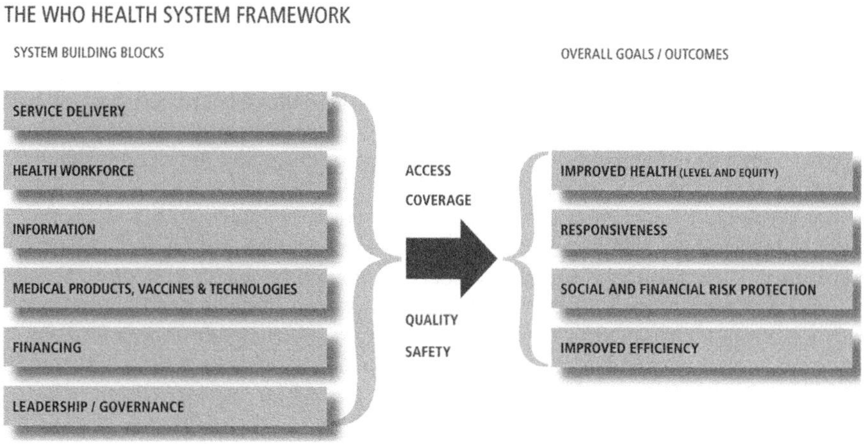

THE WHO HEALTH SYSTEM FRAMEWORK

SYSTEM BUILDING BLOCKS

OVERALL GOALS / OUTCOMES

SERVICE DELIVERY		
HEALTH WORKFORCE	ACCESS / COVERAGE	IMPROVED HEALTH (LEVEL AND EQUITY)
INFORMATION		RESPONSIVENESS
MEDICAL PRODUCTS, VACCINES & TECHNOLOGIES		SOCIAL AND FINANCIAL RISK PROTECTION
FINANCING	QUALITY / SAFETY	IMPROVED EFFICIENCY
LEADERSHIP / GOVERNANCE		

Fig. 3. The 6 building blocks of a health system that must be considered for effective, comprehensive delivery of laboratory services. (*From* World Health Organization. Everybody's business — strengthening health systems to improve health outcomes. WHO's framework for action. Geneva (Switzerland): World Health Organization; 2007. Available at: http://www.who.int/healthsystems/strategy/everybodys_business.pdf. Accessed June 5, 2017.)

corresponding diagnostic tests and therapeutic interventions is particularly important. Novel, and often expensive, targeted therapies given in the absence of accurate diagnosis increase costs and, more importantly, introduce the potential for unnecessary patient harm.

Normative guidance, such as that provided in WHO List of Priority Medical Devices for Cancer Management, can help policymakers better define the service package and associated medical devices, competencies, and infrastructure. Service should be based on health system capacity, fairness, and evidence-to-decision frameworks that are context specific and supported by stakeholder support and legislation.[9]

Population Coverage

Because laboratory medicine is an essential component of the health system, population coverage for basic services should be maximized. This includes coverage for vulnerable populations such as rural groups or those encountering geographic barriers and low-income socioeconomic groups. Currently, many countries do not have anatomic pathology services available in the public sectors. WHO data have shown that only 35% of low-income countries and 60% of lower-middle-income countries reported such services are available.[10] In the African region, 37% of countries reported generally available pathology services in the public sector. Of the 340 accredited laboratories in Africa, only 28 are in sub-Saharan Africa for a population of more than 800 million (excluding South Africa).[11] Resultantly, public health programs have encountered challenges linked to the lack of reliable laboratory support, disease diagnosis, and management of patient care resulting in large percentages of the population lacking basic coverage.[11] Significant shortages in a well-trained health workforce for pathology services contribute to gaps in services.[12] In regions where basic histopathology and anatomic pathology services do exist, these services are often limited to facilities in the capital and/or other main cities.[13]

Building capacity and population coverage in pathology requires a multisectoral approach that includes prioritizing education and training, improving coordination of services, and investing in capital expenditures in regional and peripheral facilities. With profound shortages in trained staff, increasing or augmenting current health workforce capacity is paramount to expanding population coverage. Diverse strategies can be considered ranging from telementoring to increasing output of trained providers to remote reading.[14–16] As done in the WHO List of Priority Medical Devices for Cancer, defining core interventions and services facilitates the development of competencies among relevant cadre.

Prior WHO guidance has also emphasized the value of improving the efficiency of referral mechanisms and coordination among existing staff to expand population coverage.[17–19] Regional and peripheral hospitals should be linked to central facilities through organized models of service delivery, improved efficiency of transportation, and routine communication.[13] Expanding capacity in regional/subnational facilities to offer more advanced services can also promote access and reduce delays in care.[20]

Direct Costs

The spectrum of laboratory investigations, including anatomic pathology, ranges from simple and inexpensive to sophisticated and costly. Financing mechanisms of laboratory services vary substantially between countries, as does the relative contributions of public contributions (eg, government agencies and donors) and household contributions. Overall, medicines, vaccines, and health technologies consume a significant proportion of recurrent health budgets, estimated at 50% in some settings.[5] Although the exact out-of-pocket contributions to pathology services are not well established, approximately 37% to 50% of total health expenditure in low- and lower-middle income countries are out of pocket, resulting in significant barriers to services including pathology.[21] Households may encounter double expenditures when seeking pathology services: payment directed toward the necessary supplies to perform the test as well as the service.[1] To further compound the challenge, laboratory and pathology services for NCDs including cancer have significantly lower funding streams than those for communicable diseases.[19]

There are compelling opportunities for improving the financing of laboratory and pathology services, because more than half of this expenditure has been attributed to ineffectual spending from poor planning and management.[5] Coherent and financed national laboratory policies can improve efficiency of public expenditure and also develop schemes to reduce out-of-pocket expenditures. The development of a core package of services and an essential diagnostic list can help direct rational use of resources.[8,22]

DOMAINS OF QUALITY

What good does it do to offer free maternal care and have a high proportion of babies delivered in health facilities if the quality of care is substandard or even dangerous?
— Dr Margaret Chan, former Director General, WHO[23]

This statement from the former director general of WHO reflects the importance of quality in service delivery. What good does it do to have a pathology laboratory and provide a diagnosis if that diagnosis is incorrect; the report is lost or delayed, or critical information is not included? Critical to achieving the intended outcomes of clinical and public health interventions is the assurance that services are high quality. Where pathology service does exist in less developed countries, services may be inappropriate, unreliable, and lacking quality assurance.[13] The consequences of poorly delivered pathology services are that they are inefficient, and, of greater concern, that they are harmful. An incorrect diagnosis results in delaying appropriate treatment and also incurs the risks associated with incorrect treatment.

Components of laboratory quality include that results are as accurate as possible, all aspects of the laboratory operations are reliable, and reporting is timely in order to be useful in a clinical or public health setting.[11,24] The laboratory services involve many steps of activity and personnel, resulting in a complex system with multiple processes subject to errors. The quality management system model, which looks at the entire system, is important for achieving good laboratory performance (**Table 1**).[25] Working with partners, WHO The Regional Office for Africa developed the Stepwise Laboratory Quality Improvement Process Toward Accreditation (SLIPTA).[11] At the time of initial audits, most of the laboratories had not surpassed the 3-star rating (out of 5 stars). Strategic planning with committed resources for quality improvement and mentoring is critical to quality improvement and accreditation preparedness, such as strengthening laboratory management toward accreditation (SLMTA).[26,27]

PLANNING AND IMPLEMENTING PATHOLOGY AND LABORATORY PROGRAMS TO EXPAND COVERAGE

National authorities and policymakers are encouraged to develop a sustainable and coherent national framework for laboratory services that encompasses national laboratory policies, national regulatory mechanisms, and a national laboratory plan, with a designated focal point and an oversight mechanism.[5] WHO has provided guidance on the development of national plans and systems.[19,28–30]

To successfully expand universal coverage of laboratory services, there are 4 steps: assess, plan, finance and implement. A situational analysis should include an analysis

Table 1
Summary of universal coverage dimensions, framed by quality and informed by national laboratory plans, policies and regulations

Dimension	Question	Sample Problem	Sample Solution
Service coverage	Which services are covered?	Prioritize services among expanding menu of pathology and laboratory tests for management of NCDs	Identify key interventions and ensure sufficient health system capacity (eg, devices, infrastructure, and workforce available)
Population coverage	Who is covered?	Gaps in available services for vulnerable populations or in particular regions	Multisectoral approach to coordinate services including referral networks, health workforce capacity
Direct costs	What proportion of costs is covered?	Insufficient funding for pathology and laboratory medicine, particularly for NCDs	Finance national laboratory plans according to prioritized set of interventions
Quality		Low quality resulting in poor outcomes	Develop standards, regulatory processes
National laboratory plans, policies, and regulations		Inefficient use of resources	Generate plan through cycle of assessing, planning, financing, and implementing

of the national health laboratory system including policies and the regulatory environment, and specific technical capacity at laboratory facilities. The assessment tool(s) can be appropriate for initial evaluation and routine monitoring of laboratory capacities. The WHO laboratory assessment tool can be used and adapted as needed in the field.[31] Data collected are analyzed to identify gaps and opportunities for improvement and to drive the planning for improvement.

National laboratory plans must be coordinated with other relevant health strategies including national cancer control plans and national health workforce strategies for an integrated approach. Sufficient resources and appropriate financing mechanisms to promote rational use of services should also be committed.[28] A review of plans from sub-Saharan Africa demonstrated that only 2 of 39 countries specified the percentage of health budgets earmarked for laboratory services or human resources.[32] Additionally, plans generally lacked a mechanism for monitoring and evaluation of the plan implementation and of laboratory services. No country had specified indicators to measure the performance of facilities.[32] Cooperation between governments, WHO, national professional bodies, and key partners has promoted greater emphasis on quality and international standardization.[1] However, many challenges remain in less developed settings, and further promotion of universal coverage and quality assurance in laboratory medicine is needed.

SUMMARY

Health laboratories are a fundamental component of all health systems. The WHO List of Priority Medical Devices for Cancer Management provides a framework for how to expand universal coverage by identifying set of key interventions to drive decision making on improving service and population coverage and rational allocation of resources. Furthermore, this guidance document highlights that building capacity requires alignment with the infrastructure and health workforce in a particular context.[33]

Effective implementation requires an integrated approach with an emphasis on quality and ownership by all relevant stakeholders achieved through national planning. Implementation must generally move toward a more integrated approach that prioritizes universal coverage; this will also result in more efficient use of resources and better laboratory service delivery.[5] A firm commitment is needed to improve quality through the establishment of appropriate regulatory, legal support structures, and other mechanisms.[28] An incorrect diagnosis can cause significant harm to a person, to his or her community, and to the integrity of health system.

Strengthening laboratory services will propel the global community closer to producing more resilient health systems and to achieving universal coverage. Investments in laboratory medicine and pathology can bring the world one critical step closer to realizing the UN agenda for sustainable development and to advancing health for all.

REFERENCES

1. Fleming KA, Naidoo M, Wilson M, et al. An essential pathology package for low- and middle-income countries. Am J Clin Pathol 2017;147(1):15–32.
2. The Maputo declaration on strengthening of laboratory systems. Geneva (Switzerland): World Health Organization; 2008. Available at: http://www.who.int/diagnostics_laboratory/Maputo-Declaration_2008.pdf. Accessed June 5, 2017.
3. Global health observatory: the data repository. Geneva (Switzerland): World Health Organization; 2017. Available at: http://www.who.int/gho/database/en. Accessed June 5, 2017.

4. Beastall GH. The modernisation of pathology and laboratory medicine in the UK: networking into the future. Clin Biochem Rev 2008;29(1):3–10.

5. Asia Pacific strategy for strengthening health laboratory services (2010-2015). World Health Organization regional office for the Western Pacific and regional office for South-East Asia. Manila (Philippines): World Health Organization; 2010. Available at: http://www.searo.who.int/about/administration_structure/cds/BCT_Asia_Pacific_Strategy10-15.pdf. Accessed June 5, 2017.

6. Health systems financing: the path to universal coverage. The World Health Report 2010. Geneva (Switzerland): World Health Organization; 2010. Available at: http://apps.who.int/iris/bitstream/10665/44371/1/9789241564021_eng.pdf. Accessed June 5, 2017.

7. Not merely absence of disease. Twelfth general programme of work. Geneva (Switzerland): World Health Organization; 2014. Available at. http://apps.who.int/iris/bitstream/10665/112792/1/GPW_2014-2019_eng.pdf?ua=1. Accessed June 5, 2017.

8. WHO list of priority medical devices for cancer management. Geneva (Switzerland): World Health Organization; 2017. Available at: http://www.who.int/medical_devices/publications/priority_med_dev_cancer_management/en/. Accessed June 5, 2017.

9. Bertram MY, Lauer JA, De Joncheere K, et al. Cost-effectiveness thresholds: pros and cons. Bull World Health Organ 2016;94(12):925–30.

10. Assessing national capacity for the prevention and control of noncommunicable diseases: global survey. Geneva (Switzerland): World Health Organization; 2016. Available at: http://apps.who.int/iris/bitstream/10665/246223/1/9789241565363-eng.pdf?ua=1. Accessed June 5, 2017.

11. WHO guide for the stepwise laboratory improvement process towards accreditation in the African Region (SLIPTA). Brazzaville (Congo): World Health Organization; 2015. Available at: http://www.afro.who.int/sites/default/files/2017-06/guide-for-the-slipta-in-the-african-region071115.pdf. Accessed June 5, 2017.

12. Adesina A, Chumba D, Nelson AM, et al. Improvement of pathology in sub-Saharan Africa. Lancet Oncol 2013;14(4):e152–7.

13. Basic histopathology and antomical pathology services for developing countries with variable resources. WHO Regional Publications, Eastern Mediterranean series 23. Cairo (Egypt): World Health Organization; 2003. Available at. http://apps.who.int/iris/handle/10665/119675. Accessed June 5, 2017.

14. Bennett A, Garcia E, Schulze M, et al. Building a laboratory workforce to meet the future: ASCP Task Force on the laboratory professionals workforce. Am J Clin Pathol 2014;141(2):154–67.

15. Weinstein RS, Graham AR, Lian F, et al. Reconciliation of diverse telepathology system designs. Historic issues and implications for emerging markets and new applications. APMIS 2012;120(4):256–75.

16. Hartman DJ. Mobile technology for the practice of pathology. Adv Anat Pathol 2016;23(2):118–24.

17. Laboratory quality standards and their implementation. World Health Organization regional office for the Western Pacific and regional office for South-East Asia. Manila (Philippines): World Health Organization; 2010. Available at: http://apps.who.int/medicinedocs/documents/s22409en/s22409en.pdf?ua=1. Accessed June 5, 2017.

18. Guide for national public health laboratory networking to strengthen integrated disease surveillance and response. Brazzaville (Congo): World Health Organization; 2008. Available at: http://www.afro.who.int/sites/default/files/2017-06/afro_lab_guidelines_final_doc_oct08_en.pdf. Accessed June 5, 2017.

19. Guidance for development of national laboratory strategic plans World Health Organization – regional office for Africa and United States Centers for Disease Control and Prevention (CDC), Atlanta (Georgia). Brazzaville (Congo): World Health Organization; 2009. Available at: http://www.who.int/hiv/amds/amds_guide_dev_nat_lab_strat.pdf. Accessed June 5, 2017.

20. Guide to cancer early diagnosis. Geneva (Switzerland): World Health Organization; 2017. Available at: http://apps.who.int/iris/bitstream/10665/254500/1/9789241511940-eng.pdf?ua=1. Accessed June 5, 2017.

21. The World Bank, World development indicators (2014). Fertility rate, total (births per woman), Atlas method [Data file]. Available at: http://data.worldbank.org/indicator/SP.DYN.TFRT.IN. Accessed March 1, 2015.

22. WHO to develop essential diagnostics list. Available at: http://www.who.int/medicines/news/2017/WHO_develop_essential_diagnostics_list/en/. Accessed June 5, 2017.

23. Best days for public health are ahead of us, says WHO director-general. Address to the Sixty-fifth World Health Assembly. Geneva (Switzerland). Available at: http://www.who.int/dg/speeches/2012/wha_20120521/en/. Accessed June 5, 2017.

24. Ethical practice in laboratory medicine and forensic pathology. WHO regional publications, Eastern Mediterranean series, 20. Cairo (Egypt): World Health Organization; 1999. Available at: http://www.emro.who.int/dsaf/dsa38.pdf. Acecssed June 5, 2017.

25. Laboratory quality management system handbook. Geneva (Switzerland): World Health Organization; 2011. Available at: http://www.who.int/ihr/publications/lqms_en.pdf. Accessed June 5, 2017.

26. WHO guide for the stepwise laboratory improvement process towards accreditation in the African region. Brazzaville (Congo): World Health Organization; 2011. Available at: http://wwwwhoint/tb/laboratory/afro-slipta-checklist-guidancepdf. Accessed June 5, 2017.

27. Perrone LA, Voeurng V, Sek S, et al. Implementation research: a mentoring programme to improve laboratory quality in Cambodia. Bull World Health Organ 2016;94(10):743–51.

28. Development of national health laboratory policy and plan. World Health Organization regional office for the Western Pacific and regional office for South-East Asia. Manila (Philippines): World Health Organization; 2010. Available at: http://apps.searo.who.int/PDS_DOCS/B4725.pdf?ua=1. Accessed June 5, 2017.

29. Laboratory services national strategic plan. Geneva (Switzerland): World Health Organization; 2008. Available at: http://www.who.int/hiv/amds/amds_nat_strat_plan_lab_2008.pdf?ua=1. Accessed June 5, 2017.

30. Guidance for establishing a national health laboratory system. Brazzaville (Congo): World Health Organization; 2014. Available at: http://apps.who.int/iris/bitstream/10665/148351/1/GuidLabSyst.pdf. Accessed June 5, 2017.

31. Laboratory assessment tool. Geneva (Switzerland): World Health Organization; 2012. Available at: http://apps.who.int/iris/bitstream/10665/70874/3/WHO_HSE_GCR_LYO_2012.2_eng.pdf?ua=1&ua=1. Accessed June 5, 2017.

32. Ondoa P, van der Broek A, Jansen C, et al. National laboratory policies and plans in sub-Saharan African countries: gaps and opportunities. Afr J Lab Med 2017; 6(1):578.

33. Lilford RJ, Burn SL, Diaconu KD, et al. An approach to prioritization of medical devices in low-income countries: an example based on the Republic of South Sudan. Cost Eff Resour Alloc 2015;13(1):2.

Breast Cancer in Low- and Middle-Income Countries
Why We Need Pathology Capability to Solve This Challenge

Yehoda M. Martei, MD[a], Lydia E. Pace, MD, MPH[b],
Jane E. Brock, MBBS, PhD[c], Lawrence N. Shulman, MD[a],*

KEYWORDS

- Breast cancer • Pathology • Sub-Saharan Africa
- Low- and middle-income countries • Cancer control

KEY POINTS

- Breast cancer is the leading cause of cancer mortality among women in low- and middle-income countries (LMIC). Timely and accurate histopathological diagnoses of breast cancer are critical to delivering high-quality breast cancer care to patients in LMIC.
- The most important prognostic factors in breast cancer along with tumor size and nodal status are tumor grade and estrogen receptor status. Human epidermal growth factor receptor 2 status is important in countries where specific targeted therapies are available.
- Endocrine therapy with tamoxifen is affordable and widely available in most LMIC. It is therefore critical for basic pathology evaluations to include an assessment of estrogen receptor status by immunohistochemistry to identify those women who could benefit from endocrine therapy.
- Detailed and complete cancer registry data are needed to assess a country's disease burden and specific patient population needs to guide disease prioritization and allocation of resources for breast cancer treatment.
- Innovations in leapfrog technology and low-cost point-of-care tests for molecular evaluations are needed to provide accurate and timely pathology, with the ultimate goal of improving survival outcomes for patients with breast cancer in LMIC.

Disclosure Statement: J.E. Brock received research funding from Cepheid. Y.M. Martei, L.E. Pace, and L.N. Shulman have nothing to disclose.
[a] Division of Hematology-Oncology, Department of Medicine, University of Pennsylvania, Abramson Cancer Center, 3400 Civic Center Boulevard, Philadelphia, PA 19106 USA; [b] Division of Women's Health, Department of Medicine, Brigham and Women's Hospital, 75 Francis Street, Boston, MA 02115, USA; [c] Department of Pathology, Brigham and Women's Hospital, 75 Francis Street, Boston, MA 02115, USA
* Corresponding author. University of Pennsylvania, Abramson Cancer Center, 3400 Civic Center Boulevard, Suite 12-111 South, Philadelphia, PA 19104.
E-mail address: Lawrence.shulman@uphs.upenn.edu

Clin Lab Med 38 (2018) 161–173
https://doi.org/10.1016/j.cll.2017.10.013
0272-2712/18/© 2017 Elsevier Inc. All rights reserved.

labmed.theclinics.com

INTRODUCTION

The global burden of cancer is increasing worldwide, with most new cancer cases and cancer-related mortality occurring in low- and middle-income countries (LMIC).[1] It is estimated that by 2035, two-thirds of new cancer diagnoses will occur in developing countries.[2] Breast cancer remains the leading cancer diagnosis and cause of cancer-related deaths among women globally.[1] In most LMIC, breast cancer is either the leading or the second most common cause of cancer deaths among women. Although early-stage breast cancer is potentially curable, mortality-to-incidence ratios for breast cancer are significantly worse in LMIC than in countries of high income.[3] The high mortality-to-incidence ratio means patients diagnosed with breast cancer are more likely to die from their cancer in LMIC. Some of the mortality-to-incidence ratios reported in Middle, Eastern, and West Africa are as high as 0.55, compared with 0.16 in North America.[3] These alarming figures have drawn global attention to this cancer epidemic and the socially and economically devastating consequences of breast cancer among women in the world's poorest settings.

A country's strategy for national cancer planning requires knowledge of the disease burden in the country, information that is obtained when it is possible to make an accurate cancer diagnosis and document all relevant prognostic factors for a tumor. With this information, it is then possible to allocate available resources for patient care. Accurate diagnoses require timely and adequate pathology support.[4] Current reports show a significant deficiency in both professional and technical pathology services in LMIC, with some of the lowest numbers of pathologist-to-population ratios documented in sub-Saharan Africa.[5] Ratios in sub-Saharan Africa vary from that in Mauritius, where there is approximately 1 pathologist for every 84,133 persons, to Niger where there is one pathologist to 9,264,500 persons.[5] Moreover, countries like Somalia, Benin, Eritrea, and Burundi have only one or no pathologist in-country.[6] By comparison, the pathologist-to-population ratio in North America is 1 to 17,544 persons.[7]

Most patients in sub-Saharan Africa present with advanced stage disease: stage III and IV.[8–15] Despite the advanced stage of their disease, many of these patients can benefit from surgery, chemotherapy, targeted therapies, and endocrine therapy, depending on tumor biology, with treatments aimed at improving quality of life, and in some cases, significantly prolonging life. Even advanced disease requires confirmation of the presence of breast carcinoma by pathologic diagnosis, because other benign or malignant tumors can mimic breast cancer, for example, lymphoma, phyllodes tumor, or untreated infection, and all of these merit different treatment approaches.[16] A significant proportion of breast biopsies for palpable masses in a large cohort of breast cases in Ghana and a retrospective analysis of breast presentations in Rwanda was benign.[9,16] Thus, it is unethical and unsafe to offer mastectomy, cytotoxic chemotherapy, or other systemic therapy to a woman without having a pathologically confirmed diagnosis of breast cancer at the onset, and optimal treatment depends on the elucidation of both the stage of disease and the biologic markers, hormone receptors, and Human epidermal growth factor receptor 2 (HER2).

Prognostic factors, including tumor size, grade, estrogen receptor (ER) status, and nodal involvement, drive treatment choices. These prognostic factors are obtained from gross examination of a surgical specimen and subsequent histopathological review under a microscope. Tissue samples obtained by fine-needle aspirate (FNA), core-needle biopsy, or excision biopsy can all be adequate specimens for diagnostic purposes. In the United States, initial diagnosis with core-needle biopsy is recommended. It is more likely to yield adequate tissue to assess invasive versus in situ status and hormone receptors and HER2 than FNA and is less invasive than excisional biopsy. For patients who ultimately have a benign diagnosis, it avoids surgery altogether. Obtaining a complete and timely histopathological review is a tremendous challenge in LMIC given the lack of access to high-quality tissue processing facilities and prognostic marker evaluation. Innovative approaches to breast cancer diagnostics are needed to more rapidly satisfy the demand for accurate diagnoses at the point of care in the absence of adequate tissue processing facilities, trained technicians to run those facilities, and pathologists in LMIC. The goal is to demonstrate the extent to which timely and accurate histopathological diagnoses of breast cancer are critical to delivering high-quality breast cancer care to patients in LMIC.

BREAST CANCER HISTOPATHOLOGIC FEATURES AND RELEVANCE IN CLINICAL MANAGEMENT
Tumor, Nodal Status, and Histologic Grade

Population-based cancer registries in most LMICs do not contain a high percentage of anatomically staged cancers and detailed breast cancer prognostic features, which impairs the ability to prognosticate and treat patients adequately. The most important prognostic factors in breast cancer along with tumor size and nodal status are tumor grade and ER status. HER2 status is important in countries where specific targeted therapies are available. The prognostic and predictive significance of these features have been demonstrated and validated in multiple studies. **Tables 1** and **2** summarize current American Joint Commission on Cancer staging for breast cancer, 7th edition. In the National Surgical Adjuvant Breast and Bowel Project B-06 trial, an increase in the number of positive lymph nodes was associated with a worse prognosis.[17,18] Tumor size, perimenopausal status, number of axillary lymph node metastases, poorly differentiated grade, and presence of lymphatic invasion were also identified as negative independent predictors of prognosis.[19] In a long-term follow-up of patients with breast cancer with stage I and II disease followed for a median of 18.2 years, the risk of local recurrence at 20 years for T1N0 and T1N1 (1–3 positive nodes at diagnosis) disease was estimated at 2.8% and 6.5%, respectively.[19] Tumor biology heavily influences the time course for local recurrence, with most recurrences in ER-negative tumors being within 8 years of diagnosis, and risk of recurrence in ER-positive tumors increasing annually for the lifetime of the patient. Annual recurrence risk is 1% to 2% in N1 disease and 3% to 4% annually in N2 disease (≥4 positive nodes).[20] In addition, recent studies have shown that in multivariate analyses of patients with operable breast cancer treated according to standard protocol, histologic grade remains an independent predictor of breast cancer–specific survival and disease-free survival when analyzed as a whole and within stage subsets.[21–23]

Histologic Subtypes of Breast Cancer and Their Clinical Importance

Histologic subtype can also be important in determining therapy and is an important prognostic factor. Although the most common histologic subtypes are invasive ductal carcinoma of no special type (~60%), and invasive lobular carcinoma (~15%), more than 20 different subtypes of breast carcinoma exist, each with different risk factors, patterns of spread, and response to therapy.[24] Tumor subtypes with a better prognosis include tubular and cribriform, which are always ER positive, but also mucinous carcinoma and some other rare subtypes, such as secretory carcinoma and adenoid cystic carcinoma, which have a good prognosis despite their ER-negative status.[25–27] ER-negative breast cancers typically have a worse prognosis with an early risk of recurrence compared with ER-positive tumors, and when feasible, chemotherapy is

Table 1	
American Joint Committee on Cancer TNM summary staging system for breast cancer	
Primary tumor (T)	
TX	Primary tumor cannot be assessed
T0	No evidence of primary tumor
Tis	**Carcinoma in situ**
T1	**Tumor ≤20 mm in greatest dimension**
T2	**Tumor >20 mm but ≤50 mm in greatest dimension**
T3	**Tumor >50 mm in greatest dimension**
T4	Tumor of any size with direct extension to the chest wall and/or the skin (ulceration or skin nodules)
Regional lymph nodes (N): Clinical	
NX	Regional lymph nodes cannot be assessed
N0	**No regional lymph node metastasis**
N1	**Metastases to movable ipsilateral I, II axillary lymph nodes**
N2	**Metastases in ipsilateral level I, II axillary lymph nodes that are clinically fixed or matted; or in clinically detected ipsilateral internal mammary nodes in the absence of clinically evident axillary lymph node metastases**
N3	**Metastases in ipsilateral infraclavicular (level III) axillary lymph node(s) with or without level I or II axillary lymph node involvement; or in clinically detected ipsilateral internal mammary lymph node(s) with clinically evident level I, II axillary lymph node metastases; or metastases in ipsilateral supraclavicular node(s) with or without axillary or internal mammary lymph node involvement**
Pathologic (pN)	
pNX	Regional lymph nodes cannot be assessed
pN0	**No regional lymph node metastases histologically**
pN1	**Micrometastases; metastases in 1–3 axillary lymph nodes; and/or in internal mammary nodes with metastases detected by sentinel lymph node biopsy but not clinically detected**
pN2	**Metastases in 4–9 axillary lymph nodes; or in clinically detected internal mammary lymph nodes detected in the absence of axillary lymph node metastases**
pN3	**Metastases in 10 or more axillary lymph nodes; or in infraclavicular (level III axillary) lymph nodes; or in clinically detected ipsilateral internal mammary lymph nodes in the presence of one or more positive axillary level I, II lymph nodes; or in more than 3 axillary lymph nodes and in internal mammary lymph nodes with micrometastases or macrometastases detected by sentinel lymph node biopsy but not clinically detected; or in ipsilateral supraclavicular lymph nodes**
Distant metastasis (M)	
M0	No clinical or radiographic evidence of distant metastasis
cM0(1+)	**No clinical or radiographic evidence of distant metastasis, but deposits of molecularly or microscopically detected tumor cells in circulating blood, bone marrow, or other nonregional nodal tissue that are no larger than 0.2 mm in a patient without symptoms or signs of metastases**
M1	Distant detectable metastases as determined by classic clinical and radiographic means and/or histologically proven larger than 0.2 mm

Staging in boldface represents staging information that can only be obtained via pathologic assessment. Metastatic disease at the time of initial presentation will also require pathologic assessment to confirm diagnosis.

Data from American Joint Committee on Cancer. Breast cancer staging. 7th edition. Available at: https://cancerstaging.org/references-tools/quickreferences/Documents/BreastSmall.pdf. Accessed October 19, 2017.

Table 2
Anatomic stage/prognostic groups and summary of recommended systemic therapies

						Receptor Status		
						ER and/or PR Positive	HER2 Positive	Triple-Negative Breast Cancers
Stage 0	Tis	N0	M0					
Stage IA	T1	N0	M0	Stage 1	Endocrine therapy	YES	NO	NO
Stage IB	T0	N1mi	M0		HER2-directed therapy	NO	YES	NO
	T1	N1mi	M0		Chemotherapy	+/−[a]	YES	YES
Stage IIA	T0	N1	M0	Stage 2				
	T1	N1	M0		Endocrine therapy	YES	NO	NO
	T2	N0	M0		HER2-directed therapy	NO	YES	NO
Stage IIB	T2	N1	M0		Chemotherapy	+/−[a]	YES	YES
	T3	N0	M0					
Stage IIIA	T0	N2	M0	Stage 3				
	T1	N2	M0					
	T2	N2	M0					
	T3	N1	M0		Endocrine therapy	YES	NO	NO
	T3	N2	M0		HER2-directed therapy	NO	YES	NO
Stage IIIB	T4	N0	M0		Chemotherapy	YES	YES	YES
	T4	N1	M0					
	T4	N2	M0					
Stage IIIC	Any T	N3	M0					
Stage IV	Any T	Any N	M1	Stage IV	Endocrine therapy	YES	NO	NO
					HER2-directed therapy	NO	YES	NO
					Chemotherapy	+/−[b]	YES	YES

[a] +/− is indicated for subsets for which genomic assays assist with clinical decision regarding the additional benefit of chemotherapy versus not.
[b] In the metastatic setting, chemotherapy for ER/PR-positive tumors is recommended only for patients with visceral crisis or those who have failed multiple lines of endocrine therapy.

offered to improve survival and decrease risk of recurrence if the tumors are greater than 1 cm in size. It is important to be able to recognize rare subtypes of ER-negative cancer like adenoid cystic carcinoma and secretory carcinoma to prevent overtreatment with chemotherapy when it is not indicated.

ASCERTAINMENT OF MOLECULAR PATHOLOGY AND CLINICAL RELEVANCE
Hormone Receptor Status

Thirty percent of women with ER-positive early breast cancer will eventually present with recurrent disease. All women with ER-positive disease should be offered endocrine therapy to reduce this risk. Tamoxifen is the least expensive endocrine therapy available and acts as an anti-estrogen, binding the estrogen receptor. It reduces the risk of recurrence by half and slows tumor growth in sensitive tumors, but there is no benefit from endocrine therapy in tumors not expressing ER, and therapy should be avoided in these patients given the potential side effects of hormonal therapy, which include menopausal symptoms, thrombosis, osteoporosis, and very rarely, endometrial carcinomas.[28,29] Endocrine therapy with tamoxifen is affordable and widely available in most LMIC. Furthermore, it is less toxic than intravenous and oral systemic chemotherapy and requires less frequent visits and monitoring. It is therefore critical for basic pathology evaluations to include an assessment of ER status by immunohistochemistry to identify those women who could benefit from endocrine therapy. Seventy percent of tumors in developed countries overexpress ER. The proportion of women in LMIC that have ER expression is less, around 60%, primarily because of different population demographics. The proportion of the population that is postmenopausal and/or obese is lower in LMIC compared with high-income countries, and these are clinical factors associated with hormone receptor positivity.

Accurate determination of ER status requires access to high-quality histology and immunohistochemistry facilities as part of a pathologic review. A major quality control issue in LMICs is appropriate handling of biopsy or excision specimens. Frequently, there is little control over cold ischemic time of the tissue specimen, which is often prolonged because of limited access to pathology processing facilities and even physician ignorance in handling the tissue specimen. It is also common to have a pathology specimen fixed in formalin that is either diluted and is a suboptimal volume for adequate rapid fixation, or specimens are overfixed by sitting in formalin for weeks before being processed. All of these factors influence ER evaluation and can increase the false negative rates of ER status. For many years, it was thought that African women had much higher rates of ER-negative breast carcinoma, an erroneous assumption based on poor tissue handling and poor-quality histopathology and immunohistochemical evaluation of specimens. To reduce the impact of poor tissue processing on evaluation of ER status in high-income countries, tissue handling guidelines have been issued by the American Society of Clinical Oncology and the College of American Pathologists (CAP).[30–32] Cold ischemia time, which is the time from loss of vascular blood supply to tissue to the time it is exposed to fixative such as formalin, should be less than 60 minutes.[32] Longer times lead to degradation of critical biomarker proteins and false negative results. Tissue fixation time is also critical, with an optimal time defined as a minimum of 6 hours of fixation for core biopsies, and a maximum of 72 hours for optimal hormone receptor assessment. Shorter and longer times have been linked to false negative and false positive results, although it takes several weeks of prolonged fixation for a strongly ER-positive tumor to become completely ER negative, rather than hours or days of prolonged fixation.[33,34]

In addition to guiding patient care, high-quality immunohistochemistry will permit better understanding of potential ethnic variation in the expression of breast tumor hormonal markers in sub-Saharan Africa.[35–40] The reported range in expression of ER in breast tumors ranges from 24% to 71% among black women in West Africa compared with 63% in South Africa.[41–43] Data from Rwanda and Kenya also suggest that East Africa may have higher rates of ER-positive disease and closer to that of Europe and North America at 60% to 70%, especially in places like Rwanda, where the cold ischemic time for most samples is known.[44–47] The heterogeneity of these data is more likely to be a phenomenon of tissue handling procedures and quality of histopathology and immunohistochemistry review than a significant ethnic difference, but in the absence of knowledge about tissue handling and access to quality pathology, it is not possible to know this for certain. Increasing access to high-quality immunohistochemistry will better delineate the molecular heterogeneity of breast cancer subtypes in sub-Saharan Africa and other LMICs. In addition, it will expand access to quality immunohistochemistry for use in other cancer types and subtypes.

Human Epidermal Growth Factor Receptor 2 Receptor Status

Breast cancers that overexpress HER2 are aggressive tumors with a high risk of early recurrence and death. The use of HER2-targeted therapy has greatly improved outcomes for these patients and is standard therapy in high-income countries, but HER2 therapies are costly, and are rarely available in LMIC. The most recent update of the World Health Organization's model list of essential medicines in 2015 included the HER2-targeted medicine, trastuzumab, because of its significant positive impact on survival.[48] In the absence of available therapy, HER2 testing by immunohistochemistry or fluorescence in situ hybridization is not merited. As trastuzumab goes off patent soon and biosimilars become available, this is projected to halve the cost of HER2-targeted therapy in Europe, India, and North America, and more affordable HER2-targeted therapy options can be expected, which may increase availability in LMICs.[49,50]

PATHOLOGY EVALUATION OF SURGICAL SPECIMENS AFTER PREOPERATIVE THERAPY

In LMICs where a significant majority of patients with breast cancer present with advanced stage disease, preoperative chemotherapy or endocrine therapy may be appropriate for improving surgical resectability in inoperable tumors and not just offered in the palliative setting. Preoperative (or neoadjuvant) chemotherapy does not adversely affect survival outcomes compared with adjuvant therapy.[51,52] Pathologic assessment of a completely resected tumor bed and appropriate node sampling following preoperative chemotherapy provide useful prognostic information for a patient. Patients with no residual invasive carcinoma in the breast and axillary lymph nodes after preoperative chemotherapy (called a pathologic complete response) have a superior recurrence-free survival, particularly if they are ER negative.[53] Those with residual disease after neoadjuvant chemotherapy have a higher risk of distant recurrence and a worse prognosis.[54]

PATHOLOGY TURNAROUND TIME

In addition to accurate histopathological diagnosis and biomarker assessments, it is critical to improve the timeliness of pathology results in LMIC. With current challenges in pathology services in most LMIC, the turnaround time (TAT) for pathology results is on the order of weeks to months in some countries. Because initial therapy is determined by pathologic evaluation of tumor size, nodal status, grade, ER/progesterone receptor (PR), and HER2 status, prolonged TAT can lead to either needing to choose a therapy without this critical information, which may result in inappropriate therapy, or waiting for results, which could allow disease to progress, consequently worsening prognosis. A historical analysis identified that delays in excess of 3 months before initiating therapy led to stage migration in patients with breast cancer.[55] In some cases, even more timely pathology is needed to identify patients who might benefit from more surgery, such as re-resection of positive margins and residual disease, or complete axillary lymph node dissection for patients wherein positive sentinel lymph nodes have been identified. A retrospective review of TAT from Butaro Cancer Center in Rwanda reported a median TAT from specimen receipt to reporting of 32 days.[56] Another retrospective analysis from Malawi identified median TAT for cancer specimens paid out of pocket as 43 days, and 101 days for nonpaid for specimens, which rely on state funds.[57] The CAP recommends a TAT of 2 business days for biopsy specimens.[58] Two days is likely not an attainable goal currently in most LMIC. A realistic goal of maximum TAT of 1 week will still be timely to aid in most of the clinical prognostication and management choices discussed in this article.

PATHOLOGY AND NATIONAL BREAST CANCER CONTROL

LMIC nearly alway lack detailed and complete cancer registry data, impairing ability to assess a country's disease burden and specific patient population needs to guide disease prioritization and allocation of resources for breast cancer treatment. Without adequate pathology, resources for breast cancer may be misguided and may not translate into improved survival outcomes for patients. For instance, it is imperative both in the clinical management of patients and from the national medicines procurement level to be able to ascertain the proportion and projected number of patients with breast cancer that are and will be ER positive and will benefit from endocrine therapy. Knowing the proportions of specific molecular subtypes and specifically ER positive breast cancers ultimately facilitates the procurement of adequate quantities of endocrine therapy, a medicine that can be prescribed daily for 5 years in the adjuvant setting and daily until time of tumor progression in the metastatic and palliative setting.[59,60] In addition, as HER2 biosimilars become available, there might be utility in assessing HER2 status and determining whether this is a cost-effective therapy that can be financed by LMIC governments. Breast cancer is commonly managed by a multimodality specialty team, involving surgery and radiation oncology. In countries where this is outsourced to specific public surgical centers or private radiation facilities, quality pathologic evaluation is needed to predict the utilization of these modalities and to guide future resource allocation to the different arms of breast cancer control. The elements of a pathology evaluation, including tissue handling, tissue histology, and immunohistochemical evaluations of the key prognostic factors described above, inform key holders about the distribution of disease. Quality pathology evaluation is a key factor along with access to medical and surgical therapies and interventions to increase earlier detection, with the goal of improving outcomes for women with breast cancer in LMICs.

BREAST CANCER PATHOLOGY IN LOW- AND MIDDLE-INCOME COUNTRIES: INNOVATION AND RESEARCH

Given the histopathologic and molecular heterogeneity of breast cancer, especially within sub-Saharan Africa, complete and timely pathology is needed to accurately assess the variations in disease burden and molecular subtypes. These efforts are severely impaired by the deficit of pathologists in LMIC. Innovations in leapfrog technology have been used in various LMIC by partnering with other institutions in developed countries to assist with pathology reporting. One such example is the collaboration between Ministry of Health in Rwanda, Partners in Health, and the Dana-Farber Cancer Institute in providing remote pathology assessment via telepathology to assist with breast cancer and other pathology diagnoses. The setup of whole slide image scanning and the automation of processing have helped with the provision of timely and complete pathology services for patients with cancer in Rwanda.[61] In Kenya, task shifting is being used to increase pathology capacity in-country by training pathologists to teach medical officers, who then teach other medical officers, to perform biopsies, FNAs, and bone marrow biopsies.[62]

High-quality immunohistochemistry is a challenge in LMIC hospitals, even for those hospitals that have adequate histology resources to provide quality hematoxylin and eosin stain diagnoses from pathology specimens. Inadequate IHC capacity limits the ability to provide the prognostic marker ER status for women with a cancer diagnosis. One solution is to use molecular pathology to solve this problem. Although molecular pathology remains a challenge even in countries where pathologists are able to perform histopathologic assessments, point-of-care testing could be a reality. The

GeneXpert technology is a platform for performing quantitative reverse transcription polymerase chain reaction that is already widely distributed in LMIC for a variety of tests, including rapid diagnosis of tuberculosis using a simple dedicated cartridge. A dedicated cartridge that can perform messenger RNA amplification of ER, PR, HER2, and Ki-67 and give breast cancer biomarker results from formalin-fixed paraffin-embedded is anticipated to soon be available, which can be used to provide prognostic markers in the absence of access to ER immunohistochemistry.[63]

A future need in LMIC is to have low-cost point-of-care tests for molecular evaluations like OncotypeDX, but it is not an urgent need right now because very few women present with early breast cancer (tumors <5 cm and axillary node negative), and there is less of a dilemma in most of the breast cancer population as to whether to offer chemotherapy or not. In high-income countries, additional molecular testing, such as OncotypeDX, provides prognostic information on the risk of recurrence at 10 years in ER-positive tumors that are either node negative (N0) or node positive (1–3 positive nodes). It is frequently used in a predictive manner to help in the decision-making process whether to withhold chemotherapy and offer only endocrine therapy. Tumors with low recurrence scores (RS <11) do not need chemotherapy, and those with intermediate scores (RS 11–25) are likely to have minimal benefit from chemotherapy.[64–68]

Improving clinical research and pathology capacity in LMIC will enrich the knowledge of unique variations in the molecular and genomic landscape of breast cancer among different racial and geographic populations. A recent study of the genomic alterations in breast tumors from Nigeria, West Africa compared with African American women and women of European ancestry, analysis on structural variants (SV) showed genome-wide SV counts among the 3 populations are comparable in ER-negative cancers; however, among ER-positive cancers, Nigerians had significantly more SV counts compared with African Americans or European Americans in ER-positive cancers, suggestive of a more aggressive ER-positive phenotype.[69] These data emphasize the heterogeneity of genomic landscape for breast cancer and the need to improve quality pathology, which would inform accurate prognostic risk assessment and choice of targeted therapy to specific diverse populations.

Finally, in areas where there are high burdens of infectious comorbidities, such as HIV, quality pathology reviews of tissue specimens and clinical research will help to better understand whether worse outcomes reported in HIV-positive patients with breast cancer are due to treatment-related toxicity or to interaction with the biology of their disease. In addition, there is significant potential for research to help to identify breast cancer risk factors and employ the right tools to mitigate the high cancer burden. Ultimately, increased pathology capacity will help provide timely information to guide clinical care and help narrow the survival gap between patients with breast cancer in developed and developing countries.

REFERENCES

1. Cancer IAfRo. GLOBOCAN 2012: estimated cancer incidence, mortality and prevalence worldwide in 2012. Available at: http://globocaniarcfr/Defaultaspx Accessed March 16, 2017.

2. Tefferi A, Kantarjian H, Rajkumar SV, et al. In support of a patient-driven initiative and petition to lower the high price of cancer drugs. Mayo Clin Proc 2015;90: 996–1000.

3. DeSantis CE, Bray F, Ferlay J, et al. International variation in female breast cancer incidence and mortality rates. Cancer Epidemiol Biomarkers Prev 2015;24: 1495–506.

4. African Strategies for Advancing Pathology Group Members. Quality pathology and laboratory diagnostic services are key to improving global health outcomes: improving global health outcomes is not possible without accurate disease diagnosis. Am J Clin Pathol 2015;143:325–8.

5. Nelson AM, Milner DA, Rebbeck TR, et al. Oncologic care and pathology resources in Africa: survey and recommendations. J Clin Oncol 2016;34:20–6.

6. Adesina A, Chumba D, Nelson AM, et al. Improvement of pathology in sub-Saharan Africa. Lancet Oncol 2013;14:e152–7.

7. Robboy SJ, Weintraub S, Horvath AE, et al. Pathologist workforce in the United States: I. Development of a predictive model to examine factors influencing supply. Arch Pathol Lab Med 2013;137:1723–32.

8. Pace LE, Mpunga T, Hategekimana V, et al. Delays in breast cancer presentation and diagnosis at two rural cancer referral centers in Rwanda. Oncologist 2015; 20:780–8.

9. Brinton L, Figueroa J, Adjei E, et al. Factors contributing to delays in diagnosis of breast cancers in Ghana, West Africa. Breast Cancer Res Treat 2017;162:105–14.

10. Brinton LA, Awuah B, Nat Clegg-Lamptey J, et al. Design considerations for identifying breast cancer risk factors in a population-based study in Africa. Int J Cancer 2017;140:2667–77.

11. Adebamowo CA, Adekunle OO. Case-controlled study of the epidemiological risk factors for breast cancer in Nigeria. Br J Surg 1999;86:665–8.

12. Anyanwu SN. Temporal trends in breast cancer presentation in the third world. J Exp Clin Cancer Res 2008;27:17.

13. Abdulrahman GO Jr, Rahman GA. Epidemiology of breast cancer in Europe and Africa. J Cancer Epidemiol 2012;2012:915610.

14. Othieno-Abinya NA, Nyabola LO, Abwao HO, et al. Postsurgical management of patients with breast cancer at Kenyatta National Hospital. East Afr Med J 2002; 79:156–62.

15. Zouladeny H, Dille I, Wehbi NK, et al. Epidemiologic and clinical profiles of breast diseases in Niger. Int J Cancer Oncol 2015;2.

16. Pace LE, Dusengimana JMV, Hategekimana V, et al. Benign and malignant breast disease at Rwanda's first public cancer referral center. Oncologist 2016;21: 571–5.

17. Fisher B, Redmond C, Poisson R, et al. Eight-year results of a randomized clinical trial comparing total mastectomy and lumpectomy with or without irradiation in the treatment of breast cancer. N Engl J Med 1989;320:822–8.

18. Fisher ER, Anderson S, Redmond C, et al. Pathologic findings from the National Surgical Adjuvant Breast Project protocol B-06. 10-year pathologic and clinical prognostic discriminants. Cancer 1993;71:2507–14.

19. Rosen PP, Groshen S, Saigo PE, et al. Pathological prognostic factors in stage I (T1N0M0) and stage II (T1N1M0) breast carcinoma: a study of 644 patients with median follow-up of 18 years. J Clin Oncol 1989;7:1239–51.

20. Pan H, Gray RG, Davies C, et al. Long-term recurrence risks after use of endocrine therapy for only 5 years: relevance of breast tumor characteristics. J Clin Oncol 2016;34(suppl). abstr 505.

21. Rakha EA, El-Sayed ME, Lee AH, et al. Prognostic significance of Nottingham histologic grade in invasive breast carcinoma. J Clin Oncol 2008;26:3153–8.

22. Lundin J, Lundin M, Holli K, et al. Omission of histologic grading from clinical decision making may result in overuse of adjuvant therapies in breast cancer: results from a nationwide study. J Clin Oncol 2001;19:28–36.

23. Schwartz AM, Henson DE, Chen D, et al. Histologic grade remains a prognostic factor for breast cancer regardless of the number of positive lymph nodes and tumor size: a study of 161 708 cases of breast cancer from the SEER Program. Arch Pathol Lab Med 2014;138:1048–52.
24. Weigelt B, Geyer FC, Reis-Filho JS. Histological types of breast cancer: how special are they? Mol Oncol 2010;4:192–208.
25. Rakha EA, Lee AH, Evans AJ, et al. Tubular carcinoma of the breast: further evidence to support its excellent prognosis. J Clin Oncol 2010;28:99–104.
26. Caldarella A, Buzzoni C, Crocetti E, et al. Invasive breast cancer: a significant correlation between histological types and molecular subgroups. J Cancer Res Clin Oncol 2013;139:617–23.
27. Dieci MV, Orvieto E, Dominici M, et al. Rare breast cancer subtypes: histological, molecular, and clinical peculiarities. Oncologist 2014;19:805–13.
28. Howat JM, Harris M, Swindell R, et al. The effect of oestrogen and progesterone receptors on recurrence and survival in patients with carcinoma of the breast. Br J Cancer 1985;51:263–70.
29. Early Breast Cancer Trialists' Collaborative Group. Effects of chemotherapy and hormonal therapy for early breast cancer on recurrence and 15-year survival: an overview of the randomised trials. Lancet 2005;365:1687–717.
30. Hammond ME, Hayes DF, Dowsett M, et al. American Society of Clinical Oncology/College of American Pathologists guideline recommendations for immunohistochemical testing of estrogen and progesterone receptors in breast cancer (unabridged version). Arch Pathol Lab Med 2010;134:e48–72.
31. Hammond ME, Hayes DF, Dowsett M, et al. American Society of Clinical Oncology/College of American Pathologists guideline recommendations for immunohistochemical testing of estrogen and progesterone receptors in breast cancer. J Clin Oncol 2010;28:2784–95.
32. Yildiz-Aktas IZ, Dabbs DJ, Bhargava R. The effect of cold ischemic time on the immunohistochemical evaluation of estrogen receptor, progesterone receptor, and HER2 expression in invasive breast carcinoma. Mod Pathol 2012;25:1098–105.
33. Pekmezci M, Szpaderska A, Osipo C, et al. The effect of cold ischemia time and/or formalin fixation on estrogen receptor, progesterone receptor, and human epidermal growth factor receptor-2 results in breast carcinoma. Patholog Res Int 2012;2012:947041.
34. Mohsin SK. Frozen section library: breast. New York: Springer; 2012.
35. Dietze EC, Sistrunk C, Miranda-Carboni G, et al. Triple-negative breast cancer in African-American women: disparities versus biology. Nat Rev Cancer 2015;15:248–54.
36. Der EM, Gyasi RK, Tettey Y, et al. Triple-negative breast cancer in Ghanaian women: the Korle Bu Teaching Hospital experience. Breast J 2015;21:627–33.
37. Proctor E, Kidwell KM, Jiagge E, et al. Characterizing breast cancer in a population with increased prevalence of triple-negative breast cancer: androgen receptor and ALDH1 expression in Ghanaian women. Ann Surg Oncol 2015;22:3831–5.
38. Cubasch H, Joffe M, Hanisch R, et al. Breast cancer characteristics and HIV among 1,092 women in Soweto, South Africa. Breast Cancer Res Treat 2013;140:177–86.
39. Rais G, Raissouni S, Aitelhaj M, et al. Triple negative breast cancer in Moroccan women: clinicopathological and therapeutic study at the National Institute of Oncology. BMC Womens Health 2012;12:35.

40. Eng A, McCormack V, dos-Santos-Silva I. Receptor-defined subtypes of breast cancer in indigenous populations in Africa: a systematic review and meta-analysis. PLoS Med 2014;11:e1001720.

41. Huo D, Ikpatt F, Khramtsov A, et al. Population differences in breast cancer: survey in indigenous African women reveals over-representation of triple-negative breast cancer. J Clin Oncol 2009;27:4515–21.

42. McCormack VA, Joffe M, van den Berg E, et al. Breast cancer receptor status and stage at diagnosis in over 1,200 consecutive public hospital patients in Soweto, South Africa: a case series. Breast Cancer Res 2013;15:R84.

43. Adebamowo CA, Famooto A, Ogundiran TO, et al. Immunohistochemical and molecular subtypes of breast cancer in Nigeria. Breast Cancer Res Treat 2008; 110:183–8.

44. O'Neil DS, Keating NL, Dusengimana JMV, et al. Quality of breast cancer treatment at a rural cancer center in Rwanda. J Glob Oncol 2017. [Epub ahead of print].

45. Sawe RT, Kerper M, Badve S, et al. Aggressive breast cancer in western Kenya has early onset, high proliferation, and immune cell infiltration. BMC Cancer 2016; 16:204.

46. Nyagol J, Nyong'o A, Byakika B, et al. Routine assessment of hormonal receptor and her-2/neu status underscores the need for more therapeutic targets in Kenyan women with breast cancer. Anal Quant Cytol Histol 2006;28:97–103.

47. Sayed S, Moloo Z, Wasike R, et al. Is breast cancer from Sub Saharan Africa truly receptor poor? Prevalence of ER/PR/HER2 in breast cancer from Kenya. Breast 2014;23:591–6.

48. Shulman LN, Wagner CM, Barr R, et al. Proposing essential medicines to treat cancer: methodologies, processes, and outcomes. J Clin Oncol 2016;34:69–75.

49. WHO to begin pilot prequalification of biosimilars for cancer treatment. Press Release 4 May 2017. Available at: http://wwwwhoint/mediacentre/news/releases/2017/pilot-prequalification-biosimilars/en/. Accessed May 17, 2017.

50. Rugo HS, Barve A, Waller CF, et al. Effect of a proposed trastuzumab biosimilar compared with trastuzumab on overall response rate in patients with ERBB2 (HER2)-positive metastatic breast cancer: a randomized clinical trial. JAMA 2017;317:37–47.

51. Fisher B, Bryant J, Wolmark N, et al. Effect of preoperative chemotherapy on the outcome of women with operable breast cancer. J Clin Oncol 1998;16:2672–85.

52. Bear HD, Anderson S, Smith RE, et al. Sequential preoperative or postoperative docetaxel added to preoperative doxorubicin plus cyclophosphamide for operable breast cancer:National surgical adjuvant breast and bowel project protocol B-27. J Clin Oncol 2006;24:2019–27.

53. Esserman LJ, Berry DA, DeMichele A, et al. Pathologic complete response predicts recurrence-free survival more effectively by cancer subset: results from the I-SPY 1 TRIAL–CALGB 150007/150012, ACRIN 6657. J Clin Oncol 2012;30: 3242–9.

54. Symmans WF, Wei C, Gould R, et al. Long-term prognostic risk after neoadjuvant chemotherapy associated with residual cancer burden and breast cancer subtype. J Clin Oncol 2017;35:1049–60.

55. Richards MA, Westcombe AM, Love SB, et al. Influence of delay on survival in patients with breast cancer: a systematic review. Lancet 1999;353:1119–26.

56. Mpunga T, Tapela N, Hedt-Gauthier BL, et al. Diagnosis of cancer in rural Rwanda: early outcomes of a phased approach to implement anatomic pathology services in resource-limited settings. Am J Clin Pathol 2014;142:541–5.

57. Masamba LPL, Mtonga PE, Phiri LK, et al. Cancer pathology turnaround time at Queen Elizabeth Central Hospital, the largest referral center in Malawi for oncology patients. J Glob Oncol 2017. [Epub ahead of print].

58. Zarbo RJ, Gephardt GN, Howanitz PJ. Intralaboratory timeliness of surgical pathology reports. Results of two College of American Pathologists Q-Probes studies of biopsies and complex specimens. Arch Pathol Lab Med 1996;120: 234–44.

59. Tannock IF. 10-year analysis of the ATAC trial: wrong conclusion? Lancet Oncol 2011;12:216–7 [author reply: 7].

60. Goss PE, Ingle JN, Pritchard KI, et al. Extending aromatase-inhibitor adjuvant therapy to 10 years. N Engl J Med 2016;375:209–19.

61. Mpunga T, Hedt-Gauthier BL, Tapela N, et al. Implementation and validation of telepathology triage at cancer referral center in rural Rwanda. J Glob Oncol 2016;2:76–82.

62. Topazian H, Cira M, Dawsey SM, et al. Joining forces to overcome cancer: the Kenya cancer research and control stakeholder program. J Cancer Policy 2016;7:36–41.

63. Wu NC, Wong W, Ho KE, et al. High concordance of ER, PR, HER2 and Ki67 by central IHC and FISH with mRNA measurements by GeneXpert® breast cancer stratifier assay [abstract]. In: Proceedings of the 2016 San Antonio Breast Cancer Symposium; 2016 Dec 6-10; San Antonio, TX. Cancer Res 2017;77 [abstract: P1-03-03].

64. Berry DA, Cirrincione C, Henderson IC, et al. Estrogen-receptor status and outcomes of modern chemotherapy for patients with node-positive breast cancer. JAMA 2006;295:1658–67.

65. van Tienhoven G, Voogd AC, Peterse JL, et al. Prognosis after treatment for loco-regional recurrence after mastectomy or breast conserving therapy in two randomised trials (EORTC 10801 and DBCG-82TM). EORTC Breast Cancer Cooperative Group and the Danish Breast Cancer Cooperative Group. Eur J Cancer 1999;35:32–8.

66. Paik S, Shak S, Tang G, et al. A multigene assay to predict recurrence of tamoxifen-treated, node-negative breast cancer. N Engl J Med 2004;351: 2817–26.

67. Sparano JA, Gray RJ, Makower DF, et al. Prospective validation of a 21-gene expression assay in breast cancer. N Engl J Med 2015;373:2005–14.

68. Albain KS, Barlow WE, Shak S, et al. Prognostic and predictive value of the 21-gene recurrence score assay in postmenopausal women with node-positive, oestrogen-receptor-positive breast cancer on chemotherapy: a retrospective analysis of a randomised trial. Lancet Oncol 2010;11:55–65.

69. Olopade OI, Pitt JJ, Riester M, et al. Comparative analysis of the genomic landscape of breast cancers from women of African and European ancestry. Cancer Res 2017;77.

Cytopathology in Low Medical Infrastructure Countries

Why and How to Integrate to Capacitate Health Care

Andrew S. Field, MBBS (Hons), FRCPA, FIAC, DipCytopath (RCPA)

KEYWORDS

- Cytopathology • FNA Cytology • LMIC • Teaching

KEY POINTS

- Cytopathologic assessment, particularly fine-needle aspiration cytology (FNAC), is a rapid, accurate, minimally invasive, inexpensive biopsy technique that requires minimal laboratory infrastructure and proceduralist costs.
- Cytology provides infectious and noncommunicable disease diagnoses and will play an essential role in the establishment of cancer services in low-income and middle-income countries (LMICs).
- All cytology specimens need to be handled using well-established protocols, FNAC biopsy requires specific training in the technique, and interpretation requires rigorous training.
- The use of ancillary tests on cytology material, including molecular tests, is established and rapidly expanding in high-income countries in the era of personalized medicine and will spread to LMICs.
- To establish cytology services and strengthen health services there must be a rapid increase in the training of cytopathologists and cytotechnologists, as well as increased education of clinicians in the roles and utility of diagnostic cytopathology and a commitment from governments and specialist training groups and funding.

INTRODUCTION

The major current problems with providing high-quality pathology diagnostic services in low-income and middle-income countries (LMICs) are the lack of infrastructure in pathology laboratories and equipment, as well as the lack of trained technical and medical practitioners.[1,2] There is a lack of funding for the establishment and

Disclosure Statement: The author has nothing to disclose.
Department of Anatomical Pathology, St Vincent's Hospital, Sydney, New South Wales, 2010, Australia
E-mail address: Andrew.Field@svha.org.au

Clin Lab Med 38 (2018) 175–182
https://doi.org/10.1016/j.cll.2017.10.014
0272-2712/18/© 2017 Elsevier Inc. All rights reserved.

labmed.theclinics.com

ongoing running costs of laboratories and for the ongoing costs of maintaining a pathology laboratory workforce, and for training pathologists and technologists for diagnostic work and teaching.[3] This is particularly so for cytopathologists and cytotechnologists.

There are also problems related to current clinical practice in which cytopathology and other pathologic tests are not integrated into the management protocols for patients who have cancer, are undergoing surgery, or have infectious disease because pathologic assessment has not been available up to this time. This affects the management of infectious diseases, which have traditionally been the main causes of morbidity and mortality in developing countries, and noncommunicable diseases (NCDs), which are increasingly becoming the most important causes of disease in LMICs.[4] There needs to be a strengthening of health systems. This will require political commitment and significant increases in funding to build up human resources, infrastructure, and data collection systems, and to invest in new technology and research, which will inform the best and most productive application of funding as countries attempt to reach their sustainable development goals.[5]

HOW CAN CYTOPATHOLOGY HELP?

Cytopathology covers a broad range of diagnostic and screening tests, including the cervical Papanicolaou (Pap) smear, sputum, urine, pleural and ascitic fluids, cerebrospinal fluid, and fine-needle aspiration cytology (FNAC). Cytopathology requires minimal laboratory infrastructure and, in the case of FNAC, is often able to replace more expensive core and surgical pathologic assessment.

Traditional cervical cancer screening programs using the cervical Pap smear provided a major tool to diagnose and ultimately greatly reduce the incidence of cervical cancer through screening programs in developed countries. Cervical cancer remains a significant cause of cancer-related deaths in the developing world. In LMICs there are few if any formal cervical cancer screening programs but the simple Pap smear is used in an ad hoc, mainly user-pay, system to screen and diagnose cervical cancer and its precursors. Of the exfoliative cytology tests, only examination of sputum is widely used, mainly to attempt to diagnose mycobacterial lung infections. FNAC is variably but increasingly used across LMICs and has become a major diagnostic tool in India. It can be performed in hospital inpatient and outpatient settings, as well as in doctors' surgeries and rural clinics. It has a potentially crucial role in the diagnosis of both NCDs and infections in LMICs, including adult and pediatric tuberculosis.[6–8] FNAC is routinely performed without local anesthetic, quickly and easily, using 22-gauge to 27-gauge needles and a simple alcohol skin preparation. The material is directly smeared onto slides that, through a specimen splitting process, can produce multiple slides for routine alcohol-fixed Pap and air-dried Giemsa staining, as well as specialized stains, such as the Ziehl-Neelsen stain for mycobacterial infection.[9] Rinsed material from the needle can then be placed into cell blocks, fixed in formalin, and paraffin-embedded for the full range of immunohistochemical and even molecular testing if available. The FNAC material can be used in rapid polymerase chain reaction (PCR)-based testing, such as GeneXpert, for the diagnosis of tuberculosis, or directly inoculated into culture bottles or handled in a more traditional manner by a microbiological laboratory for cultures and drug-sensitivity studies.[10] The range of targets can be extended from palpable lesions to impalpable and deep seated lesions by the use of relatively inexpensive ultrasound guidance.

The use of FNAC is greatly facilitated by rapid on-site evaluation (ROSE) in which a pathologist or a cytotechnologist attends the FNAC procedure and is able to direct the clinician performing the procedure to do further passes to ensure adequacy, as well as immediately triage, in a cost-effective manner, the material from each individual case for ancillary testing. This whole procedure is greatly facilitated if the cytopathologist actually performs the FNAC biopsy, provides ROSE using a rapid Giemsa stain to ensure adequacy, provides a provisional diagnosis in the clinical settings, and triages the case for the most cost-effective selection of further tests.[11]

FNAC preceded by only clinical history and examination provides a fundamental diagnostic tool that can be used as an FNAC biopsy-first diagnostic approach to superficial lesions in LMICs.[10,11] This can be extended to deeper lesions with the use of ultrasound. In the LMIC setting in which infection is among the major causes of disease, the FNAC biopsy-first procedure allows for the diagnostic workup of any palpable lesion, most notably lymphadenopathy. For example, when pediatric patients present with cervical lymphadenopathy, FNAC can often confirm mycobacterial infection by Pap and Ziehl-Neelsen stains on direct smears and provide material for molecular pathology such as GeneXpert.[7,8]

In NCDs, FNAC biopsy can assess, with a high degree of accuracy, any palpable lesion, including salivary glands, lymph nodes, thyroid, neck masses, breast (where the most common lesions are cysts, fibroadenomas, and abscesses as well as, carcinoma and proliferative breast lesions), soft tissue tumors, and the skin, including skin tumors, leprosy, and disseminated fungal infections.[9–11] For example, a patient presenting with a midcervical mass can have an FNAC biopsy performed in the outpatient room to differentiate between a branchial cyst, a metastatic squamous cell carcinoma, a high-grade lymphoma such as Burkitt or Hodgkin lymphoma, a lymph node involved by tuberculosis with its granulomatous inflammation and caseous necrosis, or a reactive lymph node. In many developing countries where mycobacterial infection is endemic and FNAC not widely available, the current management of such a patient is simply to provide antituberculosis treatment if there is any suggestion of mycobacterial infection and to watch and wait. If the lymphadenopathy persists, the patient is then frequently put on a waiting list for an excision biopsy, which would involve anesthetics, surgical time, and a surgical pathologic assessment report. Also, there is a shortage of surgical pathology laboratories in LMICs and surgical pathologic assessment is often expensive with a user-pay system and long waiting periods to receive results. As a result, the surgical pathologic assessment may not be performed and the cancer diagnosis not made or confirmed, undermining subsequent therapy for the individual patient and precluding data collection on disease prevalence.

HOW CAN CYTOPATHOLOGY BE INTEGRATED INTO AND INCREASE THE CAPACITY OF HEALTH CARE?

There are two major requirements to establish the use of cytopathology in the diagnosis of infections and NCDs. One key requirement is that a sufficient number of pathologists have to be trained in cytopathology and be supported by suitably trained cytotechnologists. This is the rate-limiting step.

Most LMICs have an inadequate number of pathologists and technologists, and they work in an environment in which the laboratories are inadequately funded and often poorly equipped.[1,2] There is a relative lack of access to cytology teaching, text books, journals, scientific meetings, electronic teaching aids, and continuing professional education. There is also often a lack of material for routine reporting, teaching, and study, as well as a crucial shortage of experienced cytopathologists as teachers.[12,13]

Formerly, pathologists from LMIC countries were mainly trained in developed countries with the tendency for well-trained pathologists to not return to their countries or to return only briefly because the lack of funding and laboratory infrastructure prevented them from practicing pathology in the way they had learned. Other pathologists return and move into relatively better paid nongovernmental organization positions. There is a need for a strong body of cytopathologists and cytotechnologists within pathology to build this service in LMICs.

HOW CAN THIS BE ACHIEVED?

Cytopathology needs to be built into the curricula of pathology trainees and supplemented by intensive tutorial programs provided by a range of organizations, including the International Academy of Cytology.[12,13] Experienced cytopathologists should be funded to work and teach in LMICs for periods of time, including rotation rosters from developed countries. Pathologists from LMICs can be supported to spend short periods of time, or "sandwich fellowships," in cytopathology centers in developed countries where they can have an intensive period of training using all the facets of pathology training, including multiple header sessions with cytopathologists, teaching slides sets, access to new text books and latest journals, Internet teaching, and conferences.[12,13] Enabling LMIC pathologists to travel out of country to cytopathology centers for part of their training will benefit the management of NCDs in LMICs where infection was formerly the cause of the greatest disease burden. Cancer services have an absolute requirement for a pathologic diagnosis in almost all patients.[4] Usually, this can be provided by cytopathologic assessment with surgical pathologic assessment as backup. In the developed world, this trend toward using FNAC for initial cancer diagnoses has been facilitated by the development of molecular pathology applied to smaller cytologic specimens, as exemplified by the role of endobronchial ultrasound FNAC biopsy in the management of lung cancer, and proven immunohistochemical and molecular testing will extend into LMICs over time.[14,15]

Ideally, these training programs and the various formats should be coordinated by in-country colleges and organizations such as the College of Pathologists of East, Central, and Southern Africa (COPECSA) and the various cytology societies in LMICs.

Telepathology can offer a diagnostic service by pathologists from the developed world to LMICs. More importantly for the long-term development of cytopathology services and the strengthening of the health system in LMICs, telepathology can provide a way to provide second opinions to support indigent cytopathology services in particular hospitals. Similarly, Internet training can supplement local teaching expertise; currently, however, connectivity is variable and often expensive.

A SECOND REQUIREMENT TO ESTABLISH CYTOPATHOLOGY IN LOW-INCOME AND MIDDLE-INCOME COUNTRIES

A second major requirement to establish cytopathology as a diagnostic test in LMICs is the education and encouragement of local clinicians to use cytopathology in their patient management algorithms. Local clinicians often have limited experience in using FNAC or other cytology tests in their protocols because it has not been available. Clinicians have to be made aware of the role of cytology so that they can integrate it into their diagnostic and treatment regimens and protocols. There has to be a long-term interaction between the pathologist providing the FNAC and general cytology service and the clinicians, and this has to be supported by the medical managers of hospitals and other clinicians.

This does not happen overnight and there has to be a continuing education program for clinicians to maximize the use of cytology in the diagnostic process, which often circumvents other more expensive and often unavailable tests, such as core biopsies. In the developed world, there is a constant discussion regarding the relative usefulness of FNAC and core biopsies in various sites, exemplified by breast FNAC. FNAC has a long and successful history in the workup of breast lesions, including abscesses and palpable or ultrasound-detected mass lesions such as cysts, fibrocystic change, proliferative lesions, and cancers. It is a powerful tool in the assessment of these lesions with a high degree of accuracy.[16] In LMICs, this role is a clear example of the potential impact that FNAC can have in the management of common medical problems and cancer. In developed countries where mammography is used for routine diagnostics and screening programs, FNAC and core biopsy are complementary, and core biopsy is extremely useful for the workup of ill-defined or small lesions and calcification, but core biopsy is an expensive option in an LMIC.[17]

THE WAY FORWARD

A recently completed study in Kenya, the "Resident-Driven Improvement In Fine-Needle Aspiration, Bone Marrow Aspirate, and Trephine Biopsies Study," has demonstrated the issues related to increasing FNAC services in an LMIC.[18] This was a joint project of the Aga Khan University and the University of Nairobi, supported by the Ministry of Health in Kenya and the National Cancer Institute (NCI)-USA, and funded by the NCI-Global Health Initiative.

The study aimed to assess the effectiveness of training pathology residents at the 2 hospitals in FNAC biopsy and bone marrow aspiration and terphine (BMAT) biopsy techniques. The residents then trained medical officers (MOs) and clinical officers (COs) in these techniques in large peripheral general hospitals. The aim was to develop a way to devolve these services to the general hospitals and shift the procedural load to a larger group of doctors. The MOs were in their first, second, or third year as postgraduate doctors of the university medical teaching program, whereas COs were career paramedical officers in the same hospitals. Six pathology residents underwent a 3-day intensive training program in the techniques of FNAC and BMAT biopsy techniques, and were then sent to 5 peripheral general hospitals in the Kenyan countryside to train the MOs and COs by recreating the 3-day training program, which included supervising them in FNAC clinics. Six technologists were trained in parallel and accompanied the residents to teach the technologists in the peripheral hospitals. The MOs were then visited twice over the next 4 to 6 months by audit teams, which included Kenyan pathologists and an international cytopathologist (ASF). The individual MOs were assessed in terms of their ability to perform FNACs and the audit team met with the local pathologist and the medical administrators to discuss and remedy, if possible, the ongoing problems and progression of the program.

Some 60 participants were trained in the 5 general hospitals, including 2 pathologists, 39 MOs, 5 COs, and 14 technologists. There was a 41% increase in FNAC biopsies during the project period and a significant increase in bone marrow aspirates and trephines, and new FNAC and BMAT services were initiated in 2 of the hospitals.

The project demonstrated that, in a LMIC, well trained trainee pathologists supported by senior cytopathologists and hematopathologists could train MOs and COs to provide FNAC and BMAT services in the general hospitals. Potentially, this program could be embedded into pathology and surgery specialist training curricula through COPECSA and the College of Surgeons of East, Central and Southern Africa, respectively. The project demonstrated how skills and task shifting could be achieved to allow an essential diagnostic procedural service to be augmented or established and then function with a modest degree of specialist medical staff supervision, although such supervision is beneficial and creates a better learning environment.

Involving pathology residents as trainers was of great benefit to these individuals, allowing them to improve their procedural skills, gain significant teaching experience, and learn how such projects could be managed and supervised. These future pathologists have been well-trained in the procedure and will continue to build their FNAC reporting ability based on technically better performed FNAC biopsies and more numerous cases. The project also further trained the central technologists in their processes and improved their ability to conduct quality assurance programs provided to the peripheral hospitals.

Almost all the MOs were keen to undergo the training and to perform the procedures but this inherently meant a greater workload. Initially, the MOs rosters made no allowances for the procedural time and support from some pathologists and administrations was patchy. Similarly, the general hospital pathologists, only some of whom had been invited to the pathologist trainee training program faced a potential increase in workloads to report the FNAC and BMAT biopsies. In some cases, this was not familiar diagnostic work and was challenging to the pathologists, particularly the bone marrow aspirates and trephines. So general hospital pathologists and their CEOs may have viewed the increased number of FNAC biopsies from the trained MOs and COs as an increase in workload and cost, and some pathologists may have seen the improved services in the general hospital as competition for their private FNAC clinics. However, the benefits to patient care and the more efficient diagnostic process that could decrease hospitalization time and surgical biopsy costs were recognized by pathologists and administrators, all of whom were highly supportive of the program at the final stakeholders' conference. The procedures were billable to the patients on a user-pay system, generating income for the general hospital.

The fundamental impact of the project has been that specialist diagnostic services in FNAC and BMAT have been devolved to varying degrees to each of the 5 peripheral general hospitals, and their MOs and COs have developed career enhancing technical skills that will improve patient care.

SUMMARY

Cytopathology, particularly FNAC, provides a rapid, accurate biopsy technique that is minimally invasive and well-tolerated by patients, inexpensive, and requires minimal laboratory infrastructure and proceduralist costs. FNAC biopsy does require training in the actual technique and the making of smears, and all cytology specimens need to be handled in the correct manner using well-established protocols. FNAC and the other cytology specimen types provide diagnoses in both infectious and NCD patients, and will play an essential role in the establishment of cancer services in LMIC. The use of ancillary tests on cytology material, such as PCR for infections and immunohistochemistry and molecular testing for tumors and other lesions, is established and rapidly developing in high-income countries in the era of personalized medicine.[15] These applications have started to be used in LMICs; for instance, GeneXpert in the diagnosis of tuberculosis.[10] This will provide further impetus to the use of cytopathology in LMICs.

The requirements for this "mobile telephone–moment" transition in the diagnosis of infections and NCD tumors and other lesions in LMICs are that there must be a rapid increase in the training of cytopathologists and cytotechnologists, as well as increased education of clinicians in the roles and utility of diagnostic cytopathology. Both of these requirements need support from pathologists, universities, specialist colleges, administrators, and governments. Increased funding and facilities are required for the teaching of cytopathology, with increased teaching programs, which need to be developed and supported both locally and internationally.

One immediately implementable program would be to roll out the recently completed successful pilot program based in Nairobi for teaching pathology trainees to teach FNAC biopsy techniques to MOs and COs in peripheral hospitals in Kenya. This program has been developed in an LMIC using mainly local expertise to meet local requirements and simply requires funding to be upscaled across sub-Saharan Africa.

REFERENCES

1. Adesina A, Chumba D, Nelson AM. Cancer control in Africa 2. Improvement of pathology in sub-Saharan Africa. Lancet Oncol 2013;14:e152–157.
2. Crisp N, Chen L. Global supply of health professionals. N Engl J Med 2014;370: 950–7.
3. African Strategies for Advancing Pathology Group Members. Quality pathology and laboratory diagnostic services are key to improving global health outcomes: improving global health outcomes is not possible without accurate disease diagnosis. Am J Clin Pathol 2015;143:325–8.
4. Alleyne G, Binagwaho A, Haines A, et al, The Lancet NCD Action Group. Non-communicable diseases 1. Embedding non-communicable diseases in the post-2015 development agenda. Lancet 2013;381:566–74.
5. Stenberg K, Hanssen O, Edejer TT, et al. Financing transformative health systems towards achievement of the heath sustainable development goals: a model for projected resource needs in 67 low-income and middle-income countries. Lancet Glob Health 2017;5(9):e875–87.
6. Wright CA, Pienaar JP, Marais BJ. FNAB: diagnostic utility in resource-limited settings. Ann Trop Paediatr 2008;28:65–70.
7. Wright CA, van der Burg M, Geiger D. Diagnosing mycobacterial lymphadenitis in children using FNAB: cytomorphology. ZN staining and autofluorescence—making more of less. Diagn Cytopathol 2008;36:245–51.
8. Michelow P, Omar T, Field A, et al. The cytopathology of mycobacterial infection. Diagn Cytopathol 2016;44:255–62.
9. Field AS, Geddie WR. Cytohistology of lymph nodes and spleen, Papanicolaou Society small biopsy monograph series. Cambridge (UK): Cambridge University Press; 2014.
10. Field AS, Geddie W. Role of FNAC in the diagnosis of infections. Diagn Cytopathol 2016;44:1024–38.
11. Field AS, Zarka M. Practical cytopathology: a pattern recognition diagnostic approach. New York: Elsevier; 2017.
12. Field AS. Training for cytotechnologists and cytopathologists in the developing world. Cytopathology 2016;27:313–6.
13. Field AS, Geddie W, Zarka M, et al. Assisting cytopathology training in medically under-resourced countries: defining the problems and establishing solutions. Diagn Cytopathol 2012;40:273–81.
14. Rossi ED, Gerhard R, Cirnes L, et al. Detection of common and less frequent mutations in cytological samples of lung cancer. Acta Cytol 2014;58:275–80.
15. Malapelle U, Mayo-de Las-Casas C, Molina-Vila MA, et al. Consistency and reproducibility of next-generation sequencing and other multigene mutational assays: a worldwide ring trial study on quantitative cytological molecular reference

specimens. Cancer 2017;125(8):615–26. Available at: http://www.ncbi.nlm.nih. gov/pubmed/28475299.
16. Field AS, Schmitt F, Vielh P. IAC standardized reporting of breast FNAC. Acta Cytol 2017;61(1):3–6.
17. Field AS. Breast FNA biopsy cytology: current problems and the IAC Yokohama standardized reporting system. Cancer Cytopath 2017;125:229–30.
18. Muchiri L, Sayed S, Rajab J, et al. Improving the quality of FNA, bone marrow aspirate and bone marrow trephine procedures and specimen processing at tertiary referral hospitals in Kenya. AORTIC Abstract, held at Kigali, Rwanda, November 7-10, 2017.

Biospecimens and Biobanking in Global Health

Maimuna Mendy, PhD[a], Rita T. Lawlor, PhD[b],
Anne Linda van Kappel, MSc, PhD[c], Peter H.J. Riegman, PhD[d],
Fay Betsou, PhD, HDR[e], Oliver D. Cohen, MD, PhD[f],
Marianne K. Henderson, MS[g],*

KEYWORDS

- Biobanks • Pathology • Data • Biospecimens • Tissue • Utilization • Catalogs
- Information technology

KEY POINTS

- Biobanks or Biological Resource Centres provide critical infrastructure for clinical research and biomarker discovery when samples are well annotated with preanalytic data.
- Sample collections should be encouraged from geographically and genetically diverse regions to ensure relevant clinical health data for all populations, including those in low and middle-income countries.
- Biospecimen (tissue and biofluids) collection, processing, storing, and retrieval should be carried out with strict standard operating procedures (SOPs) to ensure sample quality and fit-for-purpose use.
- The SOPs should be developed that are appropriate for the available resources, without forfeiting the quality needed to result in meaningful molecular data.
- Documentation about samples, including preanalytic data, donor consent for use, and linkage to clinical data from the donor, should be kept in a robust laboratory information system to protect the data and ensure privacy and encourage ethical use of the samples and data.

Disclosure Statement: The authors of this article have no conflicts of interest associated with the material presented.
[a] Laboratory Services and Biobank Group, International Agency for Research on Cancer, 150 Cours Albert Thomas, Lyon 69372, France; [b] ARC-Net Applied Research on Cancer Centre, University of Verona, Piazzale LA Scuro 10, Verona 37134, Italy; [c] IMV Technologies, ZI n°1 Est, l'Aigle 61300, France; [d] Department of Pathology, Tissue Bank, Erasmus MC, Dr Molewaterplein 40, Rotterdam 3015, The Netherlands; [e] Integrated BioBank of Luxembourg, 6 rue Nicolas Ernest Barble, Luxembourg L-1210, Luxembourg; [f] AGEIS EA 7407 Laboratory, Medical School of Grenoble, Joseph Fourier University, Domaine de la Merci, La Tronche 38700, France; [g] Center for Global Health, National Cancer Institute, NIH, DHHS, 9609 Medical Center Drive, Room 3W534, Bethesda, MD 20892, USA
* Corresponding author.
E-mail address: hendersm@mail.nih.gov

Clin Lab Med 38 (2018) 183–207
https://doi.org/10.1016/j.cll.2017.10.015
0272-2712/18/Published by Elsevier Inc.

labmed.theclinics.com

BACKGROUND AND INTRODUCTION

Infectious diseases continue to be a major burden of disease globally. According to the Global Burden of Disease Study 2015, although the epidemic of human immunodeficiency virus (HIV)/AIDS deaths peaked in 2005 and have annually decreased since 2015, with the scale-up of antiretroviral therapy (ART) and prevention mother to child transmission of HIV (PMTCT), particularly in Sub-Saharan Africa, there continues to be large-scale HIV/AIDS epidemics in many low and middle-income countries (LMICs).[1] Although life expectancy in many regions has risen due to the investments in interventions for infectious disease, many countries are seeing an increase in rates of noncommunicable disease burdens as their populations age. In fact, the global total of new cancer cases is projected to increase by 75% to 22.2 million annually by 2030, with an estimated 13.1 million deaths from cancer yearly. Approximately half of these cancer deaths will occur in low-income countries and more than 80% of these in African countries.[2,3]

It is crucial that appropriate interventions and infrastructure be implemented to confront this disease crisis. Biobanks play an important role in the study of infectious and noncommunicable disease etiology and identification of new potential diagnostic markers, and are central to the development of personalized drug treatment and translational research.[4–6] Investments in biobank infrastructure will enable scientific progress, on which effective disease control measures depend.

The aim of this article was to provide information on the collection, processing, and storage of biospecimens and the management of biobanks as a valuable tool for global health research in LMICs.[7] A biobank, defined as a facility for the long-term storage of biospecimens, is a key resource providing for access to high-quality human biospecimens. The combination of infrastructure, facilities, and resources is referred to as a biological resource centre (BRC). Tumor banks are BRCs; they have been defined by the Organisation for Economic Cooperation and Development (OECD) as service providers and repositories of living cells, of genomes of organisms, of cells and tissues, and of information relating to these materials.

Technological advances in molecular biology and genetics have greatly enhanced our ability to investigate the interactions among genetics, the environment, lifestyle, and health. Biobanks consisting of biospecimens from clinical and epidemiologic studies provide the opportunity to more effectively study disease causation and prognosis. At the present, analytical methods have developed to a level whereby they can be applied to large numbers of biospecimens, so biobanks play a cornerstone role in genetic and molecular epidemiology studies. The management of BRCs requires comprehensive quality management systems with appropriate controls. These are necessary to ensure that biospecimens collected for clinical or research purposes are of consistently high quality and are appropriate for the intended analyses and study goals.[8]

Despite advances in biobanking activities in high-income countries, populations in LMICs are underrepresented in sharing of these resources owing to their economic constraints and related issues. This means that studies are conducted without adequate representation of the populations that are mostly affected by the life-threatening diseases. Many research studies have been conducted in LMICs, but apart from the biobanks created in HIV treatment facilities for HIV research involving many individuals,[9–12] very few other research studies have found it necessary to establish a biobank, mainly because the sample sizes for many non-HIV studies are small, and the studies very rarely collect and store frozen plasma or DNA for further biochemical and genetic studies.[13]

When such biospecimens are collected, their collection and storage are not often planned or organized in any systematic way. Noting the absence of biobank studies in Sub-Saharan Africa, Campbell and Rudan[14] conducted a systematic review of birth cohort studies to assess the resources available to support genetic epidemiologic studies. Their results showed that fewer than 40% of the 28 studies included in the review collected biological material and fewer than 20% collected and stored DNA.

In the absence of adequate funding for and awareness of the benefits of biobanks, the challenge for LMICs to establish and maintain suitable BRC infrastructure, consisting of biospecimen cold storage facilities, databases, reliable electricity supply to maintain the equipment, and quality assurance tools continues to be a challenge. Nevertheless, the first national DNA bank in Africa was established in 2000 in the Gambia as 1 of 14 such collection sites created by the Medical Research Council to study the genetics of the complicated diseases of malaria, HIV/AIDS, and tuberculosis.[15] The facility in the Gambia has expanded over the years and has continued to support research activities.

Although there is a plethora of guidelines and protocols for biospecimen processing,[9,16–19] the tools are not easily accessible in LMICs, which makes it difficult to adhere to principles defined in international protocols and best practices. It is important therefore that alternative and cheaper options of evidence-based protocols be developed for LMICs.

The aim of this article was to promote good practices in human sample biobanking in LMICs to facilitate the appropriate collection of samples for the development of local biomedical research and international collaboration. Underpinning all this is the need to have well-trained staff to operate the facilities and manage the different processes involved in providing high-quality biospecimens, to develop appropriate technologies applicable to local settings, to handle the day-to-day activities, and to deal with issues relating to sample access and patient confidentiality. Information is provided on requirements for cold storage facilities and on the development and management of databases. The emphasis here is on presenting the basic requirements for BRCs or biobanks to store and maintain high-quality biospecimens and on providing guidelines to ensure that research is conducted with integrity and in adherence to the highest ethical standards according to international regulations and rules governing ethical, legal, and social issues.

This article provides information on the value of studies on preanalytical variability of biospecimens that are crucial in ensuring the integrity of downstream analytical results[20] and how biospecimen science research can offer the opportunity to develop and validate appropriate technology and tools for LMICs. In particular, research to help identify quality control biomarkers for assessing the quality of samples before they are included in expensive research platforms, would reduce costs and free up the limited funds to be spent elsewhere. Quality control biomarkers can also contribute to higher reproducibility of data in biomarker research.

COLLECTION AND PROCESSING OF BIOSPECIMENS

Collection, annotation, and use of human biospecimens are essential activities in biomedical care and research. Biobanking is also becoming a critical process in allowing patients access to molecular-based diagnosis, prognosis, and precision medicine. Tumor banks need to comply with strict technical requirements. The definition of a tumor bank includes not only the infrastructure for collecting, archiving, and storing biospecimens and data, but includes the entire biobank continuum beginning with the procedures and services for informing patients; obtaining consent; collecting and processing specimens for secure, potential long-term storage; appropriately accessing and retrieving specimens for analysis; and processing specimens for preparation of molecular derivatives, such as DNA, RNA, and proteins, for quality control and for distribution to researchers.

Two types of methods must be distinguished: (1) biospecimen processing methods, which include different types of biospecimen handling, such as snap-freezing, paraffin embedding, plasma and buffy coat preparation, nucleic acid extraction, and establishment of cell lines; and (2) biospecimen quality control methods, which enable characterization of the biospecimens, and include such elements as the minimal sample characterization data set.

Biospecimen Processing

The types of samples collected during clinical practice include bodily secretions, tissue, and fluids. Using samples left over from clinical diagnostic procedures for biobanking purposes is generally not an optimal practice. Where possible, dedicated specimens for biobanking and research should be collected at the same time as diagnostic specimens, but in separate containers and processed through separate standardized workflows. However, tissue sampling should occur only once diagnostic procedures have been completed, such as the evaluation of margins and sufficient tissue has been sampled for diagnostic tests. The critical steps in each processing method should be acknowledged and controlled. The biospecimen processing method may depend on the anticipated end use. It is difficult for a biobank to anticipate all the different future uses for the samples; therefore, the most stringent processing requirements should be followed, where possible, by the biobank to maximize the life span and potential uses of the samples. As the impact of freezing and thawing on future target molecules is unknown for all sample types, the number of freeze-thaw cycles should be kept at a minimum. For that reason, small volumes of aliquots should be prepared before cryostorage, approximately ≤ 200 μl for serum and plasma, and ≤ 0.5 cm^3 for frozen tissue.

Prospective biospecimen collections generally have the most added value. Longitudinal follow-up of patients allows the establishment of causal links instead of simple associations between observed clinical endpoints and candidate surrogate biomarkers. Improving such studies requires coding of samples instead of irreversible anonymization and, most importantly, adequate human resources, such as clinical research nurses, for follow-up.

Furthermore, inclusion of coded family links adds value to the collection. For biological fluids or solid tissue samples intended for immunologic, molecular biology, or proteomic analyses, critical in vitro preanalytical details should be accurately recorded. For fluids, this information includes the type of primary collection tube, pre-centrifugation time delay and temperature, centrifugation conditions, post-centrifugation time delay and temperature, and long-term storage duration and temperature. For solid tissues, this information includes warm and cold ischemia times, type and duration of fixation, and long-term storage duration and conditions.[21]

Annotation of refrigeration and short processing delays are crucial, especially for urine collected without preservatives. If the samples are intended for proteomic downstream applications, high-speed centrifugation should be used, ensuring removal of white blood cells and platelets. The "as soon as possible" recommendation for preanalytical processing is not precise enough. A simple way of tracking preanalytical information is through the Standard PREanalytical Code (SPREC), a simple 7-element code that enables all preanalytical information to be captured for the different types of specimens.[22]

This information can be added as a searchable data element in the biobank database. Finally, if metabolomic applications are anticipated, in vivo preanalytical data, including the time of day when the blood or urine samples were collected, medications taken by the patient, and food intake, also should be recorded in appropriate databases.

Best Practices and Standard Operating Procedures (SOPs) for different types of biospecimens being collected and processed in tumor banks can be found on the Web sites of the International Society for Biological and Environmental Repositories Best Practices for Repositories,[16] the Canadian Tissue Repository Network (CTRNet),[18] the US National Cancer Institute (NCI), Biorepositories and Biospecimen Research Branch,[23] and the International Agency for Research on Cancer Common Minimum Technical Standards and Protocols for Biobanks dedicated to Cancer Research.[19]

Other types of samples that can be stored include human DNA for genetic susceptibility testing, human RNA from peripheral blood for gene expression, signatures such as prognostic or predictive biomarkers of treatment outcome, and peripheral blood mononuclear cells for cell sorting and cell immunophenotyping.

Coordination of project-specific prospective collections is also possible, for example, collecting urine with protease inhibitors or plasma for peptidomics analyses.

As a general rule, tubes and kits for collecting and processing biospecimens should be obtained from commercial suppliers. The advantage of using such devices is that they have already undergone significant validation by the suppliers. However, because this validation often focuses on specific quality attributes or specific molecules in the sample, the tumor bank still must validate the collection or processing device for other target molecules as these become known.

All human specimens regardless of the known disease state of the patient should be treated as potential biohazards. This is because the patient may have a known or potentially undiagnosed contagious disease. Appropriate measures should be taken to protect laboratory workers who handle specimens and to prevent others from being exposed to the specimens during transportation. This is good laboratory practice. The most commonly collected and processed biospecimens include blood, urine, and tissue.

Blood Specimens

Whole blood samples

Whole blood does not require any special processing for storage and can be stored at $-80°C$ or room temperature or as dried blood spots (DBSs) on filter paper. Storage of whole blood samples is necessary if the end use is DNA analysis. DNA is a very stable molecule that is robust to a range of storage conditions. Whole-genome sequencing requires higher-quality DNA samples than do single-target polymerase chain reaction assays. However, whole-genome amplification can be performed to obtain large quantities of DNA from minute amounts of initial material.[24] When anticoagulated blood is centrifuged, it separates into the red blood cell (RBC) fraction and the buffy coat layer containing white blood cells (WBCs), platelets, and plasma. When coagulated blood is centrifuged, it separates into the clot (RBCs, WBCs, and platelets) and serum.

Dried blood spots

In the low resource setting context, storage of whole blood as DBSs makes sense, as this avoids technical problems related to cryostorage and logistical arrangements. DBSs can be used effectively for DNA sequence analysis for up to 3 decades of storage[25] and for cytokine measurements for up 2 decades of storage at $-20°C$. DBS testing is a powerful tool for screening programs and large population-based surveys, for detection of biomarkers such as hepatocellular carcinoma,[26] and for large-scale testing for HIV infection.[27] Special attention should be paid to card selection, collection method, and storage. The ethical concerns of long-term storage and use of DBSs should be considered when consenting for the biospecimens.[28]

Plasma is the liquid fraction of anticoagulated blood. Different anticoagulants may be used, such as ethylenediamine tetra-acetic acid (EDTA), heparin, and acid citrate dextrose (ACD). The end use of the blood influences the choice of the anticoagulant.

ACD is the preferred anticoagulant when lymphocytes from the cellular fraction of the blood are to be used to establish lymphoblastoid cell lines, but citrate interferes with future metabolomic analyses in the plasma. Heparin may inhibit nucleic acid amplification and future molecular biology analyses in the nucleic acid samples obtained either from the cellular blood fraction or plasma itself (circulating nucleic acids). Therefore, EDTA is preferred, as it allows proteomic, genomic, and metabolomic analyses to be performed in the future.[29] Platelet-poor plasma can be obtained after blood centrifugation at high speeds (>3000 g) and is more suitable for proteomic analyses because it allows less interference by circulating platelets and other coagulation factors.[30]

Time delays and temperatures to which the blood is exposed between collection and centrifugation and between centrifugation and plasma storage must be carefully documented.[22] There is no consensus about time delays and temperatures that the collected blood can tolerate, but it has been shown that pre-centrifugation delays of up to 8 hours at room temperature do not significantly alter proteomic profiles.[31] For longer pre-centrifugation delays, storage at 4°C is preferred. For specific target analytes in the context of biomedical assays, validation should be performed to deal with the impact of the time delays.[32] Storage of plasma should be at −80°C, which is the temperature that has been found to ensure stability of the vast majority of molecules examined to date.[24] Validation has not yet been performed of lyophilized plasma and its storage at different temperatures, including room temperature.

Serum is the liquid fraction of clotted blood. Preparing and storing serum instead of plasma offers 2 advantages for a tumor bank: (1) serum does not contain platelets and coagulation factors and therefore it allows proteomic analysis of a greater number of proteins, including those that cannot be identified in plasma because they are bound to plasma coagulation factors,[31] and (2) the absence of additives in serum ensures there will be no interference from such elements in downstream spectrometric analyses.[29] As with plasma, for serum, it is very important to document the time delays and storage temperatures from blood collection to centrifugation (clotting time) and from centrifugation to storage. The same considerations for storage temperatures are observed for serum as for plasma. For both types of samples, the inflammatory status of the donor is an important confounder, if the anticipated use is proteomic analysis; therefore, normalization of the samples relative to the inflammatory status may need to be performed.

Peripheral blood mononuclear cells (PBMCs) include lymphocytes and monocytes. These cells can be isolated from the buffy coat layer of centrifuged anticoagulated blood through Ficoll gradient centrifugation. PBMCs should either be stored at −80°C, preferably in lysis buffer if they are intended for gene expression analyses, or cryopreserved as viable cells in liquid nitrogen (LN2) using the cryopreservation medium dimethyl sulfoxide (DMSO) for future cell sorting, cell immunophenotyping, immortalization, and establishment of lymphoblastoid cell lines. For transcriptional analysis, commercially available RNA-stabilization blood collection tubes, such as PAXgene RNA tubes (Qiagen, Valencia, CA) or Tempus tubes (ThermoFisher, Waltham, MA), are preferred due to the potential influence of preanalytical conditions on gene expression profiles.[33] For viable lymphocyte isolation, ACD blood collection tubes are preferable. If Ficoll gradient centrifugation is not possible, whole blood can be cryopreserved and used for viable lymphocyte processing or analysis in the future. Viable lymphocytes may be recovered from whole blood held at 4°C for several hours before progressive-rate freezing in DMSO.[34]

Urine Specimens

Urine samples have become quite valuable to measure metabolites associated with human disease state.[35] Urine contains DNA, RNA, proteins, and metabolites, and it is easy to collect and store for analysis of all of these molecules. However, because urine composition lacks tight homeostasis and depends on disease status, the time of the day it was collected and donor hydration status needs to be normalized for proteomic analyses. For proteomic or metabolomic analysis, urine is centrifuged and the supernatant is aliquoted and stored at −80°C. Centrifugation is necessary to avoid interference by cell components. For DNA or RNA analysis, the pellet is stored preferably in a nucleic acid stabilization solution, such as a cell protect reagent. Filtration of the supernatant must also be performed for proteomic analysis,[36] but this step can occur after thawing and immediately before analysis. Collecting midstream, first or second morning urine is preferred, and in all cases, collection time and delays should be documented.[22] Refrigeration is preferred to avoid bacterial proliferation. Different urine preservatives, such as boric acid or sodium azide, also may be used to prolong processing delays if the urine is stored at either room temperature or 4°C.[37] Metabolomic analysis is affected by the use of preservatives so for this use, urine should be kept at 4°C or frozen within 1 hour of collection.[29] Although EDTA has been reported as a DNA stabilizer in urine, its efficiency has not been reproducible in Africa.[38] Validation of standards for urine collection, processing, and analysis have been the focus of active research and publications.[36]

Tissue Specimens

As 90% of cancers are tissue, the collection of tissue samples provides the basic material for most cancer research. Tumors are made up of cancer cells and stroma and this must be evaluated during sampling and quality control of a cancer tissue sample. Furthermore, most cancers are heterogeneous in nature, differing not only from one to another, but also within different areas of the same tumor. This heterogeneity is not always identifiable by morphologic evaluation and therefore sampling of cancer tissue for molecular classification must take this into consideration. Where possible, attempts to sample multiple areas of the cancer tissue should be done.

Dissection

An absolute rule in tumor banking is that tissue sampling locations and tissue amounts for research must not interfere with routine diagnostics, resection margins, and staging. Some samples may be sampled directly in the operating suite but pathology must be notified. Once the specimen has been excised, it should be transported to the grossing room and the time from excision to processing should be noted. Grizzle and colleagues[39] reviewed the time to processing and the effects of cold ischemia on gene expression in human surgical tissues. They noted that variability in molecular results were more affected by specimen and patient characteristics than on cold ischemia; that ischemia differed with tissue organ and tissue size; and recommended that the timing be matched with the fit-for-purpose of specific research questions to be examined.

The specimen should be weighed, measured, and photographed by the pathologist, and areas with normal and abnormal tissue portions should be sampled by gross examination following diagnostic sampling and procedures. Dissection of the specimen should be performed in a way to ensure its sterility and avoid cross-contamination during dissection, which are critical factors for downstream molecular biology analyses. For each tumor sample collected, a frozen section should be performed for quality control during sampling.

Freezing

Tissue sections are immersed into either an isopentane bath previously cooled in LN2 or directly into an LN2 dewar. Tissue should be 0.5 cm^3 or thinner for quick freezing. A minimum of 2 to 3 minutes is needed for complete freezing.

Frozen samples are then transported to the tumor bank in dry ice ($-80°$C) or colder. An optimal cutting temperature (OCT) compound can be used to embed and freeze the tissue, to allow for future cryosections and morphologic examination, or molecular extractions and analyses. However, as OCT can make frozen samples unusable for mass spectometry measurements, removal techniques need to be applied for this use. Frozen tissue specimens should never be allowed to thaw, which would not only destroy the sample's morphology but also cause severe RNA degradation.

Stabilization and fixation

Different types of tissue fixatives are available. The standard fixative for preserving morphology is 10% neutral buffered formalin (NBF). However, be aware that NBF causes molecular cross-linking and undermines the quality of DNA, RNA, and proteins that can be extracted from a formalin-fixed, paraffin-embedded (FFPE) block. For complete fixation, samples should not exceed 0.5 cm^3 in size. Samples should be fixed in 10 volumes or more of NBF. Routine fixation is typically done for approximately 12 hours overnight. After fixation, the tissue specimen is removed and placed in 70% ethanol for shipping or further processing in paraffin. PAXgene tissue fixative (Qiagen) allows for morphology preservation and at the same time ensures high quality of DNA, RNA, and proteins. The only drawback seems to be the eventual necessity to revalidate the immunohistochemical (IHC) assay parameters for PAXgene-fixed, paraffin-embedded tissue.[40] Alcohol-based fixatives also are available, including Omnifix (Omni; Xenetics Biomed, Tustin, CA) and other proprietary fixatives. A section should always be made from fixed tissue for immediate histopathological quality control.

Tissue stabilizers exist that allow stabilization of molecules but do not preserve tissue morphology. RNALater (Ambion, Austin, TX) is an aqueous nontoxic tissue storage reagent that rapidly permeates tissue and stabilizes all nucleic acids. AllProtect (Qiagen) reagent allows stabilization and subsequent extraction of both nucleic acids and proteins. These stabilizers eliminate the need to process tissue samples immediately or to freeze them; however, such methods usually do not preserve tissue morphology. Finally, heat stabilization under vacuum (Denator, Biotech Center, Gothenburg, Sweden) conditions with the subsequent storage of the heat-stabilized tissue at $-80°$C has been shown to effectively preserve tissue phosphoproteome, although it does not allow preservation of morphology or use in nucleic acid analysis.[41]

Laser capture microdissection (LCM) is a technique that allows isolation of pure cell populations from heterogeneous tissue sections through direct visualization of the cells. Automated LCM platforms combine a graphical-user interface and annotation software together with staining reagents for visualization of the tissue of interest and robotically controlled microdissection. Microdissected cells for protein analysis may be stored at $-80°$C before extraction, whereas for DNA analysis they may be stored desiccated at room temperature for up to 1 week before extraction. For RNA analysis, the RNA extraction should be performed immediately after microdissection and the RNA samples then stored at −80°C.

Tissue microarrays (TMAs) are paraffin blocks that contain an array of minute specimen cores taken from different FFPE blocks or different areas of the same FFPE block. They are usually composed of several cores for each "donor" and usually contain many donors on the same block. TMAs are ideal for efficient screening of prospective biomarkers in multiple samples by IHC, fluorescence in situ hybridization, and RNA in situ hybridization methods. They are prepared by transferring paraffin tissue cores from many "donor" blocks to one "recipient" block. TMAs should have positive controls for the anticipated IHC assays. Each slide cut from this recipient block is called a TMA slide. "Frozen" TMAs may also be prepared using frozen donor tissues embedded in the OCT compound. These samples are arrayed into a recipient OCT block. This allows high-throughput evaluation of frozen tissue with corresponding visualization of tissue morphology. To preserve antigenicity, a fresh section should be cut at the time of evaluation or the TMA sections should be stored in a vacuum, in a nitrogen gas environment or at −80°C, to avoid antigen degradation due to oxidation.

Biospecimen Quality Control

Quality control (QC) procedures are important to ensure data and sample quality. For data, this includes clinical data accuracy, whereas for biospecimens it includes assays on the authenticity, integrity, and identity of the samples.[21] Biospecimen QC is required to ensure accurate sample characterization and classification and to avoid introducing bias in downstream research due to intrinsic heterogeneity of the sample. This bias was shown in a specific African breast cancer classification study.[42] The type of QC depends on the intended end use of the sample. For example, samples to be used as reference samples in commercialized diagnostic kits must undergo mandatory testing for HIV, hepatitis B virus, and hepatitis C virus. A central QC laboratory can undertake this testing, and the critical steps in each QC assay should be acknowledged and controlled by the laboratory. Accurate characterization of the samples supplied by a biobank focuses on both the authenticity and the integrity of the biomaterial.

Authenticity

Phenotypic QC methods generally used for authentication of tissue specimens involve histopathological assessment. Trained pathologists should perform the histopathological evaluation of tissue samples (fixed and/or frozen sections), to confirm the tissue type, whether it is from a tumor or normal tissue, and the basic histopathological diagnosis and classification, based on standard hematoxylin-eosin staining. The evaluation includes assessment of cellular composition, which is of critical importance in any downstream molecular analysis. A sample with highly heterogeneous cellular composition makes any definitive molecular analysis more challenging. A general rule is cellularity higher than the detection rate of the instrument, the minimum cellularity of tumor is generally set at 40% for whole-genome sequencing.[43] For lower cellularities, enrichment processes such as microdissection may be used. The standard histologic control also includes assessment of specimen morphologic degradation. Histopathological evaluation allows identification and marking of the block areas that are the most suitable for TMA cores. There may be special advantages in developing and implementing histopathological QC by telepathology in LMICs. In October 2015, the American Society for Clinical Pathologists and a coalition of world partners launched a project to provide patients in underserved areas of Sub-Saharan Africa and Haiti with access to rapid disease diagnostics and resource-appropriate treatment.[44] Static telepathology, or microscopic photographs, is based on offline imaging without interaction between operators. Virtual microscopy and dynamic telepathology allow production of "virtual slides" using navigation tools on the Internet, allowing for experts around the world to support diagnosis of diseases in LMICs that have such systems.

Integrity

Very few data are available on the use of QC tools in assessing collection procedures, shipping, and storage conditions. However, homogeneity in these steps is key for quality multicenter research studies. Recently, the H3Africa project team published on their experiences and solutions to the challenges of intracountry biospecimen shipment logistics associated with their multisite and multi-biobank network.[45]

For effective QC of prospective collections, biobank managers can proceed in several ways. QC may be performed on every specimen received at the biobank. In some instances, this may be highly recommended and cost-effective, such as hemocytometry for all blood samples. In other instances, generalized QC for samples received at the biobank is not cost-effective, such as for specimens for DNA extraction and analysis. In that case, QC may be performed before distribution of samples to researchers, such as for verification of DNA concentration, purity, or Taq amplifiability, if such the QC does not destroy the sample.[46] Retrospective QC is always an option and 2 alternatives are available: testing either a randomly selected percentage of the collected specimens or samples considered to have undergone the most "inconsistent" processing. The first approach allows comparisons of collection sites, whereas the second allows targeted assessment of "highest-risk" samples.

There are a variety of QC tests for assessment of sample integrity and purity, shipping temperature variations, and processing and storage conditions, to assess the fitness for purpose of biospecimens in a biobank.[45–48]

Plasma and Serum Quality Control

Biospecimen research is in progress to identify appropriate QC tools for serum, plasma, and urine.[47,48] Such QC markers may be serum sCD40 L to assess the duration of exposure of the sample to room temperature, protein S activity in plasma, and matrix metalloproteases in serum or plasma. Serum sCD40 L assays are particularly relevant in Africa, where high ambient temperatures are more often observed.

Biospecimen Research in Low and Middle-Income Countries

Variability in acquisition, processing, and storage of samples may contribute to experimental variability, particularly in high-throughput analyses, and may result in false research conclusions. This is especially true for the most labile bioanalytes, like RNA, functional proteins, and metabolites. In this respect, biospecimen research is linked to biospecimen QC.

High-quality nucleic acids and adequate antigen preservation can be obtained from formalin-fixed, PAXgene-fixed, or ethanol-fixed, paraffin-embedded tissues or from DBS on filter paper. These types of biospecimen processing techniques suit the logistical conditions in low resource settings because they do not need cryostorage. Biobanks in LMICs may choose to develop expertise in these approaches of maintaining biospecimen stability and robustness in the context of novel, dried blood, room temperature technologies, including lyophilization, and in room temperature storage devices for biofluids, nucleic acids, or even for whole blood.

Choosing the Best Collection Method

Choosing the right procedures for collecting and storing samples and data is very important, and such decisions need to be carefully considered even before the samples and data are collected. A review of the optimum conditions for collection and storage of many human sample types provides evidence for specific choices.[49] The focus should be to maximize the level of quality to ensure that the sample is at least fit for its intended use(s). However, if possible and affordable, the highest possible standards should be pursued to permit wide use of the samples in future tests, applications, and collaborations.[11] Collaboration must consider not only sample sharing, where not only sample quality must be comparable, but also donor consent and access where approval by local stakeholders has been considered up-front.[50]

All samples and data used within a study must at least be collected to be "fit-for-purpose" for the planned (and anticipated) experiments and all samples must be of comparable quality. Comparable quality demands that preanalytical conditions be kept as constant as possible for every sample. Therefore, every sample should be collected in analogous manner following an SOP for the collection. The object for SOPs should be focused on the highest quality possible in the specific collection setting. The QC process should be designed to reject samples from studies that are not fit for purpose.

Changing collection or storage procedures while the collection is under way can have consequences for the results from the experiment in which these samples are used and should therefore be carefully considered. Changes implemented during sample collection should be documented. Protocols should be established for the processes to be used for the entire collection period, before initiating collection. To achieve a level of standardization of processes, it is very important to have written SOPs for at least the collection, processing, storage, and distribution of samples. In addition, it is essential to ensure that the SOPs are followed and interpreted in the same way at all collection sites for a study. Regular audits and QC are needed to check compliance with the SOPs. Any variance to the collection procedures should be documented and this documentation can be used during analyses to correlate outliers in experimental results or during cohort selection for exclusion of samples that are not fit for purpose.

It is important to include an SOP for transportation between collection site and the biobank including chain of custody procedure. Often in LMIC settings, there may be challenges in shipment of samples from remote collection locations to the biobank. Transportation of samples in warm cars before processing and storage can be detrimental for many methods, and thus cooling is often required and should be addressed in a shipment SOP, to maintain sample integrity and quality.

Quality Assurance

Certification of a biobank to international standards such as ISO 9001 (quality management systems—requirements) by an independent body is proof that the biobank is effectively organized and managed. Furthermore, subcontracting testing to laboratories that are themselves accredited to international standards such as ISO 17025 (general requirements for the competence of testing and calibration laboratories) or ISO 15189 (medical laboratories particular requirements for quality and competence) by a national accreditation body is proof of reliability of the sample characterization processes. A new ISO standard specifically for biobanks is in development (ISO/DIS 20387). Although compliance with these standards is important, it essentially remains voluntary for the biobanks and can be expensive.

BIOSPECIMEN STORAGE FACILITIES AND EQUIPMENT

Biospecimen storage facilities are the most visible part of biobanks, and storage systems are important factors in maintaining sample quality. The variety of storage systems available for specimen collection increases as technologies advance. FFPE materials must be stored at room temperature, meaning that in most countries the storage room would need air conditioning to maintain the temperature below 25°C. Mechanical freezers need to be kept in clean, cool rooms because they produce a lot of heat and must have dust removed from their filters to work efficiently.

Storage equipment should be selected based on the type of specimens to be stored, the anticipated length of storage time for the specimens, the use intended for the specimens, and the resources available for purchasing the equipment.[16] In selecting equipment, quality issues should be considered, but for a local setting with limited access to tools, the primary considerations should be the available resources, staffing requirements, and equipment support and maintenance. For the sample storage equipment, such as freezers, and for infrastructure equipment, such as electrical power and backup systems, LN2 bulk tanks, and transport pipes, compatibility with local conditions, and the capacity of the vendor to provide onsite support and maintenance for the time they are used by the biobank, should be verified. Two types of storage systems are described here: ultralow-temperature or low-temperature storage systems and ambient temperature storage systems.

Sample Storage Containers

In selecting storage containers for biospecimens, consideration should be given to the following:

1. Sample volume
2. Necessary cooling and warming rates for both the individual container and the racks, boxes, or goblets
3. Potential risk of contamination of the sample or the environment
4. Storage temperature and conditions
5. Space available for sample storage
6. Frequency of access
7. Specimen identification requirements
8. Specimen preparation and after-storage processing techniques
9. Economic aspects

Containers used in cryogenic temperatures should be rated for these temperatures. Containers used for storage in LN2 should be hermetically sealed to avoid penetration of LN2 into the container and consequent risk of contamination and explosion when the container is removed from the freezer. All human specimens should be treated as potential biohazards, and the choice of storage container should integrate minimizing the risk of contamination of laboratory workers who handle the specimens and preventing others from being exposed to the samples in the laboratory or during transportation. This is good laboratory practice. Identification labels that do not contain personal identifiers should be compatible with the storage temperature and medium and should always include eye-readable codes when access to scanners for barcodes, 2D codes, or radio frequency identification codes cannot be guaranteed by the sample processing institution or end-user.

Liquid Nitrogen Freezers

Cryogenic storage using LN2 is an effective long-term storage platform because its extreme cold temperatures slow down most chemical and physical reactions preventing biospecimen deterioration. LN2 vapor-phase containers can maintain samples below Tg (glass transition temperature; ie, −132°C) whereas submersion in LN2 guarantees a stable −196°C temperature. Where a regular supply of LN2 is available, LN2 freezers reduce reliance on mechanical freezers and electrical power and guarantee sample integrity under critical temperatures during power cuts, as closed LN2 freezers can maintain samples at below −130°C for longer periods without refilling. Initial investment together with availability and cost of LN2 can be major drawbacks. When LN2 freezers are used, oxygen level sensors should be used and calibrated regularly. Use of protective goggles and gloves should be mandatory, and easily accessible. Appropriate training in the safe handling of cryogenics and samples stored in cryogenics should be provided and part of an SOP for health hazards and safety precautions.

Mechanical Freezers

Mechanical freezers are used for a variety of storage temperature ranges and come in a wide range of sizes, configurations, and electrical voltages. Ice crystals may form in biological samples at temperatures of approximately −70°C, therefore freezer temperatures should preferably be below −80°C. Cascade compressor technologies may produce temperatures as low as −140°C. Mechanical freezers generally require a lower initial investment than LN2 freezers and provide easier and safer access to samples, and can be installed if electrical power is available. However, compressor technology requires constant electrical power to maintain subzero temperatures, so backup power and an emergency response plan are needed. Ambient temperature and humidity influence temperature stability so they should be set apart in rooms that are air-conditioned and/or have equipment for extraction of hot air generated by the compressors. Internal temperature is easily affected by open doors during sample loading. Freezers need to be periodically cleaned to remove frost and filters should be cleaned.

Refrigerators

Refrigerators are commonly used where the longevity of the material being stored is enhanced by storage below ambient temperature. Storage at 4°C can also be an intermediate step before preparation for ultralow-temperature storage. For refrigerators, as for mechanical freezers, it is important to maintain and monitor the temperature in the required operating range and to organize for a backup power plan.

Ambient Temperature Storage

In the absence of mechanical or cryogenic equipment owing to practical or financial reasons, specific biological storage matrices may be used for long-term maintenance of some biological components at room temperature. Formalin-fixed, PAXgene-fixed,[51] or ethanol-fixed, paraffin-embedded tissues and lyophilized samples can be stored at such temperatures. The storage matrices should be evaluated before use to ensure that they are appropriate for downstream applications. Temperature, humidity, and oxygen levels should be controlled at the biobank, to avoid mold growth and microbial contamination.

Information Technology in Biobanking

Information technology (IT) has a fundamental role in biobank organization. Indeed, software applications known as Laboratory Information Management Systems (LIMS) have been adapted and developed to address biobank processes, optimize workflow efficiency, drive quality assurance, and maximize the use of collections. IT systems also have been developed to manage the large amounts of resulting molecular research data and provide controlled access to the data by the research community.

IT tools are particularly important as part of quality management systems of biological resources. Documenting actions (metadata) associated sample collection, processing and preservation times, storage locations and temperatures (traceability), provide important quality indicators for both fluid and tissue samples. This sample metadata, together with sample-associated clinical annotation and consent documentation, create enriched, valuable information about the quality of the sample collections. The ISO 9001:2015 standard sets out the criteria for a quality management system. The ISO/TC276 standards in development will include specific requirements for a quality management system (QMS) for biobanks and biological resources. The standards aim to harmonize business practices and IT requirements and optimize exchanges between biobanks. As part of a QMS, LIMS tools facilitate auditing of biobank procedures, to allow for evaluation of conformity to SOPs, and continued quality process improvement.

Use of Information Technology in Tumor Biobanks

Large numbers of primary and derived samples can be easily managed with most LIMS software. Every process and procedure should time-stamped and recorded with information on operator, equipment used, and reagents and other consumables used. Digital versions of forms documenting sample collection, sample reception forms, sample processing, and anonymized/de-identified sample may be designed and completed electronically to reduce manual input of data to reduce user errors, increase workflow efficiency, and improve quality assurance.

Most LIMS software provides the ability to trace the movement of samples over time in a biobank. Storage information shows the current position and movement of samples in storage units (freezers). A storage location tool within an LIMS can suggest sample storage locations for new collections, based on the total number of samples to be stored and the collection to which it belongs. Free space in storage units can be identified to optimize the use of space in the biobank's units.

All processing and storage-related incidents also should be recorded. Each incident should be described by (1) event type, for example, a missing subject consent or deviation from protocol, and (2) event status, for example, whether corrective action is pending, is ongoing or has been taken.

LIMS can also be used to track and manage donor consent, if scanned copies of consent documents (or copy of the informed consent template) are saved, consent information is registered with the IT system and these data are permanently linked to patient and/or sample data. It is important to release samples only for the uses contained in the approved scope of the donor's consent.

When using samples, the LIMS should track the distribution of samples and therefore often permits the registration of dates, such as sample requests and transfers, parties involved, sample recipients, and sample quantities requested, transferred, or returned. Some LIMS may also store the scanned material transfer agreements or material transfer agreement (MTA) number associated with a transfer requisition. Criteria may be set in some biobank LIMS that can alert staff when a pre-established minimum sample aliquot number threshold has been reached, to ensure adequate volumes are maintained and stored for future use.

Many biobanks now include a "return of research information" policy that requires data from experiments or publication citations be returned to the biobank. These data if uploaded to the biobank database permit for continuous enrichment of the collection and increase the collections value to the research community. However, the format of the data and whether the biobank has the capacity to store and analyze raw data needs careful consideration.

Biospecimen Catalogs and Directories

A catalog is an electronic list of the biobank's collections and associated metadata. Catalogs are established as institutional, national, or regional infrastructures to promote harmonization and can provide standardized resources for enhanced utilization of collections in international collaborative studies (eg, the NCI's Specimen Resource Locator, BBMRI-ERIC [Biobanking and BioMolecular Resource Research Infrastructure – European Research Infrastructure Consortium] catalog, CTRNet and BCNet [Biobanking and Cohort Building Network]). Catalogs may be updated manually or periodically by a formatted program issued from the biobank's database. Biobank catalogs or directories are developing at a rapid pace to provide visibility for biological resources and data for secondary access to collections available once studies have completed their primary objectives and end points. A new study collection can be built up from samples (biological resources) selected for their common biological, clinical, and preanalytical characteristics, such as those in SPREC,[22] from across several collections within or among biobank catalogs. IT solutions can facilitate the selection of homogeneous or comparable resources and for research on diagnostic or therapeutic biomarkers.

For example, the BBMRI-ERIC directory[52] represents the European biobanking infrastructure for collections and biobank networks and provides information on the what sample sets and data sets are available for sharing. The NCI's funded extramural collections are listed in the Specimen Resource Locator catalog.[17] The CTRNet has a biobank locator created to increased collaboration and use of Canadian specimen collections. The locator individually lists the networked biobanks, their major collection type, and the contact information for the biobanks, across Canada.[53] The Biobank and Cohort Building Network global catalog[54] provides the ability to register, store and track biological collections held by BCNet LMIC member organizations. It is being developed to enhance research sample and data sharing to support public health research within the member's countries/regions.

Commercially available catalog solutions are becoming more widely available, as well as those integrated into biobank LIMS software.

Types of Information Technology

Biobank LIMS software must be selected or designed for its security, robustness, interoperability, and configuration features. In making the decision on software, attention also should be paid to the data items to be recorded and the quality of the data. The IT solution must ensure the security and accuracy of donor identification. Donors must be anonymized at all times. Hospital patients must be identified by their permanent ID numbers and their hospital visit numbers so that the samples can be linked to the respective hospital visits. Many systems are developed that protect and maintain patient information confidentiality per the standards of the Title 21 Code of Federal Regulations (21 CFR Part 11) of the US Food and Drug Administration. Specific security attention should be paid to systems that hold genetic data. Software solutions based on Web informatics systems are preferred for biobanks as they offer high security. They also have the advantage of interoperability with other clinical informatics systems. Selection of an LIMS should consider the ease of configuration and ability of the local administrator to customize content and functionality, extensibility, and maintenance.

The amount of preexisting specimen metadata to be imported to a new LIMS solution, will help drive specific software selection, based on the ease of data migration.

Off-the-shelf LIMS solutions include open-source software or tables. Although open-source software solutions may appear to be free to the biobank, they may have secondary costs, such as those for installation, "training," or "support," to set up the application and adapt the solution to the specific requirements of the biobank. Some open-source LIMS require expert local administration at the biobank.

OpenOffice or Excel tables are other forms of off-the-shelf IT solutions, but are most likely not the best option for biobanks with multiple collections and users. Furthermore, tables and spreadsheets do not offer data traceability, and do not have the functionality to alert or log changes in data content.

The marketplace for off-the-shelf, commercially available LIMS for small and large-scale biobanking, regardless of sample type, has exponentially increased over the past several years.

Annotation of Biospecimens

Data items that are recorded in biobank LIMS likely include the following:

1. Patient identification and demographic data, with sex and date of birth, as well as state of the vital signs.
2. Diagnostic data, with principal diagnostic endpoint and date, and clinical tumor–lymph node–metastasis (cTNM) classification.
3. Specimen data, including sample identifiers, sampling date, sample nature, organ from which sample was collected, collection method, stabilization process, and preservation details.
4. Lesion data, including histologic type, size, event nature, whether primary tumor or metastasis, lesion advancement and invasion, and pathologic tumor–lymph node–metastasis classification (pTNM), grading, and other important data, such as Gleason score for prostate cancers.
5. Sample data, type, number, size, characterization (for tissue, whether the sample is tumor [neoplastic], non-neoplastic, normal adjacent, normal distant, node, and a QC evaluation based on the percentage of tumor, necrosis, and stroma), and sample preanalytical data, such as SPREC.
6. Derivative data, including type, number, quantity, SOP used to produce derivative (eg, DNA or RNA) and its characterization (eg, concentration, purity, integrity).
7. Storage data, including temperature, location (freezer, shelf, rack, box, position in box) and events.

All data items should use standard terminology to optimize their use and to allow their future export into a specific IT system. Although many histopathology reports use free text, this does not promote good practice for the biobank and, where possible, should be translated into standardized formats, for easier comparison. All data should be entered through drop-down lists with standardized terms based on dictionaries, ontologies, and international nomenclatures like the International Classification of Diseases for Oncology[55] or the Systematized Nomenclature of Medicine.[56]

Recent publications have emphasized the importance of a common terminology for improved data sharing[57] and ISO 11179-3 conformant metadata repositories.[58]

Data Backup and Disaster Recovery

IT systems must include a required process that backs data up to an alternate database, housed in a physically distinct location (and if possible geographically distinct) for safety and disaster recovery.[59] Backup intervals could be daily, weekly, or monthly depending on the volume and nature of activity. If no IT system is available and the use of electronic tables and spreadsheets are used, backups of these should save time-stamped versions. This allows for minimal tracking of changes to the database over time as well as safety against loss.

Regulation in Biobanking

The regulations governing biobanking need to address legal and ethical issues concerning the use of biological materials and data in research. These regulations must deal with the rights and responsibilities of donors, biobank managers, and researchers. Biobank governance must respect individual donors and guarantee their privacy and confidentiality. At the same time, it must not inhibit the provision of samples for potentially beneficial research. Regulations can be found dispersed in different declarations, such as acts governing the use of human tissue and data.[60–63] Many African countries have regulatory bodies with guidelines for the use of biological samples and data for research.[64,65] Where national guidelines do not exist, international guidelines can be used to address legal and ethical aspects concerning the collection and use of biological material and data for research. However, traditional cultural values placed on human biological materials and data by local communities must be considered.

International Guidelines

The World Medical Association (WMA) Declaration of Helsinki[66] provides guidelines for medical research on human beings. It aims to promote the ethical conduct of research and to protect human subjects from associated risks. The Declaration of Helsinki was the first set of international research guidelines that required research participants to provide informed consent. Since its adoption, it was amended by the addition of the WMA Declaration of Taipei on Ethical Considerations regarding Health Databases, Big Data, and Biobanks.[67] Large collections of data and human specimens allow for the development of new research strategies and models, as well as new predictive types of research and analysis. The promise of large sample sets and genomic data create potential hazards for identifiability of donors, privacy worries, and a need for strong governance of biobanks and resulting data. The United Nations Educational, Scientific and Cultural Organization (UNESCO)[68] emphasizes the protection of human genome-derived genetic data.[41] The use of human biological resources and data for genetic research is addressed in the OECD Guidelines on human biobanks and genetic research databases[69] and the Belmont Report and US Code of Federal Regulations, 45 CFR 46 (Common Rule).[60]

Governance

The key aspects relating to biobank governance are the policies, processes, and procedures in place to ensure correct operation of the biobank. Governance should take into account the biobank ethical and legal issues of informed consent of samples, benefit sharing by donors' countries, confidentiality, ownership, and public participation.[70] These should include oversight mechanisms for the development, implementation, and use of the biobank collections; stakeholder support and accountability; and sustainability of the biobank. The responsibilities of funders, biobank developers, researchers, and the various institutions involved must be clearly spelled out. For samples and data, there must be well-defined and documented processes for initiating collections, acquiring specimens, sharing samples, and long-term support, as appropriate. Oversight mechanisms should include ethics policies to ensure the ethical collection and use of samples and data, consistent with the consent granted by the subjects. Scientific policies should control the scientific validity of sample requests and consider the availability of samples and their rarity or scarcity.

Data access policies should guide researchers' access to data and define the conditions for access and the review process for access. Access policies also guide the deposition of research data from the use of biospecimens, back to resources to provide wider use by approved users.[71] Governance processes must address the possible or eventual closure of the biobank and how samples and data will be disposed of or transferred to a third party. These processes must respect the initial consent granted by the donors, and disposal must comply with local regulations. Two documents set out the conditions for collection and use of samples: the informed consent and the MTA.

Informed Consent

Informed consent is a fundamental legal and ethical principle in sample donation and biobanking. It underlines the basic rights of autonomy, liberty, and dignity. It outlines the agreement between the donor and the custodian biobank on the provision of samples and data for research. Any deviation from a donor's consent must be authorized by a supervisory board, such as an institutional ethics review board.

The basis of informed consent is that donors understand the request being made for collection, storage, and use of their samples and data. The consent form should be simple, clear, and in the colloquial language of the donor.

Consent must be voluntary and should indicate the purpose of the biobank; possible physical risks associated with collection of the sample and risks associated with collection of personal data; procedures for maintaining privacy; methods of protecting donor identity; future use and access to the samples and data; the right to withdraw consent and request destruction of remaining samples or render them anonymous; the possibility of sharing samples and data with other institutions, exporting them across borders or using them commercially; and the right to refuse to provide samples, with clarification that such refusal will not affect the care to the donor/patient. It is also necessary to indicate the possibility that the donor might be re-contacted for follow-up or more information or for further consent. It may be unrealistic to expect researchers to re-contact individual participants to obtain specific informed consent for each access to their samples in a new research project. In addition to being expensive and impracticable, such requests also may be against the wishes of the donor.

Types of Informed Consent

Several types of informed consent exist, defined by the level of permission from donors for use of their samples. Specific consent limits the use of the sample and data to a specific research project whose details are made aware to the donor. It is used when samples and data are identifiable. Partially restricted consent is used in a specific research project but allows future unspecified use directly or indirectly related to the research. Broad consent allows unspecified future use of the sample and data and the donor is provided with general information about possible future research, but which should comply with applicable national or local regulations and policies. Layered or tiered consent permits the donor to consent to particular aspects of the research but not others. Specific consent is advisable for identifiable samples and data, whereas broad consent may be used where samples and data are anonymized and the research is approved by an ethics committee or other body.[72,73]

Community engagement before the launching of a project that involves the use of samples and data is a useful method of informing, consulting, and actively involving relevant communities that have a legitimate interest in the research process.

Individuals often take decisions in consultation with family, friends, and community members. Frequently, there are also clear authority structures that must be respected in the engagement process, such as permission from village chiefs and elders. Adhering to these principles is important to build respect and trust between research teams and the respective communities.[74]

Vulnerable Subjects

Safeguards should be put into place for the use of tissue from vulnerable donors, such as patients with mental incapacity, for example, heavily sedated people, people with dementia or impaired consciousness, and children. In the case of deceased donors, consent should be based on the views of the deceased person or of the family, if known. When research includes an ethnic minority, single community, or cultural group, a representative from that group should be involved in the consent process.[75]

Exceptions to Informed Consent

The requirement of consent may be waived by an ethics committee, in accordance with applicable laws and regulations, in cases in which the researcher will not come into possession of identifying information and the specific research has been approved by a recognized research ethics committee.

Material Transfer Agreements

An MTA is a contractual document governing the conditions under which samples and data may be used in research. It defines the rights and obligations of both the biobank and the receiving researcher. Provision of samples and data must be consistent with the given consent of the donor. Cross-border collaboration and sample export must be governed by the permission from the donor's informed consent and the local legislation, which will indicate whether biological material may be exported and what necessary permits are required.

An MTA should specify (1) the purpose of the transfer of the material and its intended use; (2) restrictions on the use of the samples, such as their redistribution to third parties or sale for commercial purposes; (3) restrictions on re-identification, where de-identified specimens are provided; (4) requirements for handling biosafety hazards; (5) disposal or return procedures for unused samples; (6) ownership of intellectual property rights; (7) acknowledgment arrangements and publication rights; (8) provision of aggregated or raw research data; (9) guarantees and waivers; and (10) other factors that may govern sample transfer and the applicable regulations and law. The specific protections for data may be included in the same MTA or a separate agreement. Such an agreement must deal with the future use of the data, including their possible redistribution, requirements for maintaining privacy and confidentiality, governance for access to data, and protection of data against unauthorized access. Most MTAs provide a time limitation and should provide guidance on the final disposition of the samples and data, whether the residual samples should be returned or destroyed. Based on the funding for the research or the regulations of the sample provider, data resulting from the use of the samples may be required to be deposited in centralized databases for open access to the research community.[71]

Data Privacy and Data Protection

Data protection is a key principle in protecting donor privacy and confidentiality.[76] The types of data collected by the biobank are (1) sample-related data on quantity, quality, and methods of collection and storage, and (2) donor-related data on clinical, pathologic, and lifestyle aspects. These data are considered sensitive because they provide information for potential identification of the donor and possible familial indicators. Therefore, procedures must be put in place to store data in a manner that protects the identity of the donor, including de-identifying or coding any identifying data, storing samples without associated identifying data, and ensuring that data are stored securely with access restricted to authorized personnel, including access to coding keys that may re-identify data or associate them with other data sets.

Sample Identification

Identifying information should not be provided to researchers unless the research specifically requires it and approval from either the donor or the ethics committee has been received. If identifiable samples are used for research, donors should be informed about any implications, for example, if they will be re-contacted by researchers or receive feedback or additional requests for access to medical records.

Genetic Data

In disease research, genetic data can be defined as somatic or germline. Somatic alterations are genomic anomalies that are confined to diseased cells and have the potential to provide valuable diagnostic, prognostic, and treatment information.

Germline variations are gene variants that increase the risk of disease either related to hereditary predisposition or promoted by lifestyle and environmental exposures. Sharing germline data requires specific consent, because they are considered as sensitive identifying material with consequences not only for donors but also for other family members.

Particular attention needs to be paid to the protection and release of these data.[77] A dedicated data access committee should make the decision about providing genetic data to the general research community. Complex ethical issues, such as whether to provide genetic and genomic research information to donors about heritable factors or disease risks, mean that ethics boards require that biobanks should choose to err on the side of caution, and these data should remain in the domain of research unless clinically validated and actionable in a clinical context. There is ongoing debate on the topic of release of genetic data directly to individuals or in research projects.[78]

Sustainability of Biobanking

Creating a successful biomolecular research program requires the creation of a quality biobank infrastructure that spans the continuum from consent of donors, through collection, processing, storage, and utilization of biospecimens. Quality biobanking infrastructure is inherently expensive and requires a long-term financial commitment. Currently, the funding of research biobanks is not uniformly regulated, mainly because of the different focuses, services, and concepts.[79] On the other hand, the samples and associated data of biobanks gain significant value over time, and therefore their long-term storage should be planned from the start.[80] The biobank must have the staffing, the equipment, processes, and QC plans to provide fit-for-purpose specimens to the research community. Sustainability of biobanking requires attention to operational, social, and financial dimensions of the process.[81] Securing the organization's commitment to support a biobank; creating a business plan that is reviewed and modified as the biobank matures and as the collections grow; planning for utilization of the collections and providing services to the research community in an ethically robust framework; are key components to long-term sustainability.[82–84]

SUMMARY

Biobanking has become a key infrastructure to study the molecular basis of disease across the world. The biobanking continuum includes the initiation of the informed consent for the sample donation, to collection, processing, storing, and retrieving the samples for research. Each of these important steps should be controlled by SOPs and documented in a robust information technology system. The SOPs should be developed to be appropriate for the available resources, without forfeiting the quality needed to result in meaningful molecular data for the research population being studied. The lack of biobanks and quality biological resources from LMIC populations should be addressed to make the largest impact on the global burden of disease.

REFERENCES

1. Wang H, Naghavi M, Allen C, et al. Global, regional, and national life expectancy, all-cause mortality, and cause-specific mortality for 249 causes of death, 1980-2015: a systematic analysis for the global burden of disease study. Lancet 2015;388(10053):1459–544.
2. WHO. GLOBOCAN 2012. 2012. Available at: http://globocan.iarc.fr/. Accessed November 16, 2017.
3. Bray F, Ren JS, Masuyer E, et al. Global estimates of cancer prevalence for 27 sites in the adult population in 2008. Int J Cancer 2013;132(5):1133–45.
4. Arbyn M, Ronco G, Cuzick J, et al. How to evaluate emerging technologies in cervical cancer screening? Int J Cancer 2009;125(11):2489–96.
5. Hainaut P, Vozar B, Rinaldi S, et al. The European prospective investigation into cancer and nutrition biobank. Methods Mol Biol 2011;675:179–91.
6. Pukkala E, Andersen A, Berglund G, et al. Nordic biological specimen banks as basis for studies of cancer causes and control–more than 2 million sample donors, 25 million person years and 100,000 prospective cancers. Acta Oncol 2007;46(3):286–307.
7. World Bank Country and Lending Groups: Available at: https://datahelpdesk. worldbank.org/knowledgebase/articles/906519-world-bank-country-and-lending-groups. Accessed November 16, 2017.
8. Vaught JB, Henderson MK. Biological sample collection, processing, storage and information management. IARC Sci Publ 2011;(163):23–42.
9. Biobank Quality Standard: Collecting, storing and providing human biological material and data for research National Cancer Research Institute UK, 13 March 2014. Available at: http://cmpath.ncri.org.uk/wp-content/uploads/2017/06/ Biobank-quality-standard-Version-1.pdf. Accessed November 17, 2017.
10. Abdur Rab M, Afzal M, Abou-Zeid A, et al. Ethical practices for health research in the Eastern Mediterranean region of the World Health Organization: a retrospective data analysis. PLoS One 2008;3(5):e2094.
11. Grizzle WE, Gunter EW, Sexton KC, et al. Quality management of biorepositories. Biopreserv Biobank 2015;13(3):183–94.
12. Thio CL, Smeaton L, Saulynas M, et al. Characterization of HIV-HBV coinfection in a multinational HIV-infected cohort. AIDS 2013;27(2):191–201.
13. Abimiku A, Mayne ES, Joloba M, et al. H3Africa biorepository program: supporting genomics research on african populations by sharing high-quality biospecimens. Biopreserv Biobank 2017;15(2):4.
14. Campbell A, Rudan I. Systematic review of birth cohort studies in Africa. J Glob Health 2011;1(1):46–58.

15. Sirugo G, Schim van der Loeff M, Sam O, et al. A national DNA bank in the Gambia, West Africa, and genomic research in developing countries. Nat Genet 2004;36(8):785–6.

16. ISBER Best Practices for Repositories; Available at: http://www.isber.org/bpr. Accessed November 16, 2017.

17. Available at: https://specimens.cancer.gov/. Accessed November 16, 2017.

18. Available at: https://www.ctrnet.ca/resources/operating-procedures. Accessed November 16, 2017.

19. Mendy M, Caboux M, Lawlor RT, et al. Common minimal technical standards and protocols for biobanks dedicated to cancer research. IARC Technical Publication No44 ISBN-13 (PDF) 978-92-832-2464-8. Available at: https://publications.iarc.fr/uploads/media/publication_inline/0001/02/818ee1c105105cacb9fa8adef64510c201fd92d3.pdf. Accessed November 16, 2017.

20. Moore HM, Compton CC, Alper J, et al. International approaches to advancing biospecimen science. Cancer Epidemiol Biomarkers Prev 2011;20(5):729–32.

21. Betsou F, Lehmann S, Ashton G, et al. Standard preanalytical coding for biospecimens: defining the sample PREanalytical code. Cancer Epidemiol Biomarkers Prev 2010;19(4):1004–11.

22. Lehmann S, Guadagni F, Moore H, et al. Standard preanalytical coding for biospecimens: review and implementation of the Sample PREanalytical Code (SPREC). Biopreserv Biobank 2012;10(4):366–74.

23. Available at: https://biospecimens.cancer.gov/resources/sops/default.asp. Accessed November 16, 2017.

24. Lasken RS, Egholm M. Whole genome amplification: abundant supplies of DNA from precious samples or clinical specimens. Trends Biotechnol 2003;21(12):531–5.

25. Sjoholm MI, Dillner J, Carlson J. Assessing quality and functionality of DNA from fresh and archival dried blood spots and recommendations for quality control guidelines. Clin Chem 2007;53(8):1401–7.

26. Mendy M, Kirk GD, van der Sande M, et al. Hepatitis B surface antigenaemia and alpha-foetoprotein detection from dried blood spots: applications to field-based studies and to clinical care in hepatitis B virus endemic areas. J Viral Hepat 2005;12(6):642–7.

27. Schim van der Loeff MF, Sarge-Njie R, Ceesay S, et al. Regional differences in HIV trends in the Gambia: results from sentinel surveillance among pregnant women. AIDS 2003;17(12):6.

28. Tarini BA. Storage and use of residual newborn screening blood spots: a public policy emergency. Genet Med 2011;13(7):3.

29. Bernini P, Bertini I, Luchinat C, et al. Standard operating procedures for preanalytical handling of blood and urine for metabolomic studies and biobanks. J Biomol NMR 2011;49(3–4):231–43.

30. Rai AJ, Gelfand CA, Haywood BC, et al. HUPO plasma proteome project specimen collection and handling: towards the standardization of parameters for plasma proteome samples. Proteomics 2005;5(13):3262–77.

31. Hsieh SY, Chen RK, Pan YH, et al. Systematical evaluation of the effects of sample collection procedures on low-molecular-weight serum/plasma proteome profiling. Proteomics 2006;6(10):3189–98.

32. Clark S, Youngman LD, Palmer A, et al. Stability of plasma analytes after delayed separation of whole blood: implications for epidemiological studies. Int J Epidemiol 2003;32(1):125–30.

33. Debey S, Schoenbeck U, Hellmich M, et al. Comparison of different isolation techniques prior gene expression profiling of blood derived cells: impact on physiological responses, on overall expression and the role of different cell types. Pharmacogenomics J 2004;4(3):193–207.

34. Stevens VL, Patel AV, Feigelson HS, et al. Cryopreservation of whole blood samples collected in the field for a large epidemiologic study. Cancer Epidemiol Biomarkers Prev 2007;16(10):2160–3.

35. Playdon MC, Sampson JN, Cross AJ, et al. Comparing metabolite profiles of habitual diet in serum and urine. Am J Clin Nutr 2016;104(3):776–89.

36. Thomas CE, Sexton W, Benson K, et al. Urine collection and processing for protein biomarker discovery and quantification. Cancer Epidemiol Biomarkers Prev 2010;19(4):953–9.

37. Vu NT, Chaturvedi AK, Canfield DV. Genotyping for DQA1 and PM loci in urine using PCR-based amplification: effects of sample volume, storage temperature, preservatives, and aging on DNA extraction and typing. Forensic Sci Int 1999; 102(1):23–34.

38. Cannas A, Kalunga G, Green C, et al. Implications of storing urinary DNA from different populations for molecular analyses. PLoS One 2009;4(9):e6985.

39. Grizzle WE, Otali D, Sexton KC, et al. Effects of cold ischemia on gene expression: a review and commentary. Biopreserv Biobank 2016;14(6):548–58.

40. Belloni B, Lambertini C, Nuciforo P, et al. Will PAXgene substitute formalin? A morphological and molecular comparative study using a new fixative system. J Clin Pathol 2013;66(2):124–35.

41. Boren M. Methodology and technology for stabilization of specific states of signal transduction proteins. Methods Mol Biol 2011;717:91–100.

42. Awadelkarim KD, Arizzi C, Elamin EO, et al. Pathological, clinical and prognostic characteristics of breast cancer in Central Sudan versus Northern Italy: implications for breast cancer in Africa. Histopathology 2008;52(4):445–56.

43. Jennings LJ, Arcila ME, Corless C, et al. Guidelines for validation of next-generation sequencing-based oncology panels: a joint consensus recommendation of the association for molecular pathology and College of American Pathologists. J Mol Diagn 2017;19(3):341–65.

44. Available at: https://www.ascp.org/content/get-involved/partners-in-cancer-diagnosis. Accessed November 16, 2017.

45. Croxton T, Swanepoel C, Musinguzi H, et al. Lessons learned from biospecimen shipping among the human heredity and health in Africa biorepositories. Biopreserv Biobank 2017;15(2):8.

46. Simbolo M, Gottardi M, Corbo V, et al. DNA qualification workflow for next generation sequencing of histopathological samples. PLoS One 2013;8(6):e62692.

47. Betsou F, Barnes R, Burke T, et al. Human biospecimen research: experimental protocol and quality control tools. Cancer Epidemiol Biomarkers Prev 2009; 18(4):1017–25.

48. Betsou F, Gunter E, Clements J, et al. Identification of evidence-based biospecimen quality-control tools: a report of the International Society for Biological and Environmental Repositories (ISBER) biospecimen science working group. J Mol Diagn 2013;15(1):3–16.

49. Hubel A, Spindler R, Skubitz AP. Storage of human biospecimens: selection of the optimal storage temperature. Biopreserv Biobank 2014;12(3):165–75.

50. Riegman PH, de Jong B, Daidone MG, et al. Optimizing sharing of hospital biobank samples. Sci Transl Med 2015;7(297):297fs31.

51. Kap M, Smedts F, Oosterhuis W, et al. Histological assessment of PAXgene tissue fixation and stabilization reagents. PLoS One 2011;6(11):e27704.
52. Available at: http://old.bbmri-eric.eu/bbmri-eric-directory. Accessed November 16, 2017.
53. Available at: http://biobanking.org/locator. Accessed November 16, 2017.
54. Available at: http://bcnet.iarc.fr/projects/biobank_catalogue.php. Accessed November 16, 2017.
55. Available at: http://codes.iarc.fr/. Accessed November 16, 2017.
56. Available at: http://www.snomed.org/snomed-ct. Accessed November 16, 2017.
57. Ellis H, Joshi MB, Lynn AJ, et al. Consensus-driven development of a terminology for biobanking, the Duke experience. Biopreserv Biobank 2017;15(2):126–33.
58. Ulrich H, Kock AK, Duhm-Harbeck P, et al. Metadata repository for improved data sharing and reuse based on HL7 FHIR. Stud Health Technol Inform 2016;228:162–6.
59. Henderson MK, Simeon-Dubach D, Zaayenga A. When bad things happen: lessons learned from effective and not so effective disaster and recovery planning for biobanks. Biopreserv Biobank 2013;11(4):193.
60. US HHS Office of Human Research Protections Regulations and Policies. (Belmont Report and 45 CFR 46). Available at: https://www.hhs.gov/ohrp/regulations-and-policy/index.html. Accessed November 16, 2017.
61. US Code of Federal Regulations, Title 45 Part 46 (45 CFR Part 46): Available at: https://www.hhs.gov/ohrp/regulations-and-policy/regulations/45-cfr-46/index.html. Accessed November 16, 2017.
62. EU General Data Protections Rule: Available at: http://www.eugdpr.org/the-regulation.html. Accessed November 16, 2017.
63. Single European Code for Tissues and Cells: Available at: http://eur-lex.europa.eu/legal-content/EN/TXT/PDF/?uri=CELEX:32015L0565&from=EN. Accessed November 16, 2017.
64. Rothstein MA, Knoppers BM. Harmonizing privacy laws to enable international biobank research. J Law Med Ethics 2015;43:2.
65. International Compilation of Human Research Standards in Africa: Available at: https://bioethicsresearchreview.tghn.org/site_media/media/medialibrary/2013/11/2014intlcomp_Africa.pdf. Accessed November 16, 2017.
66. Declaration of Helsinki. 2008. Available at: https://www.wma.net/policies-post/wma-declaration-of-helsinki-ethical-principles-for-medical-research-involving-human-subjects/. Accessed November 16, 2017.
67. WMA Declaration of Taipei on Ethical Considerations regarding Health Databases and Biobanks: Available at: https://www.wma.net/what-we-do/medical-ethics/declaration-of-taipei/. Accessed November 16, 2017.
68. UNESCO. Universal Declaration on Bioethics and Human Rights. 2005. Available at: http://portal.unesco.org/en/ev.php-URL_ID=31058&URL_DO=DO_TOPIC&URL_SECTION=201.html. Accessed November 16, 2017.
69. OECD guidelines on human biobanks and genetic research databases. Eur J Health L 2010;17:14.
70. Chen H, Pang T. A call for global governance of biobanks. Bull World Health Organ 2015;93:113–7.
71. US HHS Public Access Policy for Research Data. Available at: https://www.hhs.gov/open/plan/hhs-public-access-policy-for-research-data.html. Accessed November 16, 2017.

72. Elger BS, Caplan AL. Consent and anonymization in research involving biobanks: differing terms and norms present serious barriers to an international framework. EMBO Rep 2006;7(7):661–6.
73. Salvaterra E, Lecchi L, Giovanelli S, et al. Banking together. A unified model of informed consent for biobanking. EMBO Rep 2008;9(4):307–13.
74. Jao I, Kombe F, Mwalukore S, et al. Involving research stakeholders in developing policy on sharing public health research data in Kenya: views on fair process for informed consent, access oversight, and community engagement. J Empir Res Hum Res Ethics 2015;10(3):264–77.
75. Andanda PA. Human-tissue-related inventions: ownership and intellectual property rights in international collaborative research in developing countries. J Med Ethics 2008;34:9.
76. Malin B, Karp D, Scheuermann RH. Technical and policy approaches to balancing patient privacy and data sharing in clinical and translational research. J Investig Med 2010;58(1):11–8.
77. Kaye J, Heeney C, Hawkins N, et al. Data sharing in genomics–re-shaping scientific practice. Nat Rev Genet 2009;10(5):331–5.
78. Knoppers BM. Consent to 'personal' genomics and privacy. Direct-to-consumer genetic tests and population genome research challenge traditional notions of privacy and consent. EMBO Rep 2010;11(6):416–9.
79. Kirsten R, Hummel M. Securing the sustainability of biobanks. Bundesgesundheitsblatt Gesundheitsforschung Gesundheitsschutz 2016;59(3):390–5 [in German].
80. Watson PH, Nussbeck SY, Carter C, et al. A framework for biobank sustainability. Biopreserv Biobank 2014;12(1):60–8.
81. Henderson MK, Goldring K, Simeon-Dubach D. Achieving and maintaining sustainability in biobanking through business planning, marketing, and access. Biopreserv Biobank 2017;15(1):1–2.
82. Bledsoe MJ, Henderson MK, Sawyer SJ, et al. Ensuring biobank value through effective utilization. Biopreserv Biobank 2015;13(6):5.
83. Henderson MK, Simeon-Dubach D, Albert M. Finding the path to biobank sustainability through sound business planning. Biopreserv Biobank 2015; 13(6):2.
84. Simeon-Dubach D, Henderson MK. Sustainability in biobanking. Biopreserv Biobank 2014;12(5):287–91.

Printed and bound by CPI Group (UK) Ltd, Croydon, CR0 4YY

03/10/2024

01040495-0001